Essential Clinical Immunology

Edited by

John B. Zabriskie

The Rockefeller University

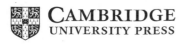

CAMBRIDGE UNIVERSITY PRESS
Cambridge, New York, Melbourne, Madrid, Cape Town, Singapore, São Paulo, Delhi

Cambridge University Press
32 Avenue of the Americas, New York, NY 10013-2473, USA

www.cambridge.org
Information on this title: www.cambridge.org/9780521704892

First published 2009

Printed in Hong Kong by Golden Cup.

A catalog record for this publication is available from the British Library.

Library of Congress Cataloging in Publication Data

Essential clinical immunology / edited by John B.
Zabriskie.
  p.   ; cm.
  Includes bibliographical references and index.
  ISBN 978-0-521-51681-5 (hardback) – ISBN 978-0-521-70489-2 (pbk.) 1. Clinical immunology.
2. Immunologic diseases. I. Zabriskie, John B.
  [DNLM: 1. Immunity. 2. Immune System Diseases. 3. Immune System.   QW 540 E783
2009]
  RC582. E85 2009
  616. 07′9–dc22   2008030935

Contents

Contributors

Dalit Ashany, M.D.
Assistant Attending Physician,
    Hospital for Special Surgery
Assistant Professor of Medicine,
    Weill Medical College of Cornell
    University
Hospital for Special Surgery
New York, NY

Jean-François Bach, M.D.
Professor of Immunology,
    Necker Hospital, Paris
Secrétaire perpétuel
Académie des sciences
Paris, France

Nina Bhardwaj, M.D., Ph.D.
Director of Tumor Vaccine Center
New York Cancer Institute
New York, NY

Frederick S. Buckner, M.D.
Associate Professor
Department of Medicine, Division of
    Infectious Diseases
University of Washington
Seattle, WA

Nicholas Chiorazzi, M.D.
Investigator and Director, Laboratory
    of Experimental Immunology
Feinstein Institute for Medical
    Research
Manhasset, NY

Mary K. Crow, M.D.
Senior Scientist

Department of Rheumatology
Hospital for Special Surgery
New York, NY

Gil Cu, M.D.
Assistant Professor and Medical
    Director
Department of Medicine, Division of
    Nephrology and Hypertension
University of Florida, Jacksonville
Jacksonville, FL

Paul M. Ehrlich, M.D.
Clinical Assistant Professor
Department of Pediatrics
New York University School of Medicine
New York, NY

Manlio Ferrarini, M.D.
Istituto Nazionale per La Ricerca sul
    Cancro, IST
Genova, Italy

Jonathan D. Field, M.D., F.A.A.A.I.
Director, Pediatric Allergy and
    Immunology Clinic
New York University/Bellevue
    Medical Center
New York, NY

Vincent A. Fischetti, Ph.D.
Head, Laboratory of Bacterial
    Pathogenesis
Rockefeller University
New York, NY

Jacqueline Friedman, M.D.
Clinical Professor
Department of Neurology
New York Harbor
    VA Medical Center
New York, NY

Allan Gibofsky, M.D.
Professor
Department of Medicine and Public
    Health
Weill Medical College of Cornell
    University
New York, NY

William W. Hall, M.D., Ph.D.
Professor
Department of Medical
    Microbiology
University College Dublin
Dublin, Ireland

Matthew Kosboth, M.D.
Rheumatology Fellow
Division of Rheumatology and Clinical
    Immunology
University of Florida
Gainesville, FL

James G. Krueger, M.D., Ph.D.
Professor/Medical Director
Rockefeller University
New York, NY

Dinakantha S. Kumararatne, M.D.
Consultant in Immunology
Department of Clinical Biochemistry
    and Immunology
Addenbrooke's Hospital
Cambridge, UK

**Christopher M. MacIsaac, M.D., Ph.D.
    Candidate**
Centre for Inflammatory Diseases
Monash Institute of Medical Research
Clayton, Victoria, Australia

Lloyd Mayer, M.D.
Professor and Chairman,
    Immunobiology Center
Dorothy and David Merksamer
    Professor of Medicine
Chief, Division of Clinical
    Immunology
Chief, Division of Gastroenterology
Mount Sinai Medical Center
New York, NY

Christine Moung, M.D.
Department of Pathology
Mount Sinai Medical Center
New York, NY

Ernesto Muñoz-Elías, Ph.D.
Postdoctoral Fellow
Department of Microbiology
Tufts University
Boston, MA

David O'Neill, M.D.
Assistant Professor of Pathology
Director, NYUCI Vaccine and Cell
    Therapy Core Facility
New York University School of
    Medicine
New York, NY

Westley H. Reeves, M.D.
Marcia Whitney Schott Professor of
    Medicine
Division of Rheumatology and Clinical
    Immunology
University of Florida
Gainesville, FL

Noel R. Rose, M.D., Ph.D.
Professor of Pathology
Professor of Molecular Microbiology
    and Immunology
Director, Johns Hopkins Center for
    Autoimmune Disease Research
Bloomberg School of Public Health
Baltimore, MD

Minoru Satoh, M.D., Ph.D.
Associate Professor
Division of Rheumatology and Clinical
    Immunology
University of Florida
Gainesville, FL

Jennifer A. Sipos, M.D.
Assistant Professor
Division of Endocrinology
University of Florida
Gainesville, FL

Anders G. Vahlne, M.D., Ph.D.
Professor of Clinical Virology
Department of Immunology,
    Microbiology, Pathology, and
    Infectious Diseases
Karolinska University Hospital,
    Huddinge
Stockholm, Sweden

Jeffrey M. Venstrom, M.D.
Fellow, Hematology-Medical
    Oncology
Department of Medicine
Memorial Sloan-Kettering Cancer
    Center
New York, NY

Kumar Visvanathan, M.D., Ph.D.
Director, Innate Immunity
    Laboratory and Infectious
    Diseases Physician
Centre for Inflammatory Diseases
Department of Medicine (Monash
    Medical Centre)
Monash University
Clayton, Victoria, Australia

Wesley C. Van Voorhis, M.D., Ph.D.
Training Program Director, Infectious
    Diseases
Professor of Medicine

Adjunct Professor of Pathobiology
University of Washington
Seattle, WA

Thomas Waldmann, M.D.
Head, Cytokine Immunology and
    Immunotherapy Section
Metabolism Branch Chief
Center for Cancer Research, National
    Cancer Institute
National Institutes of Health
Washington, DC

Robert J. Wilkinson, Ph.D., FRCP
Institute of Infectious Diseases and
    Molecular Medicine
University of Cape Town
Cape Town, South Africa

Lijun Yang, M.D.
Associate Professor
Department of Pathology,
    Immunology and Laboratory
    Medicine
University of Florida
Gainesville, FL

James W. Young, M.D.
Chief (Interim), Adult Allogeneic Bone
    Marrow Transplantation
Attending Physician and Member
Professor of Medicine, Weill Medical
    College of Cornell University
Division of Hematologic Oncology
Department of Medicine
Memorial Sloan-Kettering Cancer
    Center
New York, NY

Lisa Zaba, M.D., Ph.D.
Biomedical Fellow
Rockefeller University
Krueger Laboratory
New York, NY

John B. Zabriskie, M.D.
Professor Emeritus, Laboratory
   of Clinical Microbiology and
   Immunology
Rockefeller University
New York, NY

Haoyang Zhuang, Ph.D.
Graduate Assistant
Division of Rheumatology and Clinical
   Immunology
University of Florida
Gainesville, FL

1. Basic Components of the Immune System

John B. Zabriskie, M.D.

INTRODUCTION

This chapter is not a comprehensive review of immunology but rather a condensed version of those aspects of immunology that have particular relevance to clinical immunology. Refer to the Bibliography for a more extensive discussion of the role of each component.

It is generally believed that the immune system evolved as the host's defense against infectious agents, and it is well known that patients with deficiencies in the immune system generally succumb to these infectious diseases. However, as we shall see, it may well play a larger role in the elimination of other foreign substances, including tumor antigens or cells and antibodies that attack self.

An immune response may be conveniently divided into two parts: (1) a specific response to a given antigen and (2) a more nonspecific augmentation to that response. An important feature of the specific response is that there is a quicker response to the antigen during a second exposure to that antigen. It is the memory of the initial response that provides the booster effect.

For convenience, the specific immune response may be divided into two parts: (1) the humoral response and (2) the cellular response to a given antigen. As we shall see, however, both responses are mediated through the lymphocyte. Humoral responses are antibodies produced in response to a given antigen, and these antibodies are proteins, have similar structures, and can be divided into various classes of immunoglobulins. Cellular responses are established by cells and can only be transferred by cells. (See the Bibliography for the extraordinary beginnings of the concept of a cellular arm of the immune system.) Up to the 1940s the general dogma held that only antibodies were involved in the immune response. Dr. Merrill Chase, who began his experiments in a laboratory devoted primarily to the humoral response, clearly showed in a series of elegant experiments that immunity was not just humoral but that a cellular response by the lymphocytes could also produce immunity. Some of the best examples of the power of cellular immunity may be found in the many experiments in which transfer of cells can induce autoimmune disease in animals and humans as well as rejection of an organ graft in both animals and humans by cells.

The separation of human and cellular immunity was further advanced by the study of immunodeficient humans and animals. For example, thymectomized or congenitally athymic animals as well as humans cannot carry out graft rejection, yet they are capable of producing some antibody responses. The reverse is also true. Children (and animals) who have an immune deficit in the humoral response do not make antibodies but can reject grafts and appear to handle viral, fungal, and some bacterial infections quite well. An extraordinary finding by Good and colleagues in studying the cloacal lymphoid organ in chickens revealed that, with removal of the bursa Fabricius, these animals lost their ability to produce antibodies and yet retained the ability to reject grafts.

Out of these and many other contributions, a clearer picture of the division of efforts by lymphocytes begins to emerge. Since cellular immune responses require an intact thymus, cellular immune responses are mediated through the T lymphocytes (thymus), while antibody-producing cells, which are dependent on the bone marrow (the bursa equivalent), are known as B (bursa) cells. The pathways of both cell types are depicted in Figure 1.1.

Several types of molecules play a vital role in the immune response, and we will deal with each in detail. Antigens, both foreign and self, are substances that may or may not provoke an immune response. Both T cells and B cells have receptors that recognize these antigens. In the case of B cells, antibodies on the surface are a major source (but not the only one) of antigen recognition, and once activated, they differentiate into plasma cells that produce large quantities of antibodies that are secreted into blood and body fluids to block the harmful effects of the antigen.

T cells have similar receptors known as T-cell receptors (TCR), and in the context of the major histocompatibility complex (MHC) molecules provide a means of self-recognition and T-lymphocyte effector functions. Often these effector functions

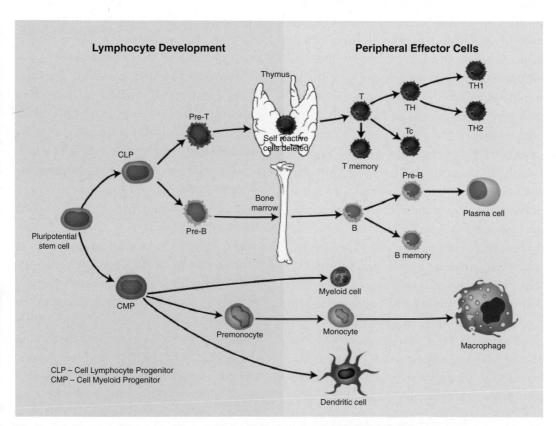

Figure 1.1 Development and differentiation of lymphocytes from pluripotential stem cells.

are carried out by messages transmitted between these cells. These soluble messengers are called *interleukins* or *cytokines*.

ANTIGENS

Antigens are any substances that are capable, under appropriate conditions, of inducing the formation of antibodies and reacting specifically with the antibodies so produced. They react with both T-cell recognition receptors and with antibodies. These antigenic molecules may have several antigenic determinants, called *epitopes*, and each epitope can bind with a specific antibody. Thus, a single antigen can bind to many different antibodies with different binding sites.

Some low-molecular-weight molecules called *haptens* are unable to evoke an immune response but can react with existing antibodies. These molecules need to be coupled to a carrier molecule to be antigenic.

For some molecules such as drugs, the molecule needs to be conjugated to a carrier. The carrier may be a host protein. The tertiary structure of the molecule as well as the amino acid sequence is important in determining antigenicity. Certain structures such as lipids and DNA are generally poor antigens.

Most antigens are either thymus-dependent or thymus-independent antigens. Thymus-dependent antigens require T-cell participation: Most proteins and foreign red cells are examples of these molecules. Thymus-independent antigens do *not* require T-cell participation for antibody production. Instead, they directly stimulate specific B lymphocytes by cross-linking antigen receptors on the surface of B cells. These molecules produce primarily IgM and IgG_2 antibodies and do not stimulate long-lasting memory cells. Most bacterial polysaccharides (found in bacterial cell walls) fall into this category. Certain polysaccharides, such as LPS (lipopolysaccharide), not only induce specific B-cell activation but also can act as a polyclonal B-cell stimulant.

ANTIBODY

The basic structure of the antibody molecule is depicted in Figures 1.2A and B. It consists of a four-chain structure divided into two identical heavy (H) chains with a molecular weight of 25 kDa. Each chain is composed of *domains* of 110 amino acids and is connected in a loop by a disulfide bond between two cysteine residues in the chain.

The amino acid N-terminal domains of the heavy and light chains include the antigen-binding site. The amino acids of these variable domains vary between different antibody molecules and are thus known as the *variable* (V) regions. Most of these differences reside in the *hypervariable* areas of the molecule and are usually only six to ten amino acid residues in length. When the hypervariable regions in each chain come together along with the counterparts on the other pair of H and L chains, they form the antigen-binding site. This part of the molecule is unique to the molecule and is known as the *idiotype determinant*. In any individual, 10^6 to 10^7 different antibody molecules can be composed from 10^3 different heavy and light chains of the variable regions. The part of the molecule next to the V region is called the constant (C) region made up of one domain in the light chain (C_1) and three or four in a heavy chain (C_H). A C_1 chain may consist of either

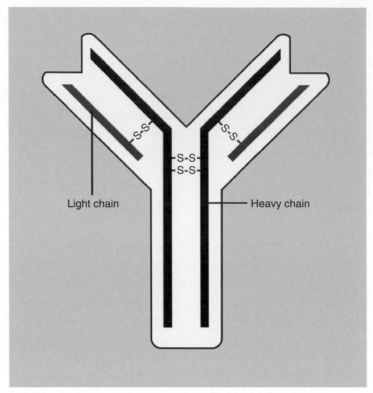

Figure 1.2A Heavy and light chains of an IgG antibody. An IgM antibody would be a pentameric structure of an IgG molecule.

two kappa (κ) or two lambda (λ) chains but *never* one of each. Of all the human antibody molecules, approximately 60%, are κ chains and 40% contain λ chains. Although there are no known differences in the functional properties of κ and λ chains, there are several different types of the C_H domain. These differences are reflected in determining the class (isotype) of the antibody and thereby the physiological function of a particular antibody molecule.

The IgM molecule is the oldest class of immunoglobulins, and it is a large molecule consisting of five basic units held together by a J chain. The major role IgM plays is the intravascular neutralization of organisms, especially viruses. The reason for this important physiological role is that it contains five complement-binding sites, resulting in excellent complement activa-

tion. This activation permits the segment removal of antigen–antibody complement complexes via complement receptors on phagocytic cells or complement-mediated lysis of the organism. However, in contrast to the IgG molecule, it has relatively low affinity binding to the antigen in question. Second, because of its size, it does not usually penetrate into tissues.

In contrast, IgG is a smaller molecule that penetrates easily into tissues. There are four major classes of IgG: IgG_1 and IgG_3 activate complement efficiently and clear most protein antigens, including the removal of microorganisms by phagocytic cells. In contrast, IgG_2 and IgG_4 react mostly with carbohydrate antigens and are relatively poor opsonins. This is the only molecule that crosses the placenta to provide immune protection to the neonate.

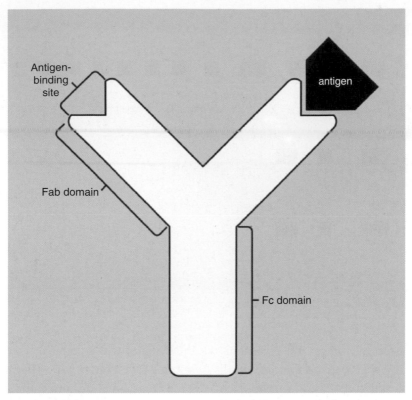

Figure 1.2B Antigen-binding sites and antigen binding in an IgG antibody. Hinge region allows for rotational and lateral movements of the two antigen-binding sites.

The major mucosal immunoglobulin, IgA, consists of two basic units joined by a J chain. The addition of a secretion molecule prevents its digestion by enzymes present in mucosal and intestinal secretions. Thus, IgA_2 is the major IgA molecule in secretions and is quite effective in neutralizing antigens that enter via these mucosal routes. IgA_1, the main IgA molecule in serum, is, however, susceptible to inactivation by serum proteases and is thus less active for defense. Its function is unclear at present.

Two other classes are worthy of note. IgD is synthesized by antigen-sensitive B cells and is involved in the activation of these cells by antigen. IgE is produced by plasma cells and binds to specific IgE receptors on most cells and basophiles. This molecule (see Chapter 9) plays an extremely important role in allergic reactions and expelling intestinal parasites, which is accomplished by increasing vascular permeability and inducing chemotactive factors following mast cell degranulation.

Given this extraordinary ability to generate large numbers of antibody molecules, how does the immune system recognize all pathogens, including past, present, and future? This diversity is achieved by the way in which the genetics of antibody production is arranged (see Figure 1.3). The light and heavy chains are carried on different chromosomes. The heavy chain genes are carried on chromosome 14. These genes are broken up into coding systems called *exons* with intervening segments of silent segments called *entrons*. The exons represent the central region of the heavy

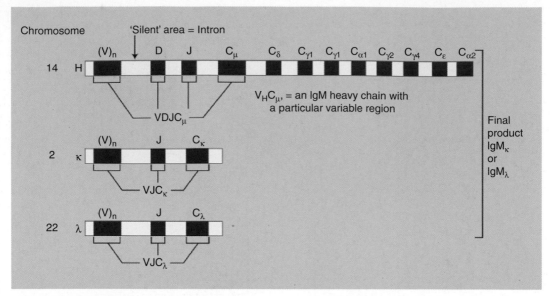

Figure 1.3 The genetics of antibody production.

chain and a large number of V regions. Between the V and D genes are two small sets of exons called the D and J. With each single B cell, one V gene is joined to one D and J in the chromosome. The product, the V_H domain, is then joined at the level of RNA processing to C_u and the B cell makes an IgM molecule. By omitting the C_u gene and joining $V_H D_J$ to a C_λ an IgG molecule is produced. This enormous versatility allows the cell to make IgM, IgD, IgG, IgA, or IgE in sequence while using the same variable regions (see Figure 1.4). The heavy chain gene recombinations are controlled by two recombination activity genes called RAG_1 and RAG_2. If these genes are eliminated by "knock-out" techniques in mice, profound immunodeficiency status occurs in these animals, characterized by absent mature B and T cells.

Thus, the diversity of antigen binding is achieved by the large number of V

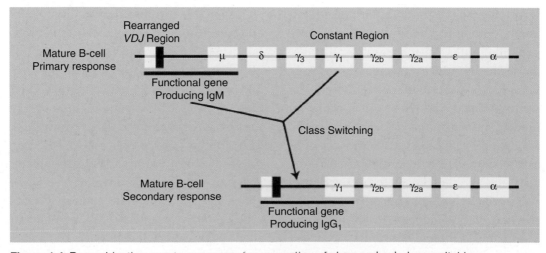

Figure 1.4 Recombination events necessary for generation of class and subclass switching.

genes available and their combination with different D and L genes to provide different antibodies. Furthermore, the inherited set of genes may be increased by somatic mutation during multiple divisions of lymphoid cells, thereby increasing the number of antibody specificities to 10^{14}, which far exceeds the number of B cells (10^{10}) in the body.

Once a given B cell is preselected to produce a particular V_H and V_L domain, all the ensuing progeny of that B cell will produce the same V_H or V_L domain. The sequence of events is as follows: initially, the B cell produces intracellular antigen-specific IgM, which becomes bound to the cell surface. The B cell is now antigen responsive with exposure to a given antigen. The committed B cell begins producing a certain isotype or class of immunoglobulins and begins dividing, and all the progeny will produce the identical immunoglobulin molecules. These B cells will later mature into either plasma cells or long-term memory B cells.

T CELLS AND THEIR RECEPTORS

Each T cell is also committed to a given antigen and recognizes it by one of two TCRs. They may have TCR2s composed of gamma (γ) and delta (δ) chains or TCR2s composed of another heterodimer of alpha (α) and beta (β) chains. These TCR2s are associated with a group of transmembrance proteins on the CD3 molecule, which takes the antigen recognition signal inside the cell. Signal transduction via the CD3 complex is regulated by a series of kinases, which are associated with the tails of the CD3–TCR complex and regulate phosphorylation. Deficiencies or blocks in the T-cell signaling pathways either at the cell-surface complex or at the level of the kinases may result in various forms of immunodeficiency. Two other important antigens present on TCR2 cells recognize histocompatibility antigens and will be discussed later. The genes for TCR chains are on different chromosomes with the β and α molecules on chromosome 7, while the α and δ are on chromosome 14. As seen in Figure 1.5, the four chains are made up of a variable region and a constant region similar to those observed with the immunoglobulins. The variable regions are also numerous and joined at D and J regions by RAG_1 and RAG_2. This permits a diversity of antigen recognition similar to that observed with immunoglobulin, but additional somatic mutation is not involved in T cells. These similarities have led to the concept that genes for antigen-specific T cells evolved in the same manner as immunoglobulin from a parent gene, and both are members of a superantigen family.

The TCR complex recognizes small peptides presented to it by the MHC class I and II and depends on the type of T cell.

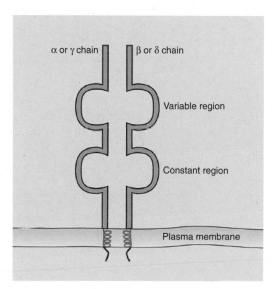

Figure 1.5 Diagram of the structure of a T-cell receptor.

Helper T cells (CD4) recognize class II antigens while suppressor cytotoxic T cells (CD8) recognize class I antigens. Because of the rather low affinity of the reactions, recognition of processed antigen alone is not sufficient to activate T cells. Soluble interleukins are needed to complete the picture and are generated during the antigen processing.

MAJOR HISTOCOMPATIBILITY COMPLEX

Human histocompatibility antigens are also known as human leucocyte antigens (HLA), a term that is synonymous with the MHC complex. These antigens are cell-surface glycoproteins classified as type I or type II. They can produce genetic polymorphism with multiple alleles at each site, thus permitting a great deal of genetic variability between given individuals (see Figure 1.6). This extensive polymorphism is important when viewed in the context of an immune system that needs to cope with an ever-increasing range of pathogens. These pathogens in turn are extremely adept at evading the immune system. Thus, the battle between invading microbe and immune recognition is constant and ever changing. Recognition of antigen by T cells is MHC restricted. Therefore, any given individual is only able to recognize antigen as part of a complex of antigenic peptide and self.

The importance of this concept is underscored by the experiments of Dougherty and Zinkernagel. Using virus-specific (virus 1) cytotoxic T cells, Figure 1.7 illustrates their remarkable discovery. If antigen-presenting cells (APCs) of mouse A are mixed with T cells of mouse A in the context of virus 1 peptides, the T cell responds and kills the virus. If the MHC complex is from mouse B and the T cells

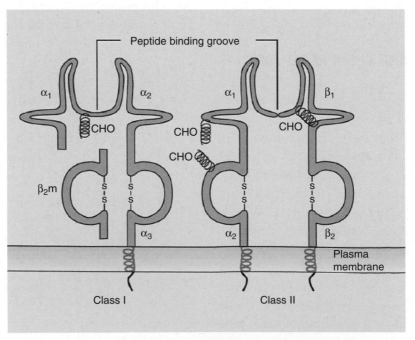

Figure 1.6 Diagrammatic representation of class I and II MHC antigens with B_2 microglobulins and CHO carbohydrate side chains.

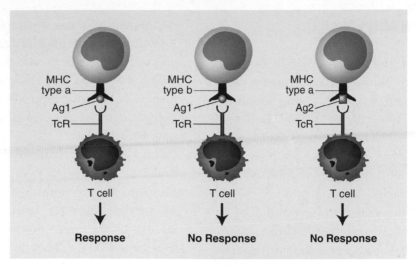

Figure 1.7 MHC restriction of antigen recognition by T cells. If APC and T cell are of the same genetic lineage as virus I, the T cell responds and kills the virus. If APC and T cell are of different lineage, no response occurs. If APC and T cell are of same lineage but virus 2 is present, no response occurs.

are from mouse A, no killing occurs. Finally, if MHC and T cells are both from mouse A but virus 2 is unrelated to virus 1, no response will occur.

The MHC class I antigens are divided into three groups (A, B, and C), and each group belongs on a different gene locus on chromosome 6. The products of all three loci are similar and are made up of a heavy chain (45 kDa) and associated β_2 microglobulin molecule (12 kDa) gene, which resides on chromosome 12. The MHC class I antigen differences are due to variations in the α chains, the β_2 microglobulin being constant. X-ray crystallography studies have shown that as few as nine amino acids can be tightly bound in the α chain groove.

MHC class II antigens also exhibit a similar structure with the groove being formed by the α_1 and β_1 chains. Unlike class I antigens present on most nucleated cells, the class II antigens are restricted to a few types: macrophages, B cells, and activated T cells. In humans, there are three groups of class II antigens: namely, HLA-DP, HLA-DQ, and HLA-DR.

Depending on the nature of the antigen (endogenous or exogenous), the MHC response is different. For example, endogenous antigens (including viral antigens) are presented by MHC class I antigen cells exclusively to CD8 cells. The endogenous antigen is first broken down into small peptides and transported by shuttle proteins called Tap I and Tap II to the endoplasmic reticulum. There they complex with MHC class I molecules and are delivered to the cell surface for further processing to the CD8 cells.

In contrast, MHC class II molecules are held in the endoplasmic reticulum and are protected from binding to peptides in the lumen (not human) by a protein called MHC class II associated invariant chain.

Finally, there are class III antigens, such as complement components C_4 and C_2, plus certain inflammatory proteins, such as tumor necrosis factor (TNF), which are encoded in adjacent areas.

ADHESION MOLECULES

In spite of the known MHC complex consisting of binding of a TCR to the processed antigen, which in turn is bound to the class II molecule of APCs, this is not enough for T-cell activation. One must have additional stimuli that are provided by a series of adhesion molecules on the two cell surfaces.

These molecules are composed of a diverse set of cell-surface glycoproteins and play a pivotal role in mediating cell-to-cell adhesion. Adhesion molecules are divided into four major groups, (a) integrins, (b) selectins, (c) immunoglobulin superfamily, and (d) caherins.

a. Integrins are heterodimers: These are divided into α and β subunits. Depending on the substructure of the β unit, there are five families, but for convenience β_1 and β_2 integrins are involved in leucocyte–endothelial interactions. β_1 integrins, also known as very late activation proteins, are so named because they appear on lymphocytes several days after antigenic stimulation and are composed of a common β chain (CD29) paired with a different α chain. They mediate lymphocyte and monocyte binding to the endothelium receptors called vascular adhesion molecule. β_2 integrins also have a common β chain (CD18), which pairs with different α chains (CD11 a, b, c) to form a number of separate molecules. These two sets of integrins mediate strong binding of leucocytes to the endothelial cell while β_3–β_5 are concerned with binding to extracellular matrix proteins such as fibronectin and vitronectin.
b. Selectins: These molecules are composed of three glycoproteins and are designated by three separate prefixes: E (endothelial), P (platelet), and L (leucocyte). The letters denote the cells on which they were first observed. These groups of selectins bind avidly to carbohydrate molecules on leucocytes and endothelial cells.
c. Immunoglobulin superfamily: The molecules in this family are so called because they contain a common immunoglobulin-like structure. They strengthen the interaction between the T cells and APCs. They include some of the most powerful molecules in the immune system, such as the CD4, CD8, CD2, lymphocyte function antigen (LFA-3 or CD58), and the intercellular adhesion molecules such as ICAM-1 through 3.
d. Cadherins: These molecules are calcium-dependent adhesion molecules and are mainly important in establishing molecular connections between epithelial cells. Their particular importance is during embryonic development.

CYTOKINES

This group of soluble molecules plays an extremely important role in clinical immunology. They are secreted by macrophages and may act as stimulatory or inhibitory signals between cells. Cytokines that initiate chemotaxis of leucocytes are called *chemokines*.

Among the group of cytokines, there are a few of particular interest because of their stimulatory activity. Interleukins 1 (IL-1) and 2 (IL-2) are of particular importance secondary to their role in amplifying the immune response. IL-1 acts on a wide range of cells including T

Basic Components of the Immune System

Table 1.1 Lymphocytes Involved in Immune Response

Cell Type	Function of Cell	Product of Cell	Function of Product
B	Antibody production	Antibody	Neutralization Opsonization Cell lysis
T_H2 cells	↑B-cell antibody production ↑Activated T_c	Cytokines IL-3, -4, -5, -10, -13	Help B and T_c
T_H1	Inflammation: Initiation Augmentation	IL-2, IFN-γ, TNF	Inflammatory mediators
T_s	↓B-cell antibody production ↓Activated T_c	Suppressor factor(s)	Suppress T_H and indirectly B and T_c
T_c	Lysis of antigenic target cells	INF-λ Perforins	Enhance MHC expression, activate NK cells, disrupt target cell membranes

T_c, cytotoxic T cell; T_H1-2, helper T-cell types; T_s, suppressor T cell.

and B cells. In contrast, IL-2 primarily acts on lymphocytes, although it has similar trophic effects on IL-receptor B cells and natural killer (NK) cells. (See Table 1.1 and functions.)

INITIATION OF THE IMMUNE RESPONSE

The effector cells are really divided into two types: B cells and T cells. B cells are primarily responsible for antibody production, whereas T cells act as effector cells and may function as both helpers and suppressors, depending on the stimulus provided by APCs.

The first step in initiation of the immune response to an antigen must necessarily involve modification of the antigen, and these specialized cells are called APCs. Without such processing, T cells cannot recognize antigen. Thus, it is the secretion of cytokines by APCs activated by antigen presentation that further activates antigen-specific T cells. This interaction between APCs and T cells is strongly influenced by a group of molecules called co-stimulators. For example, it is CD80 (B7-1) and CD86 (B7-2) on the APC cells with receptors CD28 and CTLA-4 on the T cell that provides this interaction. The absence of these co-stimulators leads to T-cell unresponsiveness. The importance of this pathway is emphasized by the fact that antagonists to these co-stimulators do interrupt the immune response in both in vitro and in vivo experiments. For example, mice with a severe form of lupus exhibit a milder disease following a CTLA-4 antagonist.

As stated before, processed antigen is presented to the T cells in the context of the MHC complex present on the surface of APCs. In this regard, the most efficient APCs are the dendritic cells. These cells have high concentrations of MHC class I and II antigens, co-stimulatory molecules, and adhesion molecules on their surface.

These cells may be divided into two major groups. The dendritic cells of the skin are called the Langerhans cells and play an important role in immune defenses since they are present in the largest protective organ of the body. Because they are mobile, Langerhans cells can capture antigen in the periphery and migrate to secondary lymph nodes where they become mature dendritic cells and interact with naïve T cells.

In contrast, the follicular dendritic cells reside in the follicular germinal center (B-cell area) of a lymph node. These cells have receptors for complement and immunoglobulins and their function is to trap immune complexes and feed them to B cells. This processed immune complex containing antigen is closely associated with MHC class II molecules on the APC surface and thus activates B cells.

ANTIBODY PRODUCTION

To achieve antibody production, at least four types of cells are required: APC, B cells, and two types of regulating cells.

B Cells

Antibodies are produced by naïve B cells and are called *plasma cells*. These cells express immunoglobulins on their surface. In the early stages, B cells first show intracellular μ-chains and then surface IgM. Through the process described earlier, these cells can later express IgG, IgA, or IgE, a phenomenon known as isotype switching. The final type of surface immunoglobulin determines the class of antibody secreted.

Isotype switching is mediated through two important protein interactions: CD40 on the B cell interacts with CD40L on activated T cells (IL-4 induced) to stimulate B cells to switch from IgM molecules to other isotypes. Deficiencies in either molecule lead to severe immunodeficiency states with only IgM produced but no IgG or IgA antibodies. This syndrome is called the hyper-IgM syndrome, and in this case of CD40L deficiency, it is an X-linked immunodeficiency.

As mentioned before, each B cell is committed to the production of antibody expressing a unique V_H–V_L combination, and the surface and excreted immunoglobulin are the same. These observations form the basis of Burnet's *clonal selection theory* in that each B cell expresses a surface immunoglobulin that acts as its antigen-receptor site. Contact with the antigen and helper T-cell factors commit each B cell to divide and differentiate to produce more of the same V_H–V_L antibody. A number of these B cells become memory cells so that a greater number of antigen-specific B cells are available on a secondary contact with the same antigen. This phenomenon is known as clonal expansion and helps to account for the greater secondary response.

Perhaps more important is that the secondary response of antibodies has a higher affinity binding for these antigens. These latter antibodies will bind to antigen even when complexed to antibody and help clear the antigen more effectively from the circulation. It is important to remember, however, that B cells alone do not respond to antigen directly, even in the presence of APC cells. They must have a second signal, normally provided by the T cells. This point was elegantly shown in a series of transfer experiments using irradiated recipient animals. As seen in Figure 1.8, antigen alone or antigen + B cells produced no antibody production in these animals. Similarly, T cells alone were ineffective. However,

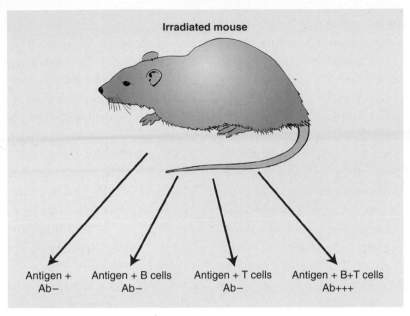

Figure 1.8 Adoptive cell transfer experiments in irradiated animals shows both T and B cells important for antibody production; Ab, antibody.

when all three were transferred into irradiated animals, this resulted in excellent antibody production.

T Cells

One must first emphasize that helper T cells can only respond to antigen presented by macrophage MHC class II antigens as a complex on APC cells. In turn, they recognize the same combination of antigen and class II MHC antigens on the corresponding B cells. It is only then that the helper T cell secretes its cytokines to activate the reaction. As seen in Figure 1.8, T cells recognize antigen in the context of their own MHC configuration. They will not cooperate with B cells and macrophages expressing antigens of a different genetic background.

When helper T cells meet an antigen for the first time, only a limited number of cells are activated to provide help for the B cells. However, when the animal is re-exposed, there is a marked increase of specific helper T cells. These cells constitute an expanded clone and the immune response is quicker and more vigorous.

This activation is also aided by two other mechanisms. First, memory cells have increased numbers of adhesion molecules (LFA-1, CD2, LFA-3, and ICAM-1) on their surface as well as a higher population of affinity receptors. Thus, memory cells produce high concentrations of IL-2 to recruit more helper cells of both types T_H1 and T_H2. The *recognition* of antigen involves several receptors on the surface of the T cells. In contrast, B cells recognize antigen by surface-bound immunoglobulin and recognize the same epitopes somewhat differently. T cells only recognize haptens (small molecules) when the haptens are coupled to a carrier protein while antibody can recognize free haptens easily.

Differentiation of T Cells

T cells have characteristic cell-surface glycoproteins that serve as markers of "differentiation" of these cells. These markers are recognized by specific monoclonal antibodies and divide them into two particular subsets.

T_H1 cells secrete TNF and INF-α and mediate cellular immunity. Conversely, T_H2 cells secrete IL-4, IL-5, IL-10, and IL-13 and are needed for stimulating antibody production by B cells. T cells secreting both cytokine profiles are designated T_H0.

What influences a naïve T cell to select which cytokine profile to secrete is not known. However, experiments in which cells are exposed to IL-1 and IL-6 promote T_H2 cells while IL-12 and IFN-α stimulate production of T_H1 T cells.

In humans, a T_H1 cytokine profile is primarily directed toward protection against intracellular pathogens while a T_H2 profile interacts with diseases characterized by overproduction of antibodies including IgE.

An elegant example of these different pathways of the T_H1 and T_H2 response is seen in the disease leprosy. Patients that develop a T_H1 response develop only limited disease (tuberculoid leprosy). In contrast, those patients mounting a T_H2 response develop debilitating and spreading lepromatous leprosy since the antibody response will not protect against an *intracellular* pathogen.

Cellular Immunity

Cell-mediated responses are implemented by T lymphocytes. The major functions of T cells can be divided into two categories: the first (cytotoxicity) is to lyse cells expressing specific antigens; the second (delayed hypersensitivity) is to release cytokines, thereby triggering an inflammatory response. These two types of cells are used to combat intracellular pathogens such as viruses, certain bacteria, and parasites inaccessible to antibodies.

Cytotoxic T cells lyse cells infected with viruses. This cytotoxicity is virus specific, and only cells expressing those proteins on the surface of the infected cell are killed. As stated before, this destruction occurs only in the presence of the same MHC class I molecules. This combination directly activates CD8+ cells and is a potent killer of virally infected cells. The induction of the cytotoxic T cell requires precursor cells and IL-2 from helper cells and is subject to regulation by other T cells.

Cytotoxic T cells also play a role in graft rejection. This was shown years ago in a mixed lymphocyte reaction in which the lymphocytes from two genetically different individuals were placed in culture. In this case, helper cells responded to a foreign MHC class II antigen, but cytotoxic T cells were able to lyse target cells carrying the MHC class I molecules of the stimulating (genetically different individual) cells. The in vivo reactions between individuals undergoing transplantation will be discussed in more detail in a later chapter.

In contrast, delayed-type hypersensitivity reactions are mediated by specific T cells that produce T_H1-type cytokines upon exposure to antigen. An example of this type of reaction is the PPD reaction, or tuberculin test. When the antigen is injected under the skin of an individual who was previously infected with *Mycobacterium tuberculosis*, a reaction in the skin evolves over 48 to 72 hours in which there is local swelling and induration >10 mm. If the site is biopsied, one finds a T-cell and macrophage infiltration. Injection of the same material in a noninfected individual produces little or no induration, and the histology is essentially negative. Whereas the cells in this case do not kill the organism, most individuals infected surround the organism in a caseous inflammatory lesion, which does not allow the organism to spread. The in vivo state of the lesions will be discussed in more detail in a later chapter.

Nonspecific Effector Molecules

There are a number of nonspecific molecules that affect the immune response, especially antibody production. These major factors are as follows: phagocytic cells such as neutrophils and macrophages, which remove antigens and bacteria, and complement, which can either destroy the organism or facilitate its destruction. The role of many of these factors will be discussed in more detail in later chapters, but a brief outline of their functions is warranted here.

COMPLEMENT

The complement component system consists of a series of heat-liable proteins, and they normally exist as inactive precursors. However, once activated each component may act as an enzyme and cleaves the next component in the sequence.

Each precursor is cleaved into two or more components, and the major fragment (designated "b") has two biologically active sites. One is for binding to cell membranes and the other is for enzymatic cleavage of the next component. The control of the sequence relies on either spontaneous decay or specific inactivation of these components. Minor fragments play a role in the fluid phase, acting as chemotactins.

The major function of the complement system is to help in the *opsonization* of microorganisms and immune complexes. These components plus antibody are more readily recognized by macrophages and more readily bound and phagocytosed through IgG: Fc and C3b receptors. Immune complexes are handled in a similar fashion, activating the classical pathway complements. Individuals who lack one of the classical pathway components are prone to immune complex disease.

The minor complement fragments contribute to the immune response by activating the inflammatory response. For example, some increase vascular permeability (C3a); others are chemotactins for neutrophils and macrophages (C5a) and not only promote leucocytosis in the bone marrow but attract these cells to the site of inflammation.

The critical step in complement activation is the cleavage of the C3 component by complement-derived enzymes called C3 convertases. This results in the presence of C3b, which mediates a number of vital biological activities. The cleavage of C3b can be initiated by three routes (classical, alternative, and lectin), but each route is in response to different stimuli. Individuals who are deficient in C3 are obviously predisposed to bacterial infections and immune complex disease.

Each of these routes will be examined in more detail (see Figure 1.9).

1. Classical pathway: As its name implies, this is the usual pathway whereby antigen–antibody complexes in the presence of complement destroy the invading organism. The antibody (either IgM or IgG) causes a conformational change in the Fc portion of the antibody to reveal a binding site for the first component of complement C1q. This component consists of six subunits and reacts with the Fc via its globular heads. The activation of this component requires the binding of two globular heads for activation. Thus, one molecule of IgM with

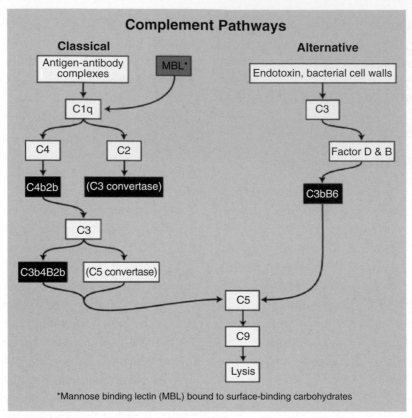

Figure 1.9 Pathways of complement activation by the classical, alternative, or lectin activation; MBL, mannose binding protein.

its pentameric conformation can easily activate C1q, while the ability of IgG, which has only two sites to activate C1q, is low. IgA, IgD, and IgE do not activate the classical pathway. C1q in turn activates C4 and C2, generating the complex C4b2b, which is the C3 "convertase" of the classical pathway. After the splitting of C3 into C3a and C3b is achieved, C3a possesses anaphylatoid and chemotactic activity. However, more important is C3b, which forms the complex C3b4b2b, which is the C5 convertase and initiates the final "lytic" attack complex.

2. The alternative pathway is phylogenetically older than the classical but was not generally accepted until the 1960s. Again, the control reaction is the activation of C3. In contrast to the classical pathway, however, this pathway bypasses antibody, C1, C4, and C2, and it is bacterial cell walls or endotoxin that activates C3. C3b here is unstable and, if an appropriate receptor is not found, it decays and the molecule becomes inactive. However, if a receptor surface is present, then the C3b molecules bind and remain active. Then C3b can use factors D and B of the alternative pathway to form the active enzyme C3bBb; this complex then becomes stabilized in the presence of properdin.

This molecule then can chose between two pathways. It can break down more C2, providing more C3b. Or it becomes stabilized to form the C5 convertase of the alternative pathway.

3. Lectin pathway: The third pathway of complement activation is created by the mannose-binding lectin MBL, a circulating protein that binds to carbohydrate on the surface of many microorganisms. MBL (structurally related to C1q) activates complement through a serine protease known as MBL-associated serine protease. Deficiencies in circulating levels of MBL are associated with frequent infections in childhood.

Once these components are activated, that is, C3b, 4b2b or C3bBb, and properdin, these molecules trigger sequentially C5, C6, C7, C8, and C9, which leads to the final lytic pathway and lysis of the target cell. The target can be a red cell, a virally infected cell, or a bacterium. Electron microscopy has shown that this complex binds to the cell membrane and actually punches a hole in the cell. Salts and water pass through the hole and the water fills the cell, eventually leading to swelling and destruction of the cell.

The control of the complement activation is important since many of its components induce inflammation. This control is executed in the following ways. First, many of the activated components are unstable and will decay rapidly if the next sequence is not present. Second, there are specific inhibitors of each component, such as C1 esterase, which inhibits factors I and H. Finally, the cells themselves contain proteins that increase the rates of breakdown of these products.

In summary, all acute phase complement components are acute phase proteins and the rate of increase occurs shortly after injury or infection. As will be seen later, there is considerable interaction between the complement system and other pathways such as clotting, fibrinolytic, and kimin pathways.

FUNCTIONAL COMPONENTS OF THE IMMUNE SYSTEM

Each of the cells in the immune response has a particular role to play. While many of these cells will be discussed in detail in subsequent chapters, a brief review of the functional capabilities is presented here.

Macrophages

These cells may be divided into two main groups: the dendritic cell and the mature macrophage. The dendritic cell's major function is to present antigen to the lymphocyte, and it is the earliest cell to recognize foreign antigen.

There are two forms of dendritic cells: *immature* and *mature*. The induction of an adaptive immune response begins when a pathogen is ingested by an immature dendritic cell. These cells reside in most tissues and are relatively long-lived. As seen in Figure 1.1, they are derived from the same cell myeloid precursor as the macrophage. This immature cell carries receptors on its surface that recognize common features of many pathogens such as cell wall carbohydrates of bacteria. Once the bacterium is in contact with these receptors, the dendritic cell is stimulated to engulf the pathogen and degrade it intracellularly. These cells also continue engulfing extracellular material (both viruses and bacteria) by a receptor-independent mechanism of *macropinocytosis*. Once accomplished, the main function of the "activated" dendritic cell is to carry pathogenic antigens to the peripheral lymphoid organs to present them to T lymphocytes. Once arrived, the dendritic cell matures into an APC, which now permits it to activate pathogen-specific lymphocytes. Another function of activated dendritic cells is to secrete cytokines that influence both the innate and adaptive immune responses (see Chapter 4).

The mature macrophage also derives from primitive stem cells in the bone marrow, but unlike the lymphocyte, it matures in the tissues. Thus monocytes, the precursors of mature macrophages, circulate for only a few hours before entering the tissues where they live for months as mature macrophages. There is great variety in the tissue macrophages; they are heterogeneous in appearance and metabolism. They include mobile alveolar and peritoneal macrophages. There are also fixed cells in the liver called Kupffer cells and skin macrophages called Langerhans cells.

The primary function of these mononuclear cells is to phagocytose invading organisms, dead cells, immune complexes, and antigens. To do this, these cells are equipped with powerful lysosomal granules containing acid hydrolases and other degrading enzymes. Macrophages need activation to carry out these functions. These include cytokines, which can bind to IgG: Fc receptors or most importantly (as we shall see later) receptors for bacterial polysaccharides. In addition, they can be activated by soluble inflammatory products such as C5a. In turn, the macrophages can release monokines, such as TNF or IL-1, which increase the inflammation in inflamed tissues.

Neutrophils

These circulating cells also play an important role in the body's defense against infection. These cells produce adhesin molecule receptors, permitting them to adhere to and migrate from the blood vessels to the site of infection. They are attracted to the site by IL-8, C3a, and C3b, cytokines released by T_H1 cells, and finally factors produced by mast cells. These cells are also phagocytic cells, and the process of phagocytosis is similar to that seen in macrophages. They are particularly effective when the invading organism becomes coated with antigen-specific antibodies (often called opsonins) along with activated complement components.

Other Functional Cells

NK cells also can kill target cells in the absence of either antigen or antibody stimulation. Their lineage is not known, but they are probably in some manner related to T cells. Unlike other cells, they can be nonspecifically activated by mitogens, interferon, and IL-12. These cells are particularly useful in the early response to viral infection. As in other cells, they have receptors on their surface that recognize particular ligands. For example, NKR-PI is a lectin-like receptor that recognizes carbohydrate moieties on target cells, which initiates killing. As in other cell systems, there is also an inhibiting receptor called KIR. This molecule binds to ligands on MHC class I ligands, and this prevents killing of the target cell.

NK cells are not immune cells, and they have a broad range of specificity and no real memory. Studies of animals with NK deficiencies indicate that they have a greater incidence of viral infections and malignancies. This suggests that they have broad "immunological surveillance" properties but the exact mechanisms whereby they exert those properties are not known.

The use of an antibody-coated target to destroy foreign target cells is called antibody-dependent cell-mediated cytotoxicity, or ADCC. This killing is dependent on the recognition by cells bearing Fc receptors and includes monocytes, neutrophils, and NK cells. These cells do not need simultaneous recognition by MHC molecules. The mechanisms of killing most likely involve the release of cytoplasmic components of the target cells and perforin, but additional factors are also probably involved.

TISSUE DAMAGE PATHWAYS

Although the major function of the components of the immune system is to neutralize or destroy the invading organisms or antigen, these reactions often cause "bystander" tissue damage as well. These are called *hypersensitivity reactions*, and Gell and Coombs conveniently divided them into five types.

Hypersensitivity Reactions

TYPE I: IMMEDIATE

These reactions are those that involve antigens that react with IgE bound to tissue mast cells or basophils. Activation of the mast cell results in the release of large amounts of pharmacologically active substances. These reactions are rapid (hence immediate) and if injected into the skin a "wheel and flare" reaction can be seen within five to ten minutes. Most antigens stimulating IgE are either inhaled or ingested. A perfect example of the inhaled antigen is ragweed pollen. The IgE production requires helper T cells and T-cell-derived cytokines. IL-4 and IL-13 stimulate IgE production while IFN-γ is inhibiting. Many factors regulate the balance between

help and suppression, including route of administration, physical nature of the substance, and the genetic background of either animals or humans. In the latter, there is a family tendency to these reactions but exact genetic factors are still ill defined.

TYPE II: CELL BOUND

These reactions are initiated by antibody reacting with antigen on the cell membranes. IgM and IgG can be involved in these reactions. Clinical examples include organ-specific autoimmune diseases and immune hemolytic anemia. The role of autosensitized T cells in some diseases such as rheumatoid arthritis and multiple sclerosis have been postulated, but the evidence for their involvement is far from clear. In Graves' disease (hyperthyroidism), autoantibodies have a primary pathogenic role but specific reactive T cells are also present. However, it is not clear whether the T cells exert a primary role in stimulating antibody production or are really secondary to the tissue damage.

TYPE III: IMMUNE COMPLEX

These reactions result from the presence of either circulating immune complexes or immune complexes in the tissues. Deposition of immune complexes depends on their size, charge, local concentration of complement, and perhaps most important the nature of the antigen. An excellent example of this type of reaction is the *arthritis reaction* in which antigen is injected into the skin of an animal previously sensitized to the same antigen and has produced antibody to that antigen. The preformed antibody goes to the site of the injected antigen and forms a complex, thereby inducing complement activation and neutrophil attraction. The result is intense local inflammation, hemorrhage, and necrosis.

There are numerous examples of this type of hypersensitivity reaction, including serum sickness, glomerulonephritis, and systemic lupus erythematosus. Many of these conditions will be described in detail in later chapters.

TYPE IV: DELAYED

T cells drive this reaction when they react with antigen and release T_H1 cytokines. The cytokines in turn attract other cells, such as macrophages, which release their lysosomal enzymes. Histologically, the lesions consist of lymphocytes, macrophages, and occasionally eosinophilic polymorphonuclear leucocytes, leading to a chronic lesion of necrosis fibrosis and granulomatosus reaction. An excellent example of this reactivity is seen when PPD is injected into the skin of a person who has been previously infected with the tuberculosis organism.

BIBLIOGRAPHY

REVIEWS

Abbas AK, Lichtman AH, Pober JS, eds. *Cellular and Molecular Immunology.* 2nd ed. Philadelphia, PA: W. B. Saunders Co.; 1994.

Janeway CA, Travers P, Walport M, Schlomchik M, eds. *Immunobiology: The Immune System in Health and Disease.* New York: Garland Publishing; 2004.

Paul WE. *Fundamental Immunology.* 2nd ed. New York: Raven Press; 1994.

LANDMARK PAPERS

Chase MW. The cellular transfer of cutaneous hypersensitivity to tuberculin. *Proc Soc Exp Biol Med.* 1942;59:134–135.

Chase MW. Hypersensitivity to simple chemicals. *Harvey Lect.* 1967;61:169–203.

Del Prete G. The concept of type 1 and type 2 helper T cells and their cytokines in humans. *Int Rev Immunol.* 1998;16:427–455.

Papermaster BW, Dalmasso AP, Martinez C, Good RA. Suppression of antibody forming capacity with thymectomy in mouse. *Proc Soc Exp Biol Med.* 1962;111:41.

Zinkernagel RM, Doherty PC. H-2 compatibility requirement for T-cell mediated lysis of target cells infected with lymphocytic choriomeningitis virus: different cytotoxic T-cell specificities are associated with structures coded for in H-2K or H-2D. *J Exp Med.* 1975;141:1427–1436.

2. Immunological Techniques

John B. Zabriskie, M.D.

INTRODUCTION

This chapter is not designed to cover all the techniques and assays used in clinical immunology. Rather, it is an introduction to various techniques commonly used in diagnosing human disease or, rather, assays to evaluate the competence or incompetence of the immune system. Finally, it will serve as an introduction to the many new techniques emerging in the past several years that have widened our knowledge of the complex relationship of microbe–host interactions in human disease.

Laboratory tests vary widely in clinical immunology. Some are essential for diagnosis while others are useful in subclassifying disorders. Finally, some are of research interest only but may add to our immunological armamentarium in the future. In this regard, it is important to understand that these tests do vary in their sensitivity and specificity.

The sensitivity of a test is defined as the number of diseased individuals that are positive for the test compared with those who are negative. The specificity of a test is the proportion of individuals without a given disease that are negative. Thus, a positive test is really restricted to the disease in question.

The various assays to be discussed later in this chapter can be conveniently divided into two main divisions. Some assays are *quantitative* in that they produce precise results. Many of these assays are automated and can be related to international standards. *Qualitative* assays are less specific and will give answers such as normal–abnormal, or positive–negative results. The problem is that interpretation of results may be subjective and require special expertise in carrying out the test. Many research tests are in this category at first, and many become quantitative assays when more fully developed.

ANTIBODY PRODUCTION

Antibodies for various tests can be produced in a number of different ways, and we will discuss the prototype of each in turn.

a. *Polyclonal antibodies*: Many mammals have been used to produce antibodies, ranging from the horse, sheep, and goat down to mice and guinea pigs. Often an animal species is selected for antibody production because it will produce less-cross-reactive antibodies to a given tissue. Larger mammals, such as goats and sheep, are used to obtain larger volumes of serum to be used therapeutically in humans. A recent fear has been that animals such as sheep or cows may have eaten animal foddage contaminated with prion disease. Thus, polyclonal antibody production for therapeutic uses has often been limited to countries like Australia or New Zealand where there have been no recorded cases of prion disease in mammals.

b. *Monoclonal antibodies*: Over the past two decades, the revolutionary experiments of Kohler and Milstein have been a major advance in the production of antigen-specific antibodies. In brief, the key to this remarkable advance was the ability to obtain spleen cells from mice that had been immunized with a given antigen and fuse these cells to a non-secreting myeloma cell line, which then produces a single antibody clone when fused with a given B cell present in the spleen cells. Antibody clones are only produced when the mouse B cell fuses with the myeloma line. Non-fused B cells are eliminated by a special factor in the medium. The beauty of the hybridoma (fused) cell is that it produces only the antibody of a single mouse B cell and is therefore identical throughout its variable and constant regions, and the antibody reacts only with a single determinant on a given antigen. Finally, it is immortal and will produce the same specificity of antibody for generations. Large-scale culture of these antibodies can provide large quantities of antibody that are precise in their reactivity.

However, a word of caution is warranted. These hybridoma clones can sometimes partially lose their antibody production so that they no longer secrete as much antibody as before and may even stop production altogether. Finally, they may also lose their specificity so that a given hybridoma line must be checked periodically against the original antigen to determine whether production or specificity

remains the same as the original clone. As will be seen in many other chapters in this book, the use of monoclonal antibodies has expanded enormously in the past ten to fifteen years. They may be "humanized" by the introduction of *human* heavy and light chains so that they can be used as therapeutic agents in many human diseases, ranging from rheumatoid arthritis to many forms of cancer.

IMMUNOLOGICAL ASSAYS

Measurements of Immunoglobulins

The introduction of automated machines to measure immunoglobulins and other proteins has proceeded rapidly in recent decades. Most clinical immunology laboratories rely almost exclusively on these machines, and research labs are also introducing these automated techniques at a rapid pace. Precise measurement of serum immunoglobulins is an essential cornerstone in this area and is important for repeated and serious infections secondary to immunosuppressive agents, immunodeficiencies, in lymphoproliferate disorders, and for detection of autoantibodies.

The main principle behind this test is related to the formation of immune complexes between the antibody and a given antigen. If the concentration of antigen–antibody complex is low, then the immune complexes remain in suspension as fine particles, which can disperse a beam of light. As the complexes increase with concentration of antibody, the complexes will precipitate, and light scattering will decrease. This degree of dispersion can be measured on a nephelometer.

Using this method, a wide variety of proteins in serum, amniotic fluid, cerebrospinal fluid, saliva, and gastrointestinal juices can be determined. The method includes a wide range of immune reactants, acute phase proteins, and tumor markers. Standard preparations are used and have been calibrated against international World Health Organization standards. These tests primarily use polyclonal antibodies for each antigen since monoclonal antibodies do not form immune precipitates because there are too few relevant epitopes.

Radioimmunoassay and Enzyme-Linked Immunosorbent Assays (ELISAs)

The use of these highly sensitive assays in human disease has virtually exploded in the past two decades. They can be used to detect the levels of a given antibody or hormone in human serum, and they are extremely sensitive methods of detecting low levels of autoantibodies.

In the radioimmunoassay, one can radiolabel a particular antigen or antibody using either ^{125}I or ^{14}C tagged to the antigen or antibody. Once the serum or purified antibody or antigen to be tested is placed in the well, a second radiolabeled antihuman IgG antibody is placed in the well. After appropriate binding and further washes, the degree of activity of the antibody to a given antigen can be determined in a γ counter (see Figure 2.1 top left).

The description of ELISAs; (Figure 2.1 top right) is similar to that described for the radioimmunoassay, but in place of the radioactively labeled antibody or antigen, various fluorochromes have been substituted in place of the radioactive label. In the presence of an appropriate substrate, the fluorochrome-labeled antibody is activated to produce a given color, and the intensity of the color is read on a spectrophotometer using a 450-nm filter. By keeping the known antigen constant and diluting the serum to be tested, one can produce a curve of decreasing optical density readings, thereby indicating the amount of antibody in a given serum when compared with a standard control.

For detection of small amounts of a given antigen or antibody in a test sample, the "capture" assay is used (Figure 2.1 bottom). In this case, an unlabeled antibody to a given molecule is laid down on the plate to "capture" the small amount of antigen or antibody present in the test sample. The second antibody to this antigen or antibody is labeled with the appropriate fluorochrome, and the rest of the tests proceed as in the direct assay described previously. While the radioimmunoassay remains the "gold" standard for many clinical laboratories, more research and clinical laboratories are turning to the ELISA since it does not present the problem of radioactivity hazards or, perhaps more important, the removal of radioactive wastes (mainly a problem of disposal sites).

Immunoblots

This immunological technique has gained great favor with both basic immunologists and clinical immunologists over the past decade. Its beauty is its simplicity and the fact that one can compare different proteins, toxins, and cellular products all at the same time and reach conclusions concerning their commonality or differences or purity. The procedure is relatively simple. The proteins to be studied are run on a standard SDS gel, the percentage of which depends on the known or estimated size of the protein: larger proteins are run in 10 percent gels, while smaller proteins are run on 15 percent gels. The gel is then

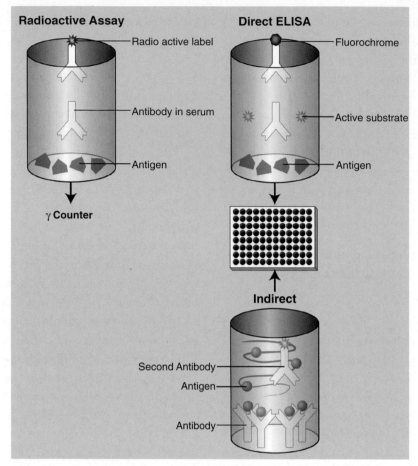

Figure 2.1 Schematic depiction of the radioimmunoassay and the direct and indirect ELISA. Both methods are extremely sensitive and will detect very small amounts of antibody in a given serum. One can label either antigen or antibody to determine amounts of antigen or antibody in a given serum or preparation. The indirect or sometimes called the "capture". ELISA is also depicted.

removed and the proteins in the gel are transferred by another electrical charge to a cellulose membrane. The membrane is treated overnight with a blocking buffer, washed, and then layered over the membrane with the antibody designed to pick up the binding to the protein (S) in question. This incubation usually lasts one hour; following washes, the membrane is treated with a species-specific second antibody tagged to an enzyme and developed with an enzyme substrate to form a colored band (see Figure 2.2).

Complement Assays

Perhaps the most useful assays for complement are the immunochemical assays of C3 and C4. As noted in Chapter 1, which outlines the alternative and classical modes of complement breakdown, a low C3 and C4 but normal factor B suggest that activation of the classical pathways has occurred. Examples would be patients with systemic lupus erythematosus or vasculitis. In contrast, if C3, C4, and factor B are all low, the alternative pathway is also activated

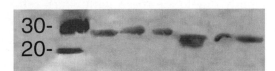

Figure 2.2 The photo is an example of an immunoblot in which the proteins in question are electrophoresed in a 15 percent SDS-gel, then transferred to nitrocellulose paper and incubated overnight in blocking buffer. This is followed by incubation with first antibody (1:1,000 dilution) followed by the species-specific second antibody tagged to alkaline phosphatase. The bands are developed using an alkaline phosphatase substrate. In this case, a single antipeptide antibody covering two sections of homology of the superantigens was used as the immunogen. Wells 2–7 contain three superantigens, each from the streptococcal and staphylococcal family of superantigens.

via either feedback loops or simultaneous activation. This would point to a gram-negative bacteremia. Normal C4 levels with low C3 and factor B levels suggest the alternative pathway alone. *Elevation* of all three components usually suggests acute or chronic infection. Acute rheumatic fever is such an example.

Assays for immune complexes are best directed toward an analysis of the immune complexes or their deposition in various human disease tissues. In most cases, the best approach is to receive freshly biopsied nonfrozen material that is then snap frozen and sections cut and stained to test for the presence of appropriate antigen or antibody (see Figure 12.3 in Chapter 12). In some cases, the antigen is still intact after formalin fixation and paraffin blocks are prepared. But in these specimens, one always runs the risk of destroying the appropriate antigen or antibody during the fixation process. Examples of the diseases studied in this manner are renal immune complex disease such as seen in SLE, acute poststreptococcal glomerulonephritis, or psoriasis.

Antibodies to common microbial antigens have been used to detect infection with different microbes for years. However, the presence of a single antibody serum specimen only tells you that the person was exposed to this microbe in the past. To diagnose an acute infection, one must have paired sera usually taken two weeks apart that demonstrate a significant rise in antibody titers in the second specimen compared to the first. One can also do these antibody tests in reverse. Normally, we are exposed to many microbial antigens during growth and development either as a result of exposure to a given microbe or after immunization with a given antigen (i.e., tetanus toxoid, pneumococcus polysaccharide, measles, or mumps viral antigen). Antibodies to the microbial products are usually found in normal individuals, but if they are not, one should suspect abnormalities of antibody production like those seen in immunodeficiency states.

LYMPHOCYTIC ASSAYS

Fluorescein-Activated Cell Sorter

With the renewed interest in the role of lymphocytes in disease states over the past thirty years, a systematic study of the markers present on B and T lymphocytes has been undertaken. The knowledge that many such markers exist on a given cell was made possible by the introduction of monoclonal antibodies specific for each marker. Thus, antibodies could quickly identify lymphocytes as B (CD19) or T lymphocytes (CD3) and later into helper (CD4) or suppressor cells (CD8) and many other markers.

The second major advance was the introduction of the flow cytometer, which measures the fluorescence of each labeled antibody. The different cell populations are aspirated into the machine, which forces the cells to flow through the chamber singly past a laser beam and light sensors. Light emitted by the excited fluorescent dye on the cell surface is detected by the sensors and analyzed by computer software. Using this system, one can divide cells into different populations, depending on their size and granularity (see Figure 2.3). Once the different cell populations are identified, a specific population can be "gated" for further study, such as identification of helper cells (CD4) and suppressor cells (CD8-PE), as well as many other lymphocyte subsets.

A variation of this technique is illustrated in Figure 2.4 in which the lymphocytes are identified with anti-CD3 labels. Of this population, the number of B cells in the population is identified by CD19-PE labeled antibodies. Finally, the number of B cells expressing a novel antigen is identified, in which the percentage of CD19+ exhibiting D8/17+ B cells is

calculated. All of these values are obtained rapidly due to the speed with which cells are counted with different labels, and the results are accurate because of the large number of cells that are counted (in the thousands). It should be emphasized that values for lymphocyte subsets will change with increasing age from children to adults, especially during the first year of life.

Using a more sophisticated machine called a fluorescein-activated cell sorter (FACS), individual subsets of lymphocytes can be separated with fluorescein-labeled antibodies into unique cell populations or even single cells. This procedure is done under sterile conditions and is useful in isolating a single cell or cell population for further cell culture, growth, and study.

Lymphocyte Proliferation Assays

This test assumes greater importance in clinical immunology both at a research level and in the clinical laboratories. These tests can be carried out in whole blood

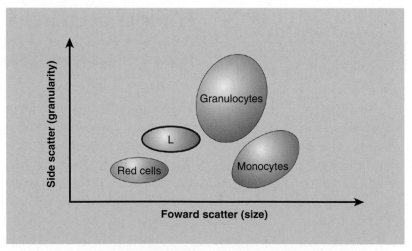

Figure 2.3 Schematic depiction of cell separation on a flow cytometry machine or fluorescein-activated cell scan. The different cell populations are separated both by size (forward scatter) and granularity (side scatter) and a given population is then separated into B or T cells and within the T cells into helper (CD4+) and suppressor (CD8+) cells. Isolation and purification of a given subset of cells can be achieved by a fluorescein-activated cell sorter.

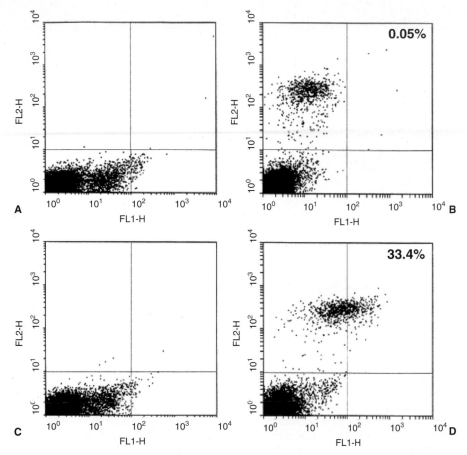

Figure 2.4 FACS analysis of D8/17-positive lymphocytes. Whole venous blood was obtained from a normal patient (panels A and B) and an obsessive-compulsive disorder (OCD) patient (panels C and D). Panels A and C are controls in which the D8/17 and CD19 antibodies were omitted. Panels B and D are dual-labeled cells from a normal individual and a patient with OCD. The D8/17 fluorescence as a percentage of total B cells was 0.5 percent in the normal and 33.4 percent in the OCD patients in panels B and D. Each point on this plot represents fluorescence recorded from an individual lymphocyte as it passes through the counter. Reprinted with permission from Elsevier; Chapman F, Visvanathan K, Carreno-Manjarrez R, Zabriskie JB. A flow cytometric assay for D8/17 B cell marker in patients with Tourette's syndrome and obsessive compulsive disorder. *J Immunol Methods.* 1998;219:181–186.

that has been anticoagulated so as to permit the use of viable cells. The preferred method is the isolation of the lymphocytes from blood using a density gradient assay method. The anticoagulated blood sample is usually diluted 1:1 with PBS (pH 7.4) and slowly layered over the density gradient solution, which has been prepared so that the cell populations will separate into different layers. As seen in Figure 2.5, neu-trophils and red blood cells are centrifuged to the bottom, while the mononuclear cell population stays in the middle of the gradient. Finally, the serum components and platelets are mainly in areas above and below the mononuclear cells. Once the mononuclear cells are removed from the gradient and washed several times, a relatively pure population of mononuclear cells is obtained.

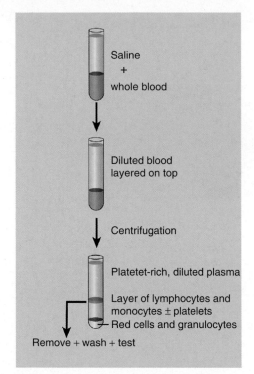

Figure 2.5 Lymphocyte and monocyte separation using a ficoll gradient. As noted, red cells and granulocytes spin to the bottom of the tube while a clear layer of lymphocytes and monocytes is separated by the gradient. These cells are counted and adjusted to a given number of cells for use in the proliferation assay.

When these cells are stimulated by a specific antigen, a few of these resting cells undergo proliferation (activated cells) and the transformation of activated cells can be measured by incorporation of radiolabeled thymidine into the DNA of the cells and the number of counts per minute measured in β-counter. More recently, these same activated cells can be measured by the number of cells expressing cell surface antigens using markers such as CD69.

DNA Technology Assays

The emergence of molecular biology and DNA technology has ushered in a whole new series of methods for the detection of microbial agents, human genetics, and analysis of tissue samples, to name but a few of the uses of DNA technology today. The analysis of blood or serum samples also has far-reaching implications in our legal system. The following is a short summary of these techniques and their importance in clinical immunology.

DNA ANALYSIS

Known unique segments of nucleic acid sequences can be used as DNA probes to determine the presence of complementary sequences of DNA in a sample from a given patient. The probe, which is a single strand of a given DNA, is presented to the target DNA, which is composed of thousands of nucleotides. The complementary strands from target and probe DNA will anneal to each other, a process known as *DNA hybridization*. The high affinity of the probe for a complementary segment in the target DNA is the most specific intermolecular interaction between biological macromolecules.

This technique may be used not only on fresh samples but also in tissues that have formalin-fixed and paraffin-embedded tissues. In this technique of *in situ hybridization,* the probes can be applied directly to tissue sections on microscope slides. However, this technique works only after deparaffinization and proteolytic digestion are performed to expose intracellular nucleic acid targets. The probe is detected in the sample either by radiolabeling the probe or radiolabeling an antibody to the probe DNA.

Another approach is the use of *restriction endonucleases* (see Figure 2.6). These are enzymes that cleave DNA at sites specifically related to the nucleotide sequences. Using enzymes with different specificities, a DNA fragment containing a particular

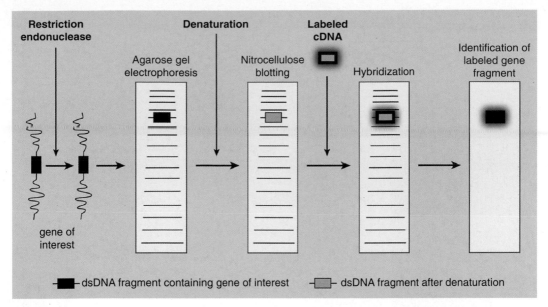

Figure 2.6 The use of restriction endonucleases to carry out gene mapping using the Southern blotting technique. DNA hybridization is the most specific intermolecular interaction between biological macromolecules.

gene can be cut out from the DNA molecule. In the Southern blot, these fragments of DNA are electophoresed on agarose gels with the smaller fragments migrating further than the larger ones. Alkaline denaturation of these fragments uncoils the fragment so that a single stranded DNA will hybridize with the complementary DNA after transfer to a special nitrocellulose filter. Blotting the gel with the nitrocellulose filter "fixes" these DNA fragments after the electrophoresis. Finally, a radiolabeled probe containing DNA known to be complementary to the DNA of interest hybridizes to it, and the fragment can be identified by autoradiography of the filter. The Northern blotting technique is very similar to the DNA experiment but uses RNA instead of DNA in the system.

POLYMERASE CHAIN REACTION (PCR) ASSAY

Although the DNA analysis systems described earlier are still used in research and clinical laboratories, a major revolution in detecting DNA material occurred with the introduction of the PCR assay. This method is particularly valuable since it can markedly amplify a small piece of DNA before cleavage with a restriction enzyme. Complementary oligonucleotide primers from either end of the target DNA are added to the denatured sample, along with a heat-resistant DNA polymerase. If the target sequence is present, the primers anneal to it and provide a starting point for the polymerase to begin the synthesis of second-strand DNA (see Figure 2.7). The newly synthesized double-stranded DNA is then denatured by heating and exposed again to the polymerase enzyme at a lower temperature. In this way, newly synthesized molecules and original DNA can reassociate with the primer and act as templates for further rounds of DNA synthesis. After completing about thirty cycles (usually two to three hours in an automated machine), the specific target sequence is amplified

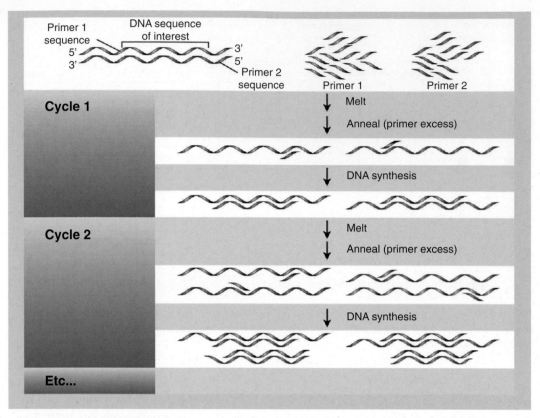

Figure 2.7 Schematic description of a PCR. To use this method, it is necessary to know the sequence of a short region of DNA on the 3′ and 5′ of the sequence. It is a very powerful tool for detecting DNA sequences in tissues, dried blood spots, and pathological specimens. The specimen must be handled carefully to avoid introduction of other DNA material, that is, the DNA of the handler of the specimen in question.

more than 1-million-fold. This powerful and sensitive technique can detect a specific DNA sequence from a single cell (e.g., lymphocyte, sperm), fixed pathological specimens, and dried blood spots. The main disadvantage is that contamination of the reaction mixture with traces of DNA from another source will lead to false positive results. Thus extreme care in handling specimens to be tested as well as in the test itself is obligatory.

MAJOR HISTOCOMPATIBILITY (MHC) ASSAYS

Using sera obtained first from multi-transfused patients and later from multiparous women (alloantigens), the early work of Dausset and others in the 1950s and 1960s identified a series of antigens present on mononuclear cells called the human leucocyte antigens (HLAs). Using a somewhat crude agglutination assay of leucocytes, they noticed that these sera agglutinated leucocytes from unrelated donors and that the patterns of such co-agglutination demonstrated definitive antigens in human populations. After extensive research and workshop meetings, it became apparent that these antigens were present on all tissues of the body, but their high concentration on peripheral blood lymphocytes enabled investigators to perform immunogenetic studies more easily on these cells. While most of the original testing for the antigens on cells and for use in transplantation relied on serological techniques using purified antibodies to detect these antigens, the introduction of the PCR assay changed the rapidity with which these antigens could be identified, and both MHC class I and class II antigens are now routinely identified by the method.

Generally, this technique is available only in centers that specialize in organ and bone marrow transplantation. In addition to the transplantation, these techniques are used for familial genetic studies as well as for specific disease states (see other chapters in this book). One example is the identification of HLA B27, which is highly associated with anklyosing spondylitis, and as the research continues one can expect that other genetic MHC markers will be identified in particular disease states. The converse is also true. It is now known that certain MHC antigens confer resistance to a given disease, while others confer susceptibility. A word of caution is warranted. These markers only suggest a susceptibility to the disease. Most disease states appear to be polygenic, and factors such as the environment and past exposure to a given microbe also play a part in establishing the full disease pattern.

MICROARRAY ASSAYS

Over the past decade, this assay system has become popular in many branches of science, including immunology. In essence, these assays have become the standard tools for gene expression profiling as the mRNA levels of a large number of genes can be measured in a single assay. Of particular interest, one can compare the levels of gene expressions across the human genome in one subset of patients in a given disease to another subset of patients with the same disease.

The method is relatively straightforward. One takes the tissues or cells to be studied and prepares them as follows:

Tissue → mRNA → cDNA → Biotinylated cRNA

The biotinylated material is layered on glass slides on which DNA fragments of the human genome have been placed (12,000 probe sets/chips). The chips are then washed, stained with streptavidin-phycoerythrin, and scanned with a probe array scanner.

As an example, Figure 2.8 represents the staining patterns seen in six psoriatic patients before and six hours after treatment with a T-cell suppression agent. Note the decreased expression of red intensity in

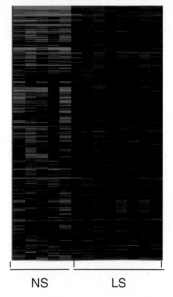

Figure 2.8 Photograph showing genomic analysis of lesional versus nonlesional skin in psoriatic skin. The heat map describes 1,119 genes that have significantly higher expression (red area) by 1.2-fold ($P < 0.05$, after BH correction) in the lesional skin versus nonlesional skin (green area).

the patterns following treatment, indicating a decrease in gene regulation.

FUTURE DIRECTIONS IN RESEARCH

The use of monoclonal antibodies, especially "humanized" ones, will play an increasingly important role in both basic immunology and clinical immunology. Their use will be in both detection of small and early tumors and in the treatment of tumors. The success of monoclonal antibodies in metastatic prostate cancer is already well established. It is believed that other tumor therapies will follow in the future.

The use of microarray assays has grown in the past decade and will continue to grow. The use of these assays has a role in diseases associated with human genetics and provides information on which cytokines or lymphokines are important in disease states.

BIBLIOGRAPHY

REVIEWS

Abbas AK, Lichtman AH, Pober JS, eds. *Cellular and Molecular Immunology.* 2nd ed. Philadelphia, PA: W. B. Saunders Co.; 1994.

Kohler G, Milstein C. Continuous cultures of fused cells secreting antibody of predefined specificity. *Nature.* 1975;256:495–497.

Rose NR, de Macario EC, Folds JD, Lane HC, Nakamura RM, eds. *Manual of Clinical Laboratory Immunology.* Washington, DC: American Society for Microbiology; 1997.

von Muhlen CA, Tan EM. Autoantibodies in the diagnosis of systemic rheumatic diseases. *Semin Arthritis Rheum.* 1995;24:323–358.

SUGGESTED READING

Alvarez-Barrientos A, Arroyo J, Canton R, Nombela C, Sanchez-Perez M. Applications of flow cytometry to clinical microbiology. *Clin Microbiol Rev.* 2000;13:167–195.

Churchill GA. Fundamentals of experimental design for cDNA microarrays. *Nat Genet Suppl.* 2007;32:490–495.

Craig FE. Flow cytometric evaluation of B cell lymphoid neoplasms. *Clin Lab Med.* 2007;27:487–512.

Dausset J. The major histocompatibility complex in man. *Science.* 1981;213:1469–1474.

Davies MA, Marstone AJ, Viza DC, Colonbani J, Dausset J. Human transplantation antigens: the HLA (Hu-1) system and its homology with the mouse H-2 system. *Transplantation.* 1968;4:571–586.

Dyer P, Middleton D. *Histocompatibility Testing: A Practical Approach.* Oxford: IRL Press; 1993.

3. Immune Regulation

*Nina Bhardwaj, M.D., Ph.D., David O'Neill, M.D.,
and Thomas Waldmann, M.D.*

INTRODUCTION

The immune system in general responds appropriately to the presence of foreign antigens. However, there are certain diseases that arise from either a defective or overresponsive immune system on the part of the host. Two major therapeutic approaches are possible: either immunosuppression or immunopotentiation of the immune system. The object of this chapter is to introduce the reader to the various approaches that have been used to either suppress or stimulate the immune response.

IMMUNOSUPPRESSION

Immunosuppressive Drugs

Several groups of drugs suppress the immune system (see Table 3.1). Among the oldest of these drugs are the *corticosteroids*, which have long been known to alter immune responses. When corticosteroids are given, the result is a transient lymphopenia peaking at four hours and lasting up to twenty-four hours. Helper T cells are predominantly affected, and at higher doses of steroids inhibition of interleukin-2 (IL-2) production by helper T cells becomes increasing important. Another major effect in humans is on resting macrophages (activated macrophages are not sensitive).

In humans, steroids are used for two main purposes. One is the prevention or reversal of graft rejection (see Chapter 18). The other is in the treatment of autoimmune and malignant diseases. Corticosteroids modulate inflammation by suppressing cytokine- and chemokine-encoding genes, which inhibits the activation and recruitment of inflammatory cells.

The side effects of steroids are numerous and often depend on both the dose used and duration of treatment. These include an increased susceptibility to infection, osteoporosis, and growth disturbances in children, as well as gastric ulcers, hypertension, acne, and hirsutism. By giving larger doses for shorter periods, many of these side effects are lessened.

The development of the *thiopurines* in the 1950s ushered in a new group of immunosuppressive agents, the most important of them being azathioprine. It is inactive until it is metabolized in the liver and takes three to four weeks to be effective. The metabolites work by inhibiting DNA synthesis in dividing cells (such as activated lymphocytes). Like many other drugs, it has side effects, mainly in bone marrow toxicity, and long-term use eventually results in granulocytopenia and thrombocytopenia.

Another group is the *alkylating agents*, of which cyclophosphamide is one of the best examples. This drug also requires activation by the liver. It inhibits cell division and can suppress antibody production, and it

Table 3.1 Monoclonal Antibodies Approved for Cancer Therapeutics

Agent	Principal Mode of Action[a]
Corticosteroids	Inhibition of activation of cytokine and chemokine genes by nuclear factor κB
Mercaptopurine	Inhibits nucleic acid synthesis in activated lymphocytes
Azathioprine	Inhibits nucleic acid synthesis in activated lymphocytes
Myocphenolate mofetil	Inhibits inosine monophosphate and lymphocyte proliferation
Methotrexate	Inhibits dihydrofolate reductase; anti-inflammatory
Leflunomide	Inhibits pyrimidine synthesis; anti-inflammatory; antiproliferative
Cyclophosphamide	Cross-links DNA; blocks cell division
Cyclosporine	Binds calcineurin, inhibits nuclear factor of activated T cells; early events in T-cell activation[b]
Tacrolimus (FK506)	Binds tacrolimus-binding protein; inhibits nuclear factor of activated T cells; early events in T-cell activation
Sirolimus FTY720	Blocks T-cell proliferation Analogue of sphingosine 1-phosphate; inhibits lymphocyte homing
Rapamycin	Interferes with cyclins; blocks mitogen-activated signals and cell cycle

[a]Nuclear factor of activated T cells is a transcription factor that regulates production of IL-2 and other cytokines; tacrolimus-binding protein is a member of a family of at least eleven proteins, some of which inhibit calcineurin.
[b]Ligation of the T-cell receptor activates calcineurin, a serine-threonine phosphatase and a member of the family of intracellular regulatory proteins termed cyclophilins. Some cyclophilins can inhibit calcineurin, regulate intracellular calcium flux, and activate the NFAT gene. Cyclosporine binds to the cyclophilin Cy^{PA}, thereby inhibiting the phosphatase activity of calcineurin.

decreases delayed-type hypersensitivity. Methotrexate, which inhibits cell division by disrupting folic acid metabolism, has similar immunomodulatory effects.

Cyclosporin, a naturally occurring fungal metabolite, also inhibits T-cell activation and cell-mediated immunity. The drug becomes active only when complexed to its intracellular receptor cyclophilin, and it inhibits early calcium-dependent events, especially the activation of several cytokine genes. Its major effect is the inhibition of IL-2 production and the $CD4^+$ proliferation responses. Cyclosporin has been extremely useful in the control of transplant rejection and is also used in several autoimmune diseases such as psoriasis and severe rheumatoid arthritis. However, long-term use has demonstrated severe toxicity such

as nephrotoxicity and hepatotoxicity and particularly lymphoma induction. Tacolimus is a newer-generation drug with a similar mechanism of action.

ANTIBODIES AND OTHER IMMUNOSUPPRESSIVE METHODS

There are a number of instances in which antibodies have been used to suppress the immune response. Among the earliest measures has been the use of anti-RHD antibodies to prevent hemolytic disease of the newborn due to incompatibility between the mother (RHD–) and an RHD+ fetus. The disease is prevented by the administration of anti-D antibodies to the mother immediately after delivery. This inhibits the formation of anti-D antibodies in the mother, thereby avoiding the development of serious disease in the infant. This therapeutic measure has virtually eliminated the incidence of RH disease in developed countries.

More recently, monoclonal antibodies are being used to suppress the immune system, and several antibodies are now approved for the treatment of autoimmune diseases. These antibodies are typically "humanized" mouse monoclonals, created by transposing the mouse antigen-binding sites onto a human antibody framework (see Figure 3.1). This technique retains the full range of effective properties of human Fc while minimizing the immunogenicity of the mouse component. Antibodies that target the immune system can target cell surface molecules on T or B cells or can target soluble mediators of inflammation such as cytokines. Among the most effective uses of monoclonal antibodies has been in treating severe rheumatoid arthritis, using monoclonal antibody directed against tumor necrosis factor (TNF-α). The drawback to this therapy is that the

infusions must be repeated frequently to sustain results.

Monoclonal antibodies can also be used as antitumor agents (see review by Reichert). Specific targeting and killing of tumor cells can be enhanced by linking tumor antigen-specific monoclonal antibodies to agents as follows: (1) a cytotoxic drug such as methotrexate, (2) a radioisotope such as iodine-131 or ytrium-90, or (3) a toxin such as ricin. Monoclonal antibodies are now approved for the treatment of non-Hodgkin's lymphoma, myeloid and lymphocytic leukemia, breast cancer, and colorectal cancer (Table 3.2).

Some new studies, still in clinical trials, are occurring in the treatment of prostate cancer, especially metastatic bone lesions, and it is hoped many more monoclonal antibodies will be forthcoming against various other tissues.

Other methods of immunosuppression are *plasmapheresis* or *plasma exchange*. In the first method, improvement may be due to removal of mediators of tissue damage, whereas in plasma exchange, it may be due to replacement of deficient factors or to

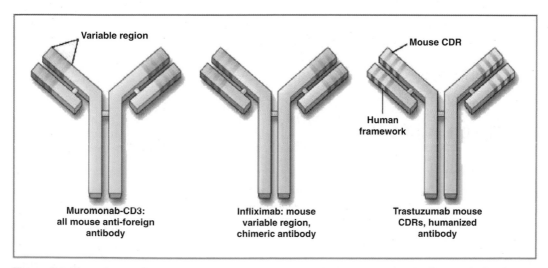

Figure 3.1 Three types of monoclonal antibodies now in clinical use. Reprinted with permission from Schwartz RS. The Shattuck Lecture: diversity of the immune repertoire and immunoregulation. *New Engl J Med*. 2003;348:1017–1026.

Table 3.2 Immunosuppressive Drugs in Clinical Use or Clinical Trials

Year Approved	Brand Name	Generic Name	Type of mAb	Target	Indication
1997	Rituxan	Rituximab	Chimeric	CD20	NHL[a]
1998	Herecptin	Trastuzumab	Humanized	HER2	Her-2/nev positive breast cancer
2000	Mylotarg	Gemtuzumab ozogamicin	Humanized	CD33	AML
2001	Campath-1	Aliemtuzumab	Humanized	CD52	B-cell CLL[b]
2002	Zevalin	Ibritumomab tiuxetan conjugated to ^{111}In or ^{90}Y	Murine	CD20	NHL
2003	Bexxar	^{31}I-tositumomab	Murine radiolabeled	CD20	NHL
2004	Avastin™	Bevacizumab	Humanized	VEGF	Colorectal cancer
2004	Erbitux	Cetuximab	Chimeric	EGFR (HER-1)	Colorectal cancer

EGFR, epidermal growth factor receptor; VEGF, vascular endothelial growth factor.
[a]NHL: Non-Hodgkin's lymphoma.
[b]CLL: Chronic lymphocytic leukemia.

the immunomodulatory effects of human immunoglobulins.

Total lymphoid irradiation produces long-term suppression of helper T cells and has been used in some severe autoimmune diseases like lupus or rheumatoid arthritis. The side effects of this treatment may be severe and sometimes fatal.

IMMUNOPOTENTIATION

Chronic infections such as HIV and hepatitis C are characterized by an inability of the host to control viral replication. The ability to potentiate the host immune response to control chronic infections is an important goal and is under active investigation. It has also been shown that at least some types of cancer can be controlled by the host immune system, so potentiation of the host immune system may prove useful in treating these cancers. There are three principal ways to potentiate the immune response in humans: through cytokines, adoptive immunotherapy, or vaccination.

Cytokine Therapy

Interferons are antiviral glycoproteins, which are secreted as a result of a viral infection and have wide-ranging antitumor and immunomodulatory effects. They have attracted much interest as immunotherapeutic agents. Interferons bind to cell surface receptors and activate secondary intracellular changes which inhibit viral replication. They can be divided into three groups: alpha (α), beta (β), and gamma (γ) interferons. All three interferons have been genetically engineered, and recombinant IFN-α, -β, and -γ are available, but IFN-α is the best studied. IFN-α is the treatment of choice for hepatitis B and C; when given systemically, it produces significant clearing of hepatitis B in chronic carriers. IFN-α has some side effects, mainly flu-like symptoms such as fever, malaise, and anorexia – all symptoms that can be tolerated. More severe effects are reversible: bone marrow depression, liver dysfunction, and cardiotoxicity.

IFN-β has been shown to be of benefit in patients with relapsing-remitting multiple sclerosis, and IFN-β1 appears to decrease the rate of progression of disability. Despite these results, the precise therapeutic role of IFN-β is still controversial.

IFN-γ is a potential activator of macrophages and is most often used in conditions in which defective macrophage function occurs. Examples of these disorders are lepromatous leprosy, leishmaniasis, and chronic granulomatous disease. IFN-γ works by increasing phagocytic bactericidal activity, but only some patients show enhanced superoxide activity, implying that IFN-γ works by several different mechanisms.

IL-2 is produced by stimulated CD4 T cells and induces clonal expansion of IL-2$^+$ T and B cells. is used in immunodeficiency states such as HIV infection where IL-2 production is defective. In patients with HIV infection and baseline counts of CD4 above 200 ml, intermittent IL-2 infusions have been shown to produce substantial and sustained increases in CD4 counts. IL-2 has side effects similar to IFN-α, with most of the effects being flu-like. The most serious side effect is IL-2 action on IL-1, IFN-γ, and TNF, all mediators of vascular permeability, resulting in marked hypotension, pulmonary edema, and neuropsychiatric symptoms.

Adoptive Immunotherapy

Adoptive immunotherapies involve the transfer of either cells or antibodies into a host. These are also referred to as passive therapies, since the host does not actively mount its own immune response. Examples include infusion of hepatitis B immune globulin and the adoptive transfer of antigen-specific T lymphocytes to treat a chronic viral infection or cancer (see Gattinoni et al. 2006).

Immunization

Prevention of infectious diseases depends on many factors. Foremost is the presence of a clean water supply, development of sanitary facilities, good nutrition, and good personal hygiene. More recently, immunization against a particular agent has been the most effective measure in controlling infectious disease. Yet, with the emergence of new infectious agents such as hepatitis C and HIV, novel approaches will be needed to generate new and effective vaccines.

IMMUNITY

The two ways to achieve immunity are actively and passively. Active immunity is achieved when exposure to a foreign stimulus triggers an immunological response to the agent by the host. The best immunity to an agent is achieved by natural infection, which evolves with a clinical or subclinical response to the agent by the host. Artificial active immunization is the administration of an immunogen as a vaccine. Vaccines may be live organisms, killed organisms, or modified toxins. Although no vaccine is ideal and each has its problems, the problems of live vaccines are generally related to their safety, while the problems of killed vaccines are related mainly to their effectiveness.

Live attenuated vaccines are useful because they infect, replicate, and immunize in a manner similar to natural infection but with milder clinical symptoms. Examples include many of the childhood infections such as measles, mumps, and rubella (MMR vaccine), chicken pox (varicella) and Bacille Calmette-Guérin (BCG) for tuberculosis. Although millions of doses have been administered with no complications, if given to an immunocompromised host (such as primary immunodeficiency or secondary to HIV infection), these live vaccines may cause serious disease.

Killed vaccines consist of suspensions of killed organisms such as typhoid, cholera, and pertussis (although there is now an acellular vaccine) or one of the products or fractions of the organism. These include toxoids of diphtheria and tetanus and subunits of viruses such as surface hepatitis B antigen. Among the most successful of these types of vaccines has been the use of polysaccharides in the pneumococcal, meningococcal, and *Haemophilus influenza* vaccines. In general, the killed vaccines are not as effective as the live viruses because they do not give long-lasting immunity as a live infection does. For example, although the tetanus toxoid vaccine is effective, it requires a booster dose every ten years.

The immunological response to the killed organism or product thereof has been enhanced by the use of adjuvants. Although the most common adjuvant for animal studies has been the complete Freund's adjuvant, it cannot be used in humans because it causes liver, skin, and spleen dysfunction. The most common adjuvant for humans is aluminum compounds, which are generally safe for human use. Others include muramyl dipeptide, biodegradable polymers, and a glycoside adjuvant called Quil A from the bark of an Amazon oak tree. However, many others are being developed or will probably be given U.S. Food and Drug Administration (FDA) acceptance in the future. The key feature will be their immunogenic enhancement and their strength of safety for use in humans.

Although we have mainly been discussing various forms of vaccination to protect against the invading organism, one of the most interesting new vaccines has not been developed to eliminate the infectious agent but rather to prevent the development of another far more serious disease – a complication of the initial infection. This is the Gardisal vaccine manufactured by Merck to protect against human papilloma virus (HPV). HPV infection is usually sexually acquired, and it is estimated that currently 20 million people are infected in the United States. The infection has no real signs or symptoms, and HPV may lead to cervical cancer. It is estimated that ten of the thirty different serotypes of the virus can induce cervical cancer, so the vaccine has been directed at eliminating those serotypes. Thus, if 10,000 women are infected with one of the high-risk viral serotypes, approximately 3,900 of them will die of cervical cancer. The new vaccine, if given before active sexual activity in women, can prevent the viral infection and thereby markedly diminish the risk of cervical cancer. Because of the possible success of this vaccine, it may be worthwhile to look at how to prevent the Epstein-Barr virus in at-risk children to prevent or diminish the risk of Burkett's lymphoma in children infected with the virus.

CYTOKINE IMMUNOMODULATION

Although many of the immunoregulation techniques revolve around the humoral arm of the immune response, there is increasing interest in targeting T cells or the cytokine regulators to regulate the elimination of autoreactive T cells, tumor cells, and the maintenance of a specific memory response to these pathogens. Such immune responses are normally regulated by cytokines, and the activities of the cytokines have a high degree of redundancy. The common cytokine receptor γ chain is used by IL-2, IL-4, IL-7, IL-9, IL-15, and IL-21 (see Figure 3.2). The IL-2R and the IL-15R have a second (β chain) subunit in common as well, but have unique α subunits (see Figure 3.3). These two cytokine receptors use a common signaling pathway that involves JAK1, JAK3, and STAT5. The signaling involves the phosphorylation of STAT5 that results in the dissociation of STAT5 from the receptor and the subsequent dimerization of STAT5. The dimers then translocate to the nucleus and promote transcription of target genes (see Figure 3.2).

There are several distinct differences in the functions of IL-2 and IL-15. IL-2 is involved in checkpoints or brakes on the immune system. IL-2 is required to maintain the competitiveness of forkhead box P3- (FoxP3-) expressing regulatory T cells, and plays a crucial role in activation-induced cell death (AICD), a process that leads to the elimination of self-reactive T cells. Thus, the unique feature of IL-2 is to prevent T-cell immune response to self that would lead to autoimmunity. In contrast, IL-15 expression has no effect on regulatory T cells but is an anti-apoptotic factor in several systems. Furthermore, IL-15 promotes the maintenance of CD8$^+$ CD44 memory T cells. Thus, IL-15 has as its primary role the maintenance of a robust memory response to invading pathogens.

These observations from ex vivo functional studies are supported by studies in mice deficient in cytokine or cytokine receptor genes. For example, IL-2-deficient and IL-2Rα-deficient mice develop a marked

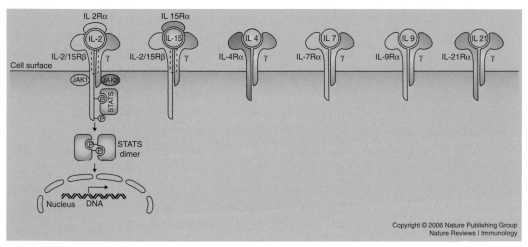

Figure 3.2 The structure and signaling pathways of the common cytokine-receptor γ chain family of receptors. Reprinted by permission from Macmillan Publishers: Waldmann T. The biology of interleukin-2 and interleukin-15: implications for cancer therapy and vaccine design. *Nat Rev Immunol.* 2006;6:595.

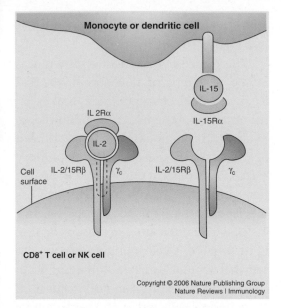

Figure 3.3 The mode of interaction of IL-2 and IL-15 with the subunits of their receptors. Reprinted by permission from Macmillan Publishers: Waldmann T. The biology of interleukin-2 and interleukin-15: implications for cancer therapy and vaccine design. *Nat Rev Immunol.* 2006;6:595.

enlargement of the peripheral lymphoid organs and polyclonal expansion of T and B cells, and this proliferation reflects the impairment of regulatory T cells and AICD. These mice develop autoimmune diseases such as hemolytic anemia and inflammatory bowel disease.

In contrast, mice that are deficient in IL-15, or its receptor IL-15Rα, do not develop enlarged lymphoid tissues, increased serum immunoglobulin, or autoimmune disease. Rather they have a marked reduction in the number of thymic and peripheral natural killer (NK) cells, NK T cells, and intestinal intraepithelial lymphocytes. Thus, IL-15Rα-deficient mice show a marked reduction in CD8+CD44hi memory T cells. The differences in the functions of IL-2 and IL-15 reflect the distinct modes of actions of these two cytokines.

IL-2 functions as a secreted cytokine, acting on preformed heterotrimeric receptors expressed on activated T and NK cells (Figure 3.3). In contrast, IL-15 acts as part of an immunological synapse. IL-15 and IL-15Rα expressed on the surface of antigen-presenting cells are presented in trans to CD8 T cells and NK cells that express only the β and γ chain of the IL-15 receptor (Figures 3.3 and 3.4).

The unique IL-2 and IL-2Rα system has been a valuable target for immunotherapy because IL-2Rα is not expressed by any resting cells with the exception of T regulatory cells. Yet, it is expressed by many malignant cells of various T- and B-cell leukemias, T cells that participate in organ-allograft rejection, and finally by T cells involved in autoimmune diseases. Thus, antibodies directed against IL-2Rα (several such antibodies have been approved by FDA for use in humans) specifically destroy those cells that are IL-2 dependent. One of these antibodies (daclizumab by Hoffmann–La Roche) is in phase II trials in patients with uveitis, in certain multiple sclerosis patients, and in asthma patients. Finally, it was shown to be effective in a subset of patients with adult T-cell leukemia due to human T-cell lymphotropic virus I.

It is believed that IL-15 might contribute to autoimmune diseases by inducing the expression of TNF-α, by inhibiting self-tolerance mediated by IL-2-induced AICD, and by facilitating the maintenance of CD8+ memory T-cell survival, including that of self-reactive memory cells. For example, dysregulated IL-15 expression has been reported in patients with a range of autoimmune diseases such as multiple sclerosis, inflammatory bowel disease, and psoriasis. In this context, cytokine-directed blockade of TNF with specific monoclonal

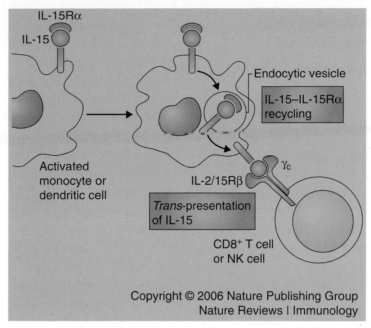

Figure 3.4 Following their co-induction on antigen-presenting cells by addition of an interferon, the interleukin receptor α chain presents IL-15 to neighboring natural killer cells and memory phenotype CD8 T cells that express the other IL-15 receptors beta and gamma. Reprinted by permission from Macmillan Publishers: Waldmann T. The biology of interleukin-2 and interleukin-15: implications for cancer therapy and vaccine design. *Nat Rev Immunol*. 2006;6:595.

antibodies or soluble TNF receptors has been an important target for many of the diseases mentioned previously. Yet TNF-directed therapies do not provide effective therapy for all these patients, and new therapeutic targets are needed. Furthermore, although TNF-directed therapy has an anti-inflammatory effect, it does not have an effect on self-reactive memory T cells that might play a role in the pathogenesis and maintenance of auto-immune diseases. Thus, it is hoped that by targeting IL-15 it might be possible to both achieve the anti-inflammatory effects and reduce the number of CD8[+] self-reactive memory T cells.

Several agents that inhibit IL-15 activity have been developed, including soluble IL-15Rα, mutant IL-15 molecules, and antibodies specific for IL-2/IL-15Rβ.

For example, in vivo, the IL-15 mutant markedly diminished antigen-specific delayed-type hypersensitivity responses in Balb/c mice and increased survival of pancreatic islet cell allografts. The use of soluble high-affinity IL-15Rα inhibited the development of mouse collagen-induced arthritis and inhibited allograft rejection. An antibody specific for IL-15 has been efficacious in mouse models of psoriasis. This antibody is now in a phase I/II clinical trial in patients with rheumatoid arthritis. Finally, a humanized antibody specific for IL-2/IL-15Rβ when administered as a single agent prolonged cardiac-allograft survival in cynomolgus monkeys, and only minimal toxicity was noted when this antibody was given in a phase I trial to patients with T-cell large granular lymphocytic leukemia.

CELLULAR VACCINES AND MODULATIONS THEREOF

Dendritic Cell Vaccines

Recently, much attention has focused on the area of dendritic cell (DC) vaccines in the treatment of cancers. The immunological basis of current approaches to therapeutic cancer vaccination (often called "vacci-treatment") has been established over the past decade or longer. These new developments are mainly based on the lessons learned from the clinical testing of these approaches. In particular, three lessons are worthy of note: First, recent randomized phase III trials suggest that vacci-treatment with autologous DCs expressing prostatic acid phosphatase or with autologous tumor-derived heat shock protein (HSP gp96) peptide complexes are showing progress in cancer patient survivals. Second, immunological monitoring of many clinical trials has failed to identify a surrogate marker for clinical outcomes. Third, many articles and reviews suggest that protective immunity to human cancer is elicited by the mutated antigenic repertoire unique to each cancer.

Focusing more closely on the type of DC needed to achieve its vaccine potential, the subsets of DCs could prove critical. Much of the current research is being carried out with monocyte-derived DCs, which are potent and homogeneous stimulators of immunity. Monocyte-derived DCs can be readily generated within a few days in large numbers (300 million–500 million mature DCs per apheresis) from precursors in the blood without the need for pretreating patients with various cytokines such GM-CSF or FLT 3-L. Rather, one obtains populations of immature DCs by exposing monocytes to GM-CSF and IL-4, and then they are differentiated into mature DCs by various stimuli such as toll-like receptor (TLR) ligands (LPS or poly I:C), inflammatory cytokines (IL-1β, TNF-α, IL-6, and PGE$_2$), or CD40L. The use of DCs that have received a maturation stimulus is likely to be important to induce strong immunity. It has become clear that antigen delivered on immature or incompletely matured DCs can even induce tolerance. However, the type and the duration of the maturation stimulus remain to be determined and may influence efficacy. At this time, monocyte-derived DCs are the most accessible and homogeneous populations of DCs.

Monocyte-derived DCs were the first to be used for treating melanoma patients, and several pilot studies have been published. Most used defined antigens in the form of peptides, but in some studies, tumor lysates or autologous DC tumor hybrids were also employed. The first trial, published in 1998 by Nestle and colleagues, aroused great interest given an overall response rate of 30 percent in stage IV patients (i.e., distant metastases), including complete responses. An important point in the first study by Nestle and colleagues was that they use fetal calf serum (FCS) during DC generation, and this might have contributed to the observed effects by providing nonspecific helper epitopes and by promoting the maturation of DCs.

Jonuleit and colleagues directly compared within each of eight patients the immunogenicity of immature DCs (generated according to Nestle and colleagues in FCS-containing media using GM-CSF and IL-4) to mature DCs generated in the absence of FCS and matured by a cocktail consisting of TNF-α, IL-1β, IL-6, and PGE$_2$ mimicking the composition of monocyte-conditioned medium. These two different DC populations were administered intranodally into opposite inguinal lymph nodes. FCS-free mature DCs induced stronger T-cell responses, both to the two recall antigens used (tetanus toxoid and PPD/tuberculin) and to tumor peptides. Interestingly, however, both immature and mature DCs showed an expansion of peptide-specific T cells by tetramer staining; yet, only mature DCs induced IFN-γ-producing and lytic CD8$^+$ T cells. These findings suggest the interesting possibility that the immature DCs might have induced regulatory T cells rather than effector T cells, an observation previously noted in studies with normal volunteers.

Cancer patients and healthy subjects often harbor a repertoire of self-reactive T cells and antibodies. This led to the idea that if one could break immunological tolerance to these self-antigens in a controllable manner one would find a "therapeutic window" in which an autoimmune response might damage cancers more than normal tissues. This approach has worked reasonably well with chemotherapies, which, although not cancer specific, can confer clinical benefit with acceptable morbidities.

The efforts to create cancer vaccines using allogeneic cell lines, differentiation antigens (such as gp100 and MART1), cancer testes (CT) antigens (such as MAGE, NY-ESO-1), or other common molecules (such as carcinoembryonic antigen, mucins, prostate-specific antigen, and prostatic acid phosphatase) represent this approach. Within this approach lie several subthemes. Thus, CT antigens, which are not expressed on normal somatic tissues but only on cancers or gonads, might be a better target for breaking tolerance than are differentiation antigens expressed on somatic tissues. Another subtheme is the idea that artificially mutated differentiation or CT antigens as vaccines might be better

at breaking tolerance than their wild-type counterparts. Finally, there is a multiplicity of choices of delivery agents for these antigens – whole proteins, peptides, RNA, DNA, viral vectors, DCs, and so on.

The importance of innate immunity and the emergence of the toll-like receptors have led to the recognition that immune modifiers must be an essential component of any cancer vaccine. The inclusion of QS21, ISCOMS, Montanide, heat shock proteins, CpG, BCG, and granulocyte-macrophage colony-stimulating factor with cancer vaccines reflects this. Of interest in this respect are the anecdotal success of Coley's toxin at the turn of the nineteenth century (a heat-killed mixture of streptococcal cells and probably superantigen broths), which may now be reinterpreted in the light of the newly identified immune response modifiers.

Finally, a better understanding of the controls that act on T cells to stimulate or inhibit them has led to the use of reagents to enhance antitumor T-cell activity. For example, blocking antibodies to the inhibitory T-lymphocyte antigen CTLA-4, manipulation of regulatory T cells, antibodies to PDL or its ligand PDLI, and enhancement of co-stimulating molecules like B7 on antigen-presenting cells are a few examples of reagents that are being used in this manner in conjunction with vacci-treatments.

BIBLIOGRAPHY

REVIEWS

Barnes P. Molecular mechanisms and cellular effects of glucosteroids. *Immunol Allergy Clin North Am.* 2005;25: 451–468.

Berzofsky JA, Ahlers JD, Belyakov IM. Strategies for designing and optimizing new generation vaccines. *Nat Rev Immunol*. 2001;1(3):209–219.

Fehniger TA, Caligiuri MA. Interleukin 15: biology and relevance to human disease. *Blood*. 2001;97:14–32.

Gattinoni L, Powell DJ Jr, Rosenberg SA, Restifo NP. Adoptive immunotherapy for cancer: building on success. *Nat Rev Immunol*. 2006;6(5):383–393.

Schwartz RS. The Shattuck Lecture: diversity of the immune repertoire and immunoregulation. *New Engl J Med*. 2003;348:1017–1026.

Strand V, Kimberly R, Isaacs JD. Biologic therapies in rheumatology: lessons learned, future directions. *Nat Rev Drug Discov*. 2007;6:74–92.

SUGGESTED READING

Blachére NE, Darnell RB, Albert ML. Apoptotic cells deliver processed antigen to dendritic cells for cross-presentation. *PloS Biol*. 2005;3:e185.

Dubois S, Mariner J, Waldmann TA, Tagaya Y. IL-15R alpha recycles and presents IL-15 in *trans* to neighboring cells. *Immunity*. 2002;17:537–547.

Jonuleit H, Giesecke-Tuettenberg A, Tüting T, et al. A comparison of two types of dendritic cell as adjuvants for the induction of melanoma-specific T-cell responses in humans following intranodal injection. *Int J Cancer*. 2001(2):243–251.

Nestle FO, Alijagic S, Gilliet M, et al. Vaccination of melanoma patients with peptide or tumor lysate-pulsed dendritic cells. *Nat Med*. 1998;4:328–332.

Steinman RM, Palucka K, Bancherceau J, Schuler-Thurner B, Schuler G. Active immunization with dendritic cells bearing melanoma antigens. In: Levine MM, Kaper JB, Rappuoli R, Liu MA, Good MF, eds. *New Generation Vaccines*. 3rd ed. New York: Marcel Dekker; 2004:987–995.

Vincenti F, Kirkman R, Light S, et al. Interleukin-2-receptor blockade with daclizumab to prevent acute rejection in renal transplantation. *N Engl J Med*. 1998;338:161–165.

Waldmann TA. The biology of interleukin-2 and interleukin-15: implications for cancer therapy and vaccine design. *Nat Rev Immunol*. 2006;6:595–601.

4. Immunological Aspects of Infection

Kumar Visvanathan, M.D., Ph.D., Christopher M. MacIsaac, M.D., Ph.D.,
William W. Hall, M.D., Ph.D., and Vincent A. Fischetti, Ph.D.

INTRODUCTION

From the moment of birth, the host is constantly exposed to a wide variety of bacteria and viruses. In general, the host manages to either eliminate or ward off these invading organisms, and a symbiosis is achieved between microbes and the host. How does this occur? There are two major pathways to achieve this resistance: nonspecific and adaptive.

NONSPECIFIC RESISTANCE

Nonspecific or natural resistance refers to barriers, secretions, and normal flora that make up our external defenses. Phagocytes and complement are also involved. Mechanical barriers are highly effective, and the skin (our largest organ) is highly suited to this protection (see Figure 4.1); loss of a major part of the skin (secondary to burns, acids, etc.) immediately exposes the host to marked susceptibility to infection. The mucosal lining of mouth and respiratory tract is another excellent defense mechanism. Yet, a defect in the mucosal lining of the respiratory tract, which occurs in cystic fibrosis, results in a heightened susceptibility to many infections. These are examples of a defect in the epithelium or epithelial lining. In general, however, it is the mobilization of the phagocytic cells such as monocytes/mac-rophages and polymorphonuclear leukocytes that ingest invading microorganisms and kill them.

The polymorpholeukocytes are a large pool of phagocytic cells that are both circulatory and in the bone marrow. Invading organisms trigger an inflammatory cascade, which stimulates these cells to adhere to vascular epithelium and actively migrate toward the infection. Phagocytosis is promoted by *opsonins* (usually IgG antibody) and complement.

The macrophages reside in the subepithelial tissues of the skin and intestine and line the alveoli of the lungs. Microbes that penetrate an epithelial surface will encounter local tissue macrophages called *histocytes*. If the organism enters via blood or lymph, then defense is provided by fixed macrophages called *Kupffer cells*, which line the sinusoids of the liver. Similarly fixed macrophages called *Langerhans cells* are also present in the epidermis of the skin. Once engaged with the organism, these macrophages release a number of macrophage-derived cytokines, which nonspecifically amplify the immunological and inflammatory reactions to the invading microbe.

Most pathogenic microorganisms have evolved methods of resisting phagocytosis. For example, group A streptococci have cell surface structures called M proteins of which there are now more than 120 antigenically distinct molecules that

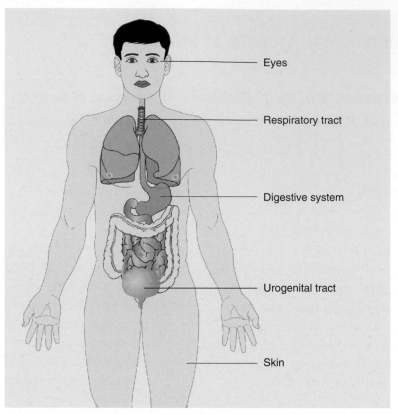

Figure 4.1 Schematic drawing of the body showing the various organs and systems that offer nonspecific resistance to infection.

inhibit direct phagocytosis, mainly by preventing deposition of complement on the organism. Another example is the pneumococcal polysaccharide capsule of which there are thirty to forty distinct polysaccharides. Another approach (taken by both group A streptococci and staphylococci) is the release of potent extracellular toxins, which kill phagocytes with the formation of pus. An intriguing bacterium, *Mycobacterium tuberculosis,* can be ingested by phagocytes but resists intracellular killing, often persisting for years in the macrophage.

Over the past decade, our knowledge of how we sense the microbial world (innate or adaptive) has fundamentally changed. It has been known for decades that microbial products such as lipopoly-saccharides, lipoproteins or peptidoglycans have profound effects on human cells. Although the structures of many different pathogenic microbial compounds have been extensively studied, the molecular basis of their recognition by the cells of the innate immune system remained elusive. Charles Janeway first developed the concept of microbial structures forming pathogen-associated molecular patterns (PAMPs), which would be recognized by pattern recognition receptors. The discovery of a family of toll receptors (toll refers to the toll gene of *Drosophila*, initially identified as an essential receptor controlling dorsoventral polarization during embryonic development of the fly larvae) in species as diverse as *Drosophila* fly and humans and the recognition of their role in distinguishing molecular patterns that are common to microorganisms led to a renewed appreciation of the innate immune system.

From these humble beginnings, the field of mammalian toll-like receptors (TLR) quickly evolved as a crucial system for alerting the host to the presence of numerous infectious agents. Infectious microbes display certain molecular patterns that are necessary for microbial virulence (see Table 4.1). Many of these molecular patterns such as lipopolysaccharide in the outer membranes of gram-negative bacteria seem to be particularly potent activators of mammalian cells. The mammalian receptors responsible for recognition of PAMPs are called *pattern recognition receptors*. The failure of the immune system to recognize a pathogen's PAMP could lead to a delay or blunting of the immune response, resulting in unchecked invasion by the microbe.

Perhaps the best example of an incomplete recognition by the TLR system is a gram-negative bacterial infection in the C3H/HeJ mouse. As few as two colony-forming units of *Salmonella typhimurium* can kill this mouse. Further exploration of this extraordinary virulence revealed that the mouse harbored a point mutation (P712H) in the TLR4, which results in defective signal transduction in response to LPS and a heightened susceptibility to gram-negative infections.

The family of TLRs is a highly specialized system that can identify a number of microbial and endogenous ligands and activate the immune system to respond. The body must be able to respond differently to various challenges. Thus, the specificity in the immune response via TLRs is becoming increasingly complex. Currently, probes of the TLR family have been described, and it is expected that many more receptors will be discovered in the future.

ADAPTIVE IMMUNITY

A specific immune response to invading microbes is conveniently divided into humoral and cellular immunity. The importance of each arm of the specific response varies from infection to infection. Experimental animal models and naturally occurring immunodeficiency states clearly demonstrate that certain components of the immune response are crucial for controlling a particular infection.

For example, individuals with antibody deficiencies are particularly prone to repeated infections with pyrogenic bacteria. Yet, replacement therapy with immunoglobulin greatly reduces the number of infections. Interestingly, these individuals can mount a normal response to most viruses (varicella, measles, mumps, etc.). Yet the absence of mucosal antibody does make them susceptible to some enteroviruses.

Although it is clear that innate immunity is the first line of defense against invading organisms, the TLRs are also playing a role in adaptive immunity, and the dendritic cell (DC) appears to be playing a key role in linking the innate and adaptive immune responses. As immature cells, they are present in the peripheral tissues. However, with the appearance of invading organisms, DCs recognize these pathogens through their TLRs. Fortunately, they express the full repertoire of TLRs. After activation of the TLRs, the DCs are transformed into more mature cells with a high expression of major histocompatibility complex (MHC) and the co-stimulatory molecules CD80 and CD86. The DCs then

Table 4.1 List of Known Toll-like Receptors, What Cells Express Them, and What the Ligand Is for Each Receptor

Receptors	Cells	Ligand
TLR1	Platelets, atherosclerotic plaques, monocytes, neutrophils, germinal center B cells, natural killer cells, DCs, B cells	Lipoprotein from *Mycobacterium tuberculosis* Soluble factors from *Neisseria meningitidis*
TLR2	Atherosclerotic plaques, monocytes, neutrophils, natural killer cells, B cells, spleen, lymph nodes	Peptidoglycan Lipoteichoic acid Triacyl lipoproteins Diacyl lipoproteins (with TLR6)
TLR3	DCs, natural killer cells	dsRNA
TLR4	Atherosclerotic plaques, neutrophils, monocytes, B cells	LPS Fusion protein from respiratory syncytial virus
TLR5	DCs, natural killer cells, monocytes, T cells	Flagellin
TLR6	Platelets, resting B cells, germinal center B cells, natural killer cells, monocytes, DCs	Diacyl lipoproteins (with TLR2)
TLR7	Monocytes, resting B cells, germinal center B cells, DCs	ssRNA
TLR8	DCs, monocytes	ssRNA
TLR9	Resting B cells, germinal center B cells, natural killer cells, monocytes, spleen	Bacterial CpG DNA
TLR10	Resting B cells, germinal center B cells, natural killer cells, DCs	Unknown
TLR11	? not expressed in humans murine kidney and bladder	Unknown

migrate to the lymph nodes to activate antigen-specific naïve T cells. The cytokine milieu being expressed around the cells determines their fate; that is, the production of IL-12 drives these cells to T_H1 cells, which produce interferon-δ, whereas IL-4 drives them toward T_H2 cells producing IL-4, IL-5, Il-10, and IL-13. These latter cytokines are of interest as they are also responsible for the development of allergic diseases such as asthma and account for the regulation of antigen-specific IgE production, accumulation of eosinophils, and activation of mast cells. In this connection, the incidence of allergic disease and atopy has markedly increased in the industrialized countries compared with developing countries over the past decades, and one hypothesis is that this increase is linked to the reduction of bacterial infections, which occurs in a cleaner environment, a hypothesis known as the "hygiene hypothesis" (see Chapter 15). The discovery that TLR signaling might be crucially involved in the establishment of T_H1/T_H2 pathways opens up the field to look for new strategies against diseases such as asthma and atopy.

In summary, the fields of both innate and adaptive immunity have experienced a new and rapid growth in interest in the past eight to ten years. Concomitant with this growth, the number of genomes that have been sequenced is expanding, thus enabling researchers to identify and to characterize the receptors and adaptors involved in the recognition.

Although much of the work over the past years has focused on defining ligands for the different TLRs, the molecular basis for this recognition is not known for a single ligand. Furthermore, the characterization of TLR-dependent signaling for the instruction of adaptive immune responses has just started to be explored. Because TLRs play such a crucial role in innate and adaptive immune responses to distinct virulence factors, the development of selective inhibitors/activators may be a worthwhile endeavor to help manage a number of infectious and immunologic diseases.

BACTERIAL INFECTION

The immune system responds to bacterial infections in two major ways. First, it may respond to soluble products of the cell such as toxins or released structural antigens like LPS of a given gram-negative bacterial cell. Most bacterial antigens are T-cell dependent and require helper T cells for initiation of the immune response. Yet certain cell antigens, such as the pneumococcal polysaccharides, are T-cell independent. They are large-molecular-weight molecules, and in children, antibody response to these antigens may take four to six years. Thus, younger children are susceptible to these infections.

An interesting sidelight to protection against these infections can be seen in breast-fed infants who are less susceptible to infection than non-breast-fed babies. It now appears that it is not polysaccharides or antibodies that are responsible for this protection but rather a multimeric form of lactoalbumin (present in high concentrations in human breast milk (see "Suggested Reading"). A broader approach to protection has been the production of pneumococcal polysaccharide vaccines specially designed to induce antibody induction in the young child.

In the following discussion, streptococci, particularly *S. pyogenes,* are used as the example of a bacterial infection, but many other organisms produce a similar response. Streptococcal antigens include specific toxins such as streptolysins O and S that lyse blood and tissue cells and pyrogenic exotoxins, which act as superantigens to overstimulate the host responses. There are also specific enzymes such as hyaluronidase and streptokinase, which help promote the spread of infecting streptococcus. Perhaps most important is the M protein (Figure 4.2), a cell surface antigen of the group A streptococcus that allows the bacteria to evade immune defenses (especially neutrophils and complement). One way in which M protein functions is to bind host factor H, which prevents complement C3 from depositing on the streptococcal surface. Since efficient phagocytosis by neutrophils requires interaction with its C3 receptor, factor H prevents this interaction.

Antibodies to streptococcal antigens other than M protein are slow to appear, and most likely do not play a role in limiting the infection. However, antibodies to streptolysin O and deoxyribonuclease B have become important clinical tools to determine whether a given individual has had a recent streptococcal infection. This is partially true if a blood sample drawn

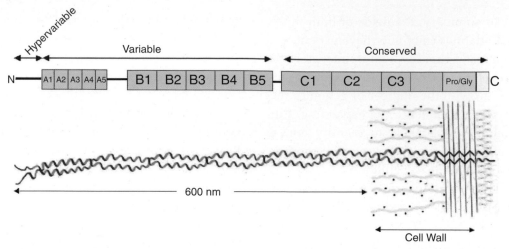

Figure 4.2 Coiled-coil structure of the M protein. The streptococcal M protein is a coiled-coil molecule that extends about 600 nm from the bacterial cell surface. The C-terminal region is embedded within the cell wall and the C-terminus is located in the cytoplasmic membrane in the nascent molecule. The coding region for the M protein is distributed in repeat blocks designated A–C in which the C-repeat region is conserved among M-protein serotypes, and the A and B repeats are variable among these serotypes. The N-terminus is the hypervariable, type-specific region for the M proteins. Pro/Gly designates the region of the M protein that is rich in proline and glycine.

at the onset and one drawn 10 to 14 days later show a marked rise in the titer. Contrary to the dogma, both skin infection and pharyngeal infection with group A streptococci can stimulate the production of both antibodies.

Some bacterial antigens such as endotoxins can be powerful stimulators of the immune response and lead to polyclonal activation of B lymphocytes. This rise in immunoglobulin levels is believed to be nonspecific since only a small portion of the total immunoglobulin level is directed to the endotoxin.

BACTERIAL SUPERANTIGENS

Among the toxins secreted by bacteria is a special group from the streptococcal and staphylococcal family of toxins called *superantigens* (SAg). Instead of binding to the specific antigen receptor known for most antigens, these toxins bind to the lateral surface of both the T-cell receptor and the MHC (see Figure 4.3). Thus, in contrast to a conventional peptide antigen, which stimulates only one in 10^4 to 10^8 T cells, the superantigen may bind up to approximately 1:50 T cells. The result is a veritable explosion of cytokines resulting in high fever, hypotension, and multiorgan shock. Death often occurs within 24 hours of the release of these toxins. The most widely studied superantigens are produced by *Staphylococcus aureus* and group A streptococcus. These superantigens bind the T-cell receptor at its β region, and that exact Vβ region is different for each superantigen. Table 4.2 lists the known superantigens and their Vβ specificities.

The role of SAg has also been explored in a number of disease states, including atopic dermatitis, psoriasis, Kawasaki disease, rheumatic fever, and tuberculosis.

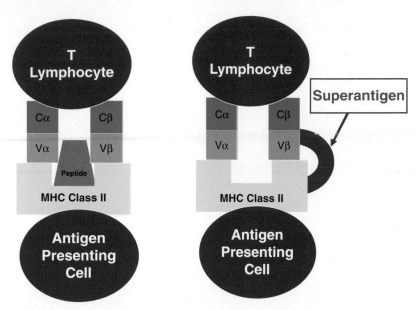

Figure 4.3 Binding of conventional (left) and superantigen (right) antigens to the T-cell receptor and antigen-presenting cell. Note that the conventional antigen binding is associated with the T-cell receptor and the major histocompatibility complex (MHC) directly and only a small proportion of T cells are activated. In contrast, the superantigen binds to the lateral sides of the T-cell receptor and MHC molecule, thereby triggering a much larger group of activated T cells (up to 25 percent of the cells).

BACTERIAL EVASION OF IMMUNE DEFENSE

There are several ways in which bacteria can survive in the host by evasion of the immune defenses. These mechanisms will be briefly summarized here, but the list of evasive mechanisms used by each bacterial species may be much longer in nature.

Capsules play an important role for long-term survival of pathogens. For example, group A streptococci have a hyaluronic acid capsule that is identical to hyaluronic acid in humans. While antibodies can be obtained following immunization with the streptococcal hyaluronic acid, they are nonprecipitating antibodies and are not effective in eliminating the organism. Polysaccharide antigens of both the pneumococcus and the meningococcus capsules can inhibit phagocytosis of the organism and mucoid secretions of these polysaccharides can block the activation of the alternate pathway of complement.

Antigenic variation or drift is another mechanism whereby bacteria evade the immune system. The M protein (the most important virulence factor of the group A streptococcus) has been shown to exhibit antigen variation in the environment, and new M protein molecules appear regularly in human isolates of group A streptococci.

Another example is the relapsing fever by *Borrelia*. During the first episode, antibodies kill the bacteria and the fever subsides. However, some antigenic variants of the bacteria persist, and after five to seven days these new variants can cause a relapse in the patient with fever reappearing. Other examples of evasion of the immune response are bacteria such as *N. gonorrhea*, *N. meningitidis*, *Haemophilus*

Table 4.2 List of All the Known Superantigens and Their Vβ Specificities

Superantigen	Human Vβ specificity
Staphylococcal enterotoxins	
SEA	1, 5.3, 6, 7, 9, 16, 22, 21.3
SEB	3, 9, 12, 14, 15, 17, 20
SEC1	3, 6, 12, 15
C2	12, 13.2, 14, 15, 17, 20
C3	3, 5, 8, 12, 13.2
SED	5, 12
SEE	5.1, 6, 8, 18
SEG	3, 7, 9, 12, 13.1, 13.2, 13.6, 14, 15
SEH	Nil? Vα10
SEI	1.1, 3, 5.1, 5.3, 13, 23
SEJ	?
SEK	5.1, 5.2, 6.7
SEL	5.1, 5.2, 6.7, 16, 22
SEM	?
SEN	?
SEO	?
SEP	?
SEQ	2.1, 5.1, 21.3
TSST-1	2
Streptococcal exotoxins	
SPE-A	2, 12, 14, 15
SPE-C	1, 2, 5.1, 10
SPE-F	2, 4, 8, 15, 19
SPE-G	2.1, 4.1, 6.9, 9.1, 12.3
SPE-H	2.1, 7.3, 9.1, 23.1
SPE-I	6.9, 9.1, 18.1, 22
SPE-J	2.1
SPE-K/L	1.1, 5.1, 23.1
SPE-M	1.1
SMEZ1	2.1, 4.1, 7.3, 8.1
SMEZ2	4.1, 8.1

influenza, and others that secrete proteases that hydrolyze IgA antibody. Some strains of staphylococci secrete catalase, which prevents them from being killed inside phagocytic cells.

One must also consider that some bacteria sequester themselves in nonphagocytic cells where they are not exposed to the immune system. An excellent example is *M. tuberculosis,* which can lie dormant for years inside a granulomatous, caseous lesion called the Ghon complex. Once ground up, live *M. tuberculosis* organism can be extracted from this complex.

Finally, a number of organisms display antigens on their surface that are cross-reactive with human antigens. This could result in an enhanced immune response to host tissue antigens or a diminished response secondary to similarities between bacterial and self-antigens.

VIRAL INFECTIONS

The clinical spectrum of viral disease is wide, and because there is such variation, we will use the template of herpes viruses as an example. In general, viral infections are self-limited and usually produce long-term immunity, and secondary attacks by the same virus are uncommon. Of the large number of herpes viruses, only eight infect humans, and each will be discussed in some detail. However, two general features of pathogens of these viruses are important. First, there must be close contact between infected and noninfected individuals for transmission to occur and no intermediate host is involved. Second, after the primary infection, herpes virus will persist in the host for life.

To eliminate virions from entering noninfected cells and to eliminate virus-infected cells, two major pathways of the immune response are initiated. The humoral response is primarily directed against virions, while the T-cell response is primarily directed against infected cells. The humoral response may directly neutralize the virus, but complement-dependent enhancement of viral phagocytosis or complement lysis of virus also may occur.

Epstein-Barr Infection

Infectious mononucleosis is caused by the Epstein-Barr virus (EBV), and in developing countries, 99 percent of children demonstrate antibodies to the virus by age 3. In developed countries, the age is much later and clinical infection usually occurs in the age group of 15 to 25 years. The virus is excreted in the oropharyngeal fluids for some months after the infection and is responsible for person-to-person transmission.

Hoagland observed that a female college student traveling from New York to Boston met several different male students on the train and exchanged kisses with all of them. All of these contacts came down with infectious mononucleosis, which is often referred to as the "kissing disease."

The pattern of antibody response to different EBV antigens helps distinguish acute or subclinical infections from postinfections with the virus. IgM antibodies to viral capsid antigen (VCA) appear early in the course of the infection, but at the time of clinical symptoms, IgG levels to VCA are quite high. Thus, paired sera at the time of clinical infection do not help diagnose the disease. In contrast, antibodies to EB nuclear antigen appear months after the infection. Antibodies to early antigen appear in about 70 percent of primary infections and are usually indicative of an acute infection.

The clinical signs of fever, such as enlarged cervical lymph nodes, and reddened pharynx with whitish exudates (also seen with other viruses) are often mistaken for group A streptococcal pharyngitis. Thus, culture and antibody tests are used to distinguish between the two.

EBV has one unique feature compared with other viruses in that it produces disease by infecting and *transforming* B lymphocytes via the CD21 molecule on the surface of B cells. These infected cells multiply like tumor cells, and up to half of the lymphoid cells from the tonsils of EBV-infected patients may be transformed.

The infection is stopped by a T-cell response that kills virus-infected cells and a humoral response that neutralizes free virions. The characteristic "atypical lymphocytes" seen in this disease are CD8$^+$ cytotoxic T cells that kill EBV-infected B cells.

Most individuals handle EBV infection quite well. However, rare individuals have a specific defect that fails to handle EBV infections and usually die of the disease. More important is the failure to contain EBV infections secondary to immunosuppressive therapy. For example, the x-linked *lymphoproliferative syndrome* that affects males from age 6 months to 20 years is in this category. These patients die of lymphomas, aplastic anemia, or immunodeficiency.

Immunosuppressive therapy may result in EBV reactivation, and about 1 to 10 percent of certain transplants may be complicated by EBV-induced lymphoproliferative disease. Similar results are also seen in patients infected with the HIV virus. One of the most interesting effects of EBV infection and transformation has been the occurrence of Burkitt's lymphoma. It is endemic in certain African countries (especially in regions of mosquito-borne disease), where it represents 90 percent of childhood cancers in contrast to 3 percent in developed countries. The link between EBV and Burkitt's lymphoma was established when it was found that EBV antigens and genome were present in the tumor cells. Since the incidence of Burkitt's lymphoma follows the same belt as the chronic malaria belt of the region, it has been suggested that the chronic malaria of these children induces EBV-infected lymphoproliferation, leading to chromosomal translocation in the long arms of chromosomes 8 and 14 and eventually to the activation and translocation of the *c-myc* oncogene to the active region of the cellular genome (see Figure 4.4).

Viruses have evolved many mechanisms to evade the immune response, but one of the key elements in these evasive mechanisms has been their ability to induce a latent status within the cells of the host. Thus, all herpes viruses can remain latent, and no viral antigen is expressed. When there is a change in the host-virus equilibrium secondary to certain other infections, metabolic disturbances, immunosuppression, or aging, only then does the virus reactivate and cause disease. Examples are herpes simplex in the trigeminal ganglia, which causes recurrent "cold sores," or herpes zoster in a dorsal root ganglion, which causes "shingles."

A second example is antigenic variation or drift in certain viruses. The best example is influenza A, an RNA virus surrounded by a lipid envelope into which two important proteins (hemagglutinin and neuraminidase) are inserted. The virus evades the neutralizing antibodies to this virus by constantly modifying the structure of these two proteins by either antigenic drift or antigenic shift. In the former, the change is minor and accounts for minor epidemics of flu during each winter. Antigenic shift is a major change in the structure of those proteins, which can cause a major pandemic of devastating proportions. Viewed in this light, the influenza vaccine currently in use is generally protective against common flu epidemics in the world but would not be protective against a major antigenic shift.

A third mechanism is viral persistence in which the virus is *not* cleared and a chronic

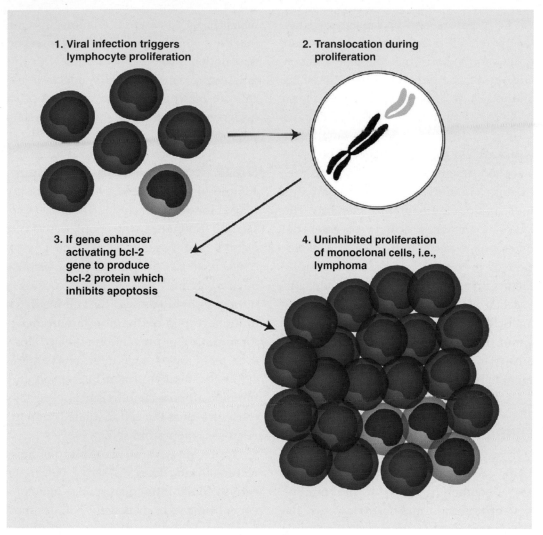

1. Viral infection triggers lymphocyte proliferation

2. Translocation during proliferation

3. If gene enhancer activating bcl-2 gene to produce bcl-2 protein which inhibits apoptosis

4. Uninhibited proliferation of monoclonal cells, i.e., lymphoma

Figure 4.4 A schematic presentation of the steps involved in the transformation of Epstein-Barr virus–infected B cells into a B-cell lymphoma.

infection with persisting virus occurs. For example, HIV persists because it eventually destroys the CD4 T cells needed to kill the virus. Hepatitis C also may persist for years with continuous carriage of the virus in the liver.

While immunological reactions to the virus are generally beneficial to the host, they may also initiate or aggravate tissue damage in the host inadvertently. For example, EBV is a polyclonal B-cell activator, and the virus may combine with host antigens to form new antigens. Antibodies

to these antigens will not only recognize viral antigens, but some will bind to host antigens as well, thereby possibly initiating an autoimmune response and disease. An example of this type of reaction is the appearance of chronic autoimmune liver disease following chronic hepatitis B infection or immune complex disease such as vasculitis or glomerulonephritis.

Another example of viral bystander damage is dengue fever in which immune enhancement plays an important part. Here, the dengue virus can infect macrophages via Fc receptors, and its capacity to enter the target cell is enhanced if it is bound to IgG antibodies. Thus, the first infection with a specific dengue virus type elicits antibodies to that specific virus. However, cross immunity to the other dengue serotypes is fleeting and lasts only a few weeks. When the individual is exposed to a second dengue virus serotype, the pre-existing antibody to the first type binds to it but does not neutralize the virus. The antibody-enhanced second virus enters the macrophage, setting off a veritable explosion of proteases, lymphokines complement activation, coagulation cascade, and vascular permeability factors. The result is a much more severe disease called dengue hemorrhagic fever, whose mortality rate in areas with poor medical facilities and treatment may be as high as 50 percent.

FUNGAL INFECTION

Fungi cause many diseases, most of which are adequately handled by the immune system of the normal host. However, the increased use of immunosuppressive drugs – the immunosuppression secondary to HIV infection – has raised our awareness of these infections. For example, *Candida albicans* can cause superficial infections in the normal host and is found throughout the intestinal tract and commonly in the vagina. The organism is usually kept under control by the bacterial flora, but changes in these flora secondary to overuse of antibiotics or changes in hormone balance will favor a chronic superficial infection. All of this is exacerbated in the immunocompromised host.

Another organism that is receiving wide attention is the fungus *Pneumocystis carinii* (now called *Pneumocystis jiroveci*),

which has a commensal relationship with the lung in the normal host. However, the sudden onset of pneumonia with this organism secondary to HIV infection in a child or adult is often the first sign of an underlying suppressed immune system caused by HIV.

In contrast to the superficial infections of fungi, systemic infections in the immunocompromised host have a higher mortality rate. This category includes *Histoplasma capsulatum* (pulmonary infection), *Coccidiodes immitis* (acute pneumonitis), and *Cryptococcus neoformas* (meningitis, lung lesions). Such systemic infections may occur in normal individuals, and the cell-mediated immune response is the more important factor in control or prevention of them. However, all of these fungal infections (superficial and systemic) are more likely to occur in immunosuppressed individuals, especially those in which the cell-mediated immune response is compromised.

There are several plausible outcomes to fungal infections. As stated before, an active cellular immune response plus topical antifungal drugs usually handles most superficial infections. Systemic infections, especially in the immunocompromised host, carry a high mortality rate, and even the use of newer prophylactic and therapeutic agents only partially decreases the mortality.

As with viruses, there is a third possible outcome. If the fungal infection is not eliminated or causes persistent infection, then the host response may trigger a hypersensitivity reaction. As an example, *Aspergillus fumigatus* infections can persist as an aspergilloma in preexisting lung cavities secondary to tuberculosis or bronchiectasis following childhood pertussis (whooping cough). Allergic bronchopulmonary aspergillosis may occur and is due to

IgE-mediated hypersensitivity to the aspergillus antigens. Clinically, the condition presents as recurrent episodes of increased wheezing and coughing, fever, and pleuritic pain similar to that seen in asthmatics. Another example is farmer's lung in which antigen-antibody complexes of *Micropolyspora faeni* cause a hypersensitivity reaction on the part of the host. The name farmer's lung indicates that this particular fungus is found in moldy hay.

PARASITIC INFECTION

Protozoa are a diverse group of parasites, but malaria, leishmaniasis, and trypanosomiasis globally account for most of the problems encountered in parasitic diseases. The balance between host and parasite is twofold. The parasite may be too virulent for the host or may evade the immune surveillance and thus kills the host. Conversely, the immune response may be vigorous and kill the parasite, thereby jeopardizing its survival. Thus, the survival of any parasite depends on a balance between induction of immunity and escape from surveillance.

Malaria

The worldwide incidence of malaria is estimated at 300 million–500 million people, and at least 1 million die each year of the disease, mostly of cerebral malaria and usually young children. Cerebral malaria is usually associated with infection with *Plasmodium falciparum* and not *Plasmodium vivax*. Patients react to protozoal infection with activation of macrophages and monocytes with the release of cytokines TNF, IL-1, and IL-6. Clinically, they produce fever, leukocytosis, and acute phase reactants.

Although most protozoa stimulate the production of IgG and IgM antibodies, these antibodies are probably not protective, and thus vaccines have not yet been successful in the control or prevention of malaria. Also in the case of malaria, protozoa invade erythrocytes and hepatocytes and thus are hidden from the immune response. Clinically, many of the signs and symptoms of these patients are related to the destruction of red blood cells and hepatocytes; therefore, anemia, jaundice, splenomegaly, hypostasis, hypotension, tender hepatomegaly, and biphasic fever are hallmarks of the disease.

Interestingly, there have been several mutations in the host that help provide resistance to malarial infection. Most striking has been the appearance of the heterozygous sickle cell trait (Hbas), which confers a survival advantage in endemic disease. Second, the absence of the red cell Duffy antigen (receptor for plasmodium vivax) is quite protective. Finally, the presence of HLA-B53 in individuals is associated with resistance to the disease.

Evasion mechanisms of protozoa fall into three major categories. The first is entrance of the organism into the host cell, where it avoids immune surveillance. One example is malaria, as noted previously. Others include toxoplasma, leishmania, and *Trypanosoma cruzi*, which enter and can grow inside macrophages. For example, leishmania binds C3 avidly and thus serves as a ligand for the CR3 receptor on macrophages. If one uses monoclonal antibodies to the CR3 receptor, this inhibits the uptake of the parasite into macrophage. Another approach is used by toxoplasma in which they prevent fusion of phagocytic vacuoles containing the parasite with lysosomes and thus are not destroyed. Finally, trypanosomes need *activated* macrophages for killing; thus they are resistant to intracellular killing in *nonactivated* macrophages.

A second mechanism for evasion is antigenic variation. *Trypanosoma brucei* is an excellent example of this. In this scenario, the trypanosomes are initially destroyed by host antibody. However, the organism resurfaces in the body with a different set of antigens or glycoproteins. The process continues, and the parasite possesses a number of genes that code for these antigens and can vary the genes used. Eventually, the parasite succeeds and avoids host elimination. This type of variation is known as phenotypic variation and differs from the genotypic variation seen in influenza epidemics.

As in bacteria, protozoa can also suppress the immune response. Malaria and leishmania organisms release soluble antigens that nonspecifically suppress the immune response by acting on lymphocytes or the reticuloendothelial system. Several parasites undergo development stages that are resistant to complement-mediated lysis. Finally, leishmania can down-regulate expression of MHC class II expression of parasitized macrophages, which reduces the effectiveness of CD8$^+$ T cells.

In summary, protozoa have developed a wide variety of techniques to evade the immune system. This makes it extremely difficult both to eliminate these protozoa and to produce vaccines that are effective against them. Thus, the field is wide open to new and innovative approaches to eliminate this class of organisms.

BIBLIOGRAPHY

REVIEWS

Alcami A, Koszinowski UH. Viral mechanisms of immune evasion. *Immunol Today*. 2000;21(9):447–455.

Fischetti VA. Streptococcal M protein. *Sci Am*. 1991;264(6):58–65.

Heine H, Lien E. Toll-like receptors and their function in innate and adaptive immunity. *Int Arch Allergy Immunol*. 2003;130:180–192.

Lavoie PM, Thibodeau J, Erard F, Sekaly RP. Understanding the mechanism of action of bacterial superantigens from a decade of research. *Immunol Rev*. 1999;168:257–269.

Wetzler LM. 2003. The role of Toll-like receptor 2 in microbial disease and immunity. *Vaccine*. 2003;21 (suppl 2):55–60.

SUGGESTED READING

Bunikowski R, Mielke ME, Skarabis H, et al. Evidence for a disease-promoting effect of *Staphylococcus aureus*-derived exotoxins in atopic dermatitis. *J Allergy Clin Immunol*. 2000;105(4):814–819.

Davison SC, Allen MH, Mallon E, Barker JN. Contrasting patterns of streptococcal superantigen-induced T-cell proliferation in guttate vs. chronic plaque psoriasis. *Br J Dermatol*. 2001;145(2): 245–251.

Hoagland RS. The transmission of infectious mononucleosis. *Am J Med Sci*. 1955;229:262–266.

Hoshino K, Takeuchi O, Kawai T, et al. Cutting edge: toll-like receptor 4 (TLR4)-deficient mice are hyporesponsive to lipopolysaccharide: evidence for TLR4 as the Lps gene product. *J Immunol*. 1999;162:3749–3752.

Janeway CA Jr. Approaching the asymptote? Evolution and revolution in immunology. *Cold Spring Harb Symp Quant Biol*. 1989;54:1–13.

Kaisho T, Akira S. 2000. Critical roles of Toll-like receptors in host defense. *Crit Rev Immunol*. 2000;20:393–405.

Meissner HC, Leung DY. Superantigens, conventional antigens and the etiology of Kawasaki syndrome. *Pediatr Infect Dis J*. 2000;19(2):91–94.

Smoot LM, McCormick JK, Smoot JC, et al. Characterization of two novel pyrogenic toxin superantigens made by an acute rheumatic fever clone of *Streptococcus pyogenes* associated with multiple disease outbreaks. *Infect Immun*. 2002;70(12):7095–7104.

Ohmen JD, Barnes PF, Grisso CL, Bloom BR, Modlin RL. Evidence for a superantigen in human tuberculosis. *Immunity*. 1994;1(1):35–43.

Poltorak A, He X, Smirnova I, et al. Defective LPS signaling in C3H/HeJ and C57BL/10ScCr mice: mutations in Tlr4 gene. *Science*. 1988;282:2085–2088.

Visvanathan K, Charles A, Bannan J, Pugach P, Kashfi K, Zabriskie JB. Inhibition of bacterial superantigens by peptides and antibodies. *Infect Immun*. 2001;69:875–884.

5. Immunological Aspects of Immunodeficiency Diseases

Dinakantha S. Kumararatne, M.D.

INTRODUCTION

The principal function of the immune system is to prevent microbial infection. Therefore, disorders resulting in impaired function of the immune system (immunodeficiency) result in increased susceptibility to infection. Immunodeficiency can arise from an intrinsic defect of a component of the immune system (primary immunodeficiency, or PID). Alternatively, immunodeficiency may be secondary to another pathological condition, which adversely affects immune function (Table 5.1). Both primary and secondary immunodeficiencies result in increased susceptibility to infection. The precise pattern of infection depends on the specific component of the immune system that is affected. Most PIDs are caused by defects in single genes and are hence heritable. Others may represent the consequence of an interaction between the genetic phenotype and an environmental influence, like viral infections. Primary immunodeficiencies are rare and based on information from national registers; these diseases are estimated to occur between 1 in 2,000 to 1 in 10,000 live births. In contrast, secondary immunodeficiencies are more commonly seen in clinical practice. (See Table 5.1 for examples of secondary immunodeficiency.)

From a clinical perspective, immunodeficiencies can be classified into eight categories (Table 5.2). Each category has a characteristic pattern of clinical presentation (Table 5.3), which will be elaborated on later.

DEFECTS IN ANATOMICAL OR PHYSIOLOGICAL BARRIERS TO INFECTION

One of the commonest predisposing causes of infection is a defect in an anatomical or physiological barrier to infection. Intact epithelial membranes, especially stratified squamous epithelial surfaces such as the skin, constitute an extremely effective barrier to infection. Thus, integumentary damage caused by burns, eczema, and trauma (including surgery), predisposes to infection. Skull fractures, particularly damage of the cribriform plate, may result in recurrent episodes of pyogenic meningitis. The existence of sinus tracts between deeper tissues and the skin surface or alternatively, the presence of foreign bodies or avascular areas (e.g., within bone) predisposes to infection. Obstruction to the drainage of hollow tubes and viscera also predisposes to infection, for example, obstruction of the biliary tract, urinary tract, or bronchi. Impaired vascular perfusion of the tissues due to edema and angiopathy (including microvascular changes following diabetes mellitus) also predisposes to infection. Alteration of the normal commensal flora by broad-spectrum antibiotic

Table 5.1 Secondary Immunodeficiency

Causes of Secondary Immunodeficiency	Defect
Defects in anatomical and physical barriers to infection (see text for explanation)	Various
Malignancies of the B-cell system Myelomatosis Non-Hodgkin's lymphoma Chronic lymphocytic leukemia	Antibody

Therapeutic agents
 Biological agents
   Anti-B-cell antibodies: e.g., Rituximab
   Anti-TNF agents
	
	 Antibody
	
	 Innate immunity and CMI

Cytotoxic drugs: Alkylating agents, cytotoxic antibiotics, antimetabolites, Vinca alkaloids, etc.	Myelosupression and CMI
Immunosuppressive drugs: Corticosteroids, calcineurin Inhibitors, antiproliferative Immunosuppressants (azathioprine, mycophenelate)	CMI
Radiotherapy, metabolic/ nutritional deficiencies Renal failure Liver failure Protein calorie malnutrition	CMI CMI and innate immunity CMI and innate immunity CMI
Increased loss of immunoglobulin Protein-losing enteropathy Nephrotic syndrome	Antibody
Virus infections HIV	CMI

CMI, cell-mediated immunity.

therapy predisposes to colonization by antibiotic-resistant potential pathogens, which may cause infectious or toxin-induced complications, for example, pseudomembranous colitis caused by *Clostridium difficile* toxin, multidrug-resistant *Staphylococcus aureus* infection. Surgical instruments, perfusion lines, and catheters may promote microbial invasion past the anatomical or physiological barriers.

Finally, damaged tissues, for example, damaged cardiac valves, provide a nidus for the establishment of infection.

Infections that recur in the same anatomical site are often due to defective anatomical or physiological barriers and hence should induce a diligent search for such factors. Microorganisms that cause infection in patients with this category of defects comprise pyogenic bacteria such

Table 5.2 Operational Classification of Imunodeficiency States

1. Immunodeficiency due to defective anatomical or physiological barriers to infection
2. Deficiency of opsonins: (a) antibody deficiency, (b) complement deficiency
3. T-cell deficiency
4. Combined T- and B-cell deficiency
5. Phagocyte deficiency
6. Defects in macrophage activation
7. Defects in immunoregulation
8. Defects in homeostasis of inflammation

as staphylococci and commensal organisms from the skin or intestinal tract. Fungi, especially *Candida*, may be another pathogen under these circumstances.

DISORDERS CHARACTERIZED BY ANTIBODY DEFICIENCY

Antibody deficiency can be defined as a condition characterized by a reduction in serum immunoglobulin concentrations below the fifth centile for age. Antibody deficiency may affect all classes of immunoglobulins or may be confined to a single isotype.

Clinical Manifestations of Antibody Deficiency

KEY CONCEPTS

1. Patients with antibody deficiency typically develop recurrent infection with encapsulated bacteria such as *Streptococcus pneumoniae* and *Haemophilus influenzae* type B. The common sites affected are the upper and lower respiratory tracts and the middle ear. From these sites, infection can spread via the bloodstream to produce metastatic infections, for example, meningitis or bone and joint infection.

2. Structural lung damage (bronchiectasis, pulmonary fibrosis) can be a consequence of recurrent respiratory tract infections in inadequately treated, antibody-deficient patients, and contributes to morbidity and mortality.

3. Once respiratory tract damage is established, patients are prone to sinopulmonary sepsis caused by nontypeable *Haemophilus influenzae* strains.

4. Overgrowth of commensal bacteria in the small intestines or chronic infection by intestine pathogens (*Giardia, Salmonella, Campylobacter*) may give rise to diarrhea or malabsorption secondary to villous atrophy.

5. In general, the course of uncomplicated viral infection (chicken pox, measles, etc.) is not significantly different from those in normal individuals, indicating that antibody production is not essential for recovery from acute viral infections. However, long-term immunity, which depends on the ability to develop neutralizing antibodies does not develop and the infections can recur.

6. Fungal and intracellular bacterial infections are not a feature of antibody deficiency.

7. About a fifth of patients with antibody deficiency due to common variable immune deficiency (which is described in a later section) develop autoimmune disorders. These include autoimmune hematological disorders (hemolytic anemia, autoimmune thrombocytopenia, pernicious anemia), autoimmune endocrinopathies (e.g., thyroid disease) or neurological diseases such as Guillain-Barré syndrome, and, rarely, a lupus-like syndrome.

Table 5.3 Pattern of Microbial Infection in Immunodeficiency

Defect	Microorganism	Site
Antibody	Encapsulated bacteria: *Streptococcus pneumoniae*, Hib, *Mycoplasma, Giardia, Salmonella, Campylobacter*	Upper and lower respiratory tract Less commonly systemic infection: meningitis, bone and joint infection Localized or disseminated Gastrointestinal tract
Complement C3/Factor I	Pyogenic bacteria, especially *Streptococcus pneumoniae*	Septicemia, meningitis, pyoderma
C5, C6, C7, C8, C2, C4	*Neisseria meningitidis* No infections or occasionally infections with *S. pneumoniae*	Meningitis, septicemia
Properdin, factor D	Encapsulated bacterial sepsis	
Phagocyte deficiency Neutropenia	Staphylococci, enteric bacteria, fungi	Systemic
Chronic granulomatous disease	*Staphylococcus aureus, Salmonella,* enteric bacteria, *Burkholderia cepacea*, fungi: *Aspergillus*	Skin, visceral abscesses: lymph nodes, lung, liver
Leucocyte adhesin deficiency	Pyogenic bacteria	Skin; any site, localized or systemic
T-cell deficiency	Viruses, fungi, protozoa, intracellular bacteria: *Mycobacteria, Listeria, Salmonella*	Any site, localized or systemic; mucocutaneous candidiasis
Defects in macrophage activation: Type I cytokine deficiency	Intracellular bacteria: *Mycobacteria, Listeria, Salmonella*	Lymph node; bone; disseminated
Combined T- and B-cell deficiency	As for antibody and T-cell deficiency	As for antibody and T-cell deficiency

Hib, *Haemophilus influenzae type B*

Major Categories of Antibody Deficiency

These are summarized in Table 5.4.

ANTIBODY DEFICIENCY ASSOCIATED WITH ABSENT B CELLS

B-cell maturation beyond the pre-B-cell stage found in the bone marrow, requires signals received through the pre-B-cell receptor complex. The pre-B-cell receptor is composed of the μ chains, surrogate light chains (heterodimers of λ constant region with V pre-β), and the signal-transducing components Igα and Igβ. The activities of the protein BTK (Bruton's tyrosine kinase) and BLNK (B-cell linker protein) are also essential for the transduction of signals received via the B-cell (and pre-B-cell) receptors. Therefore, it is not surprising that mutations in each of these elements causes early-onset antibody deficiency associated with lack of circulating B cells.

Ninety percent of all such cases occur in boys due to mutation of the *BTK* gene, which maps to the X chromosome

Table 5.4 Major Antibody and/or T-cell Deficiencies

Antibody Deficiency Diseases	Mutated Gene/Pathogenesis	Associated Features
X-linked agammaglobulinemia	*BTK*	Antibody deficiency and B lymphopenia
Autosomal recessive agammaglobulinemia	Mutations in genes for μ, Igα, Igβ, 5, or BLNK	Antibody deficiency and B lymphopenia
X-linked hyper IgM syndrome	CD40 ligand	Lack of CD40 ligand on activated T cells. Failure of Ig class-switching and affinity maturation; low IgG/IgA, raised or normal IgM; may develop neutropenia, autoimmune cytopenias, opportunistic infections, and gastrointestinal and liver pathologies
CD40 deficiency (a type of autosomal recessive hyper IgM syndrome)	*CD40*	Lack of CD40 expression on B cells. Other features similar to CD40L deficiency
Hyper-IgM syndrome (autosomal recessive)	*UNG* or *AID*	Low IgG and IgA, raised IgM
Common variable immunodeficiency	Unknown in most; *TACI* in ~10%, rarely *ICOS*, *CD19*, or *BAFFR*	Antibody deficiency; may have autoimmunity, lymphoproliferation, systemic granulomata
Selective IgA deficiency	Most unknown; few due to *TACI* mutations	Most remain healthy; increase in autoimmunity, atopy, celiac disease
IgG subclass deficiency	Unknown	If associated with specific antibody deficiency, (see text) may have recurrent sinopulmonary infections
T- and B-cell Immunodeficiencies	**Mutated Gene/Pathogenesis**	**Associated Features**
Severe combined immunodeficiency (SCID)	See Table 5.6 for details	Lymphopenia, low serum Igs, failure to thrive, severe recurrent infections by viruses, bacteria, and parasites; fatal without bone marrow transplant (BMT)
Omenn's syndrome	Hypomorphic mutation of *RAG1*, *RAG2*, *Artemis*, or *IL7Ra*	Variant of SCID; some T and B cells may develop but are oligoclonal. Features include erythroderma, lymphadenopathy, hepatosplenomegaly, eosinophilia. Outcome poor without BMT

(continued)

Table 5.4 *(continued)*

Antibody Deficiency Diseases	Mutated Gene/Pathogenesis	Associated Features
MHC class II deficiency	*MHC2TA, RFXANK, RFX5, RFXAP*: SCID due to defective MHC class II transcription	Lack of MHC class II expression resulting in CD4 lymphopenia and severe failure of T-cell and B-cell function
MHC class I deficiency	*TAP1 or TAP2*	Lack of MHC class I expression on cells; CD8 Lymphopenia; present with bronchiectasis or vasculitis

(Xp22). This condition is called X-linked agammaglobulinemia, which was the first immunodeficiency to be described in 1952 by Colonel Ogden Bruton. Mutations in the genes, encoding μ, 5, Igα, Igβ, and BLNK cause rare autosomal recessive forms of early-onset antibody deficiency with severe B lymphopenia.

ANTIBODY DEFICIENCY DUE TO DEFECT IN IMMUNOGLOBULIN ISOTOPE SWITCHING

During primary antibody responses, B cells initially produce IgM and later on in the response switch to the production of IgG, IgA, and IgE.

During the so-called immunoglobulin class-switching process, the heavy chain constant region changes while antigen specificity is maintained. Immunoglobulin class switch takes place within germinal centers contained within B-cell follicles of the secondary lymphoid organs. Another process that occurs within germinal centers is somatic hypermutation, which results in the sequential accumulation of point mutations in the Ig variable region gene. If the point mutation(s) result in increased binding affinity to the inducing antigen, the B-cell blasts (centrocytes) survive, proliferate, and eventually give rise to memory B cells and plasma cells that secrete high-affinity

antibody (this process is called affinity maturation). Through these processes, memory B cells are generated within germina centers.

Defects in genes encoding molecules required for the above processes, which operate within germinal centers, result in a form of antibody deficiency with elevated (or normal) IgM levels but lacking IgG, IgA, and IgE. These conditions are called hyper-IgM (HIGM) syndromes. A key requirement for germinal center formation and function is the interaction of CD40 (belonging to the TNF-receptor superfamily) found on the surface of B cells with an "activation induced," CD40-ligand (CD40L) protein expressed on the surface of CD4 lymphocytes. Mutations in the *CD40L* gene or the *CD40* gene result in X-linked (relatively common) and autosomal recessive (rare) HIGM, respectively. Patients with the CD40L deficiency suffer from recurrent bacterial infections typical of antibody deficiency. However, because CD40L function is required for optimal T-cell immunity, they also suffer from opportunistic infections characteristic of T-cell deficiency. About a third of patients with CD40L deficiency develop *Pneumocystis pneumonia*. Infections with cryptosporiodosis, toxoplasmosis, and nontuberculous mycobacteria also occur in this condition. These opportunistic infections can be explained on the basis that the interaction of CD40L on activated T cells with CD40 expressed on the surface of macrophages and dendritic cells, which in turn undergo maturation and activation, is required for the optimum expression of antimicrobial immunity.

A high proportion of CD40L-deficient patients develop progressive liver damage (sclerosing cholangitis), probably the result of cryptosporidial infection of the bile ducts.

Defects in the RNA-editing enzymes, activation-induced cytidine deaminase (AID), and uracil-DNA glycosylase (UNG) result in two further types of HIGM syndromes, which are defective class switching and affinity maturation.

Signaling through CD40, which belongs to the TNF-receptor superfamily, depends on the activation of the inhibitor of κ kinase (IKK) complex, resulting in the induction of NFκB. Hypomorphic mutations of the gamma subunit of the IKK complex, which is called *NEMO* (NFκB essential modulator), impairs NFκB activation. Patients with mutations in *NEMO* develop a complex immunodeficiency, which includes features of the HIGM syndrome.

COMMON VARIABLE IMMUNE DEFICIENCY

Most patients with primary antibody deficiency are collected under the heading "common variable immune deficiency," which is a condition characterized by low serum IgG and IgA and a variable decrease in IgM and the impaired production of specific antibodies following natural microbial exposure or immunization. The estimated prevalence of CVID is between 1 in 10,000 and 1 in 50,000. Clinically, CVID is dominated by the effects of antibody deficiency. About 20 percent of patients with CVID develop autoimmune disorders (arthritis, cytopenias, endocrinopathies). Some patients with CVID develop noncaseating sarcoidlike granulomata infiltrating various organs (lungs, liver, spleen, skin). The mechanisms underlying autoimmunity and granulomatous disease in CVID are unknown.

The immunological phenotype of CVID is heterogeneous with documented defects in B-cell survival, generation of B memory cells, and in vitro B- and T-cell activation. About 10 percent of cases of CVID are familial, with a predominance of autosomal dominant or autosomal recessive inheritance. CVID or selective IgA deficiency can affect different members of the same kindred. Recently, a number of gene defects have been identified in CVID patients, accounting for about 10–15 percent of the total patient pool.

The commonest defect (in approximately 10% of CVID patients) is a mutation of the gene *TACI* (transmembrane activator and calcium modulator and cyclophilin ligand interacter). *TACI*, which belongs to the TNF-receptor superfamily, is a ligand for the cytokines, BAFF (B-cell-activating factor of the TNF family) and APRIL (a proliferation-induced ligand), which induce immunoglobulin class-switch recombination.

Mice deficient in BAFF or its receptor have impaired B-cell development and antibody deficiency. TACI−/− mice have reduced serum IgA and IgM levels, reduced antibody responses to T-cell-independent antigens, and tend to develop autoimmunity and B lymphoproliferation. Mutations in *TACI* have been found in CVID patients and their relatives, with selective IgA deficiency, indicating variable penetrance of this gene defect. In the majority of currently documented patients, *TACI* mutations affect only one allele, indicating a dominant negative effect of the mutated gene. A possible explanation is that *TACI*, like other members of the TNF-receptor family, undergoes ligand-independent preassociation and function as multimeric units. Thus, incorporation of a mutated *TACI* chain in this multimeric complex may disrupt ligand binding or signal-transducing capacity. Recent studies have found that family members of CVID patients possessing heterozygous *TACI* mutations may have completely normal serum immunoglobulin levels and "in vitro" B-cell function. This leads to the conclusion that the development of antibody deficiency in those carrying heterozygous *TACI* mutations may depend on modifier genes or environmental factors.

ICOS (inducible co-stimulating receptor) is a co-stimulatory T-cell molecule that induces cytokines required for supporting class-switch recombination, Ig production and terminal B-cell differentiation. ICOS−/− and ICOS ligand−/− mice exhibit defective germinal center formation and antibody production. Mutations in the *ICOS* gene account for about 1 percent of CVID patients.

A single CVID patient was identified to have a mutation on the gene encoding the BAFF receptor, a finding that could be predicted from observations in BAFF−/− mice.

Finally, CD19 deficiency has been described in two families with CVID. CD19 is a B-cell accessory molecule that is required for B-cell activation, proliferation, and hence B-cell development. CD19−/− mice exhibit hypogammaglobulinemia and poor antibody responses to protein antigens.

In the case of the large majority of patients with CVID, the underlying molecular defect is unknown.

IgA DEFICIENCY

IgA deficiency is characterized by reduced (<0.07 g/L) or absent serum IgA levels. IgA deficiency is the commonest form of primary antibody deficiency and affects about 1 in 700 Caucasians. IgA deficiency is rare in some racial groups (Japanese, Africans). The majority of IgA-deficient individuals remain free of infection due to the ability of IgG and IgM to compensate for the lack of IgA. Long-term studies have shown that a small proportion of IgA-deficient patients develop recurrent sinopulmonary or gastrointestinal infections. Most infection-prone IgA-deficient patients have concomitant IgG2 subclass deficiency and a selective inability to produce antibodies against bacterial capsular polysaccharides. IgA deficiency is associated with an increased incidence of atopy, celiac disease, and a range of autoimmune diseases, including arthritis, "lupus-like" syndrome, autoimmune endocrinopathies, and autoimmune cytopenias.

IgA-deficient patients with serum levels below 0.07 g/L are at the risk of developing anti-IgA antibodies after receiving blood products. Such individuals are at risk of developing anaphylaxis on receiving blood products.

IgA deficiency and CVID can differentially affect members of the same kindred. Rarely, IgA deficiency can precede the development of CVID. Therefore, in some instances, the molecular mechanisms underlying CVID and IgA deficiency may be identical. TACI deficiency can cause IgA deficiency in some family members while others develop CVID. However, the molecular basis of IgA deficiency in most cases is largely unknown.

Genetic analysis of kindred with CVID and IgA deficiency have highlighted the existence of susceptibility loci within the MHC region of chromosome 6. The strongest linkage lies within the DR/DQ within the MHC class II region.

IgG SUBCLASS DEFICIENCY

Serum IgG comprises four subclasses called IgG1, IgG2, IgG3, and IgG4, respectively reflecting the relative abundance of these isotypes in the serum. IgG subclass deficiency is diagnosed on finding a reduction in the serum concentration of IgG subclasses, of more than two standard deviations below the mean value for age, despite the total IgG level being normal. In practice, IgG subclass assays are difficult to standardize due to the lack of an internationally accepted reference preparation. Furthermore, genetic variations that influence serum IgG subclass levels exist among different ethnic groups. Hence, age- and population-related normal ranges are not always available.

Some individuals with IgG subclass deficiencies are asymptomatic. Others with IgG subclass deficiencies are prone to recurrent sinopulmonary infections. Such infection-prone patients exhibit reduced antibody responses to bacterial capsular polysaccharides. Defective anti-polysaccharide antibody responses are most often seen in individuals with IgG2 subclass deficiency with or without concomitant IgA deficiency. The molecular mechanisms underlying IgG subclass deficiencies are unknown.

TREATMENT OF ANTIBODY DEFICIENCY

Prospective clinical studies have shown that optimal IgG replacement therapy reduces the incidence of sepsis and complications like structural lung damage. If replacement therapy is introduced early before organ damage is established,

antibody-deficient individuals are likely to have a normal life span. Replacement immunoglobulin is prepared from plasma pooled from large cohorts of normal donors. Current practice of prescreening donors for infection and multiple antiviral steps employed during the manufacture of plasma have eliminated the risk of HIV and hepatitis B and C transmission. Different immunoglobulin products are licensed for administration via the intravenous or subcutaneous route. Detailed management of a patient's antibody deficiency is discussed in the references on the diagnosis and management of antibody deficiency (see list of references at end of chapter).

DEFECTS IN CELL-MEDIATED IMMUNITY (T-CELL DEPENDENT IMMUNITY)

These may be inherited (primary) conditions, which are rare or secondary to other pathologies (Table 5.5). HIV infection, which is an important cause of secondarily impaired T-cell immunity is discussed in Chapter 8.

Manifestations of T-Cell Deficiency

KEY CONCEPTS

Patients with impaired T-cell function may develop the following:

1. They show increased susceptibility to infections with intracellular microbial pathogens (viruses, intracellular bacteria, and protozoa).
2. Viral infections: Infections with exanthematous viruses (measles, chicken pox) can be fatal in children with

Table 5.5 Causes of T-Cell Deficiency

Primary (inherited)	See Table 5.6 and text

Secondary	(a) Viral-induced
	  HIV
	  Measles (transient)
	(b) Iatrogenic
	  Irradiation
	  BMT until engraftment is complete
	  Chemotherapy for malignancy
	  Immunosuppressive therapy
	(c) Thymoma
	(d) Lymphoma
	(e) Severe renal or liver failure

Idiopathic	Idiopathic CD4 cell deficiency (cause unknown)

T-cell deficiency. These viruses are not a problem in adults as they have residual protective antibody responses generated by primary infection or immunization. Adults with T-cell deficiency are typically affected by the reactivation of latent viruses (e.g., cytomegalovirus, *Herpes simplex*), which can produce life-threatening disseminated infections.

3. Fungal infections: T-cell-deficient patients are typically susceptible to fungal infections.
   a. *Pneumocystis giroveci* causes interstitial pneumonia, which is pathognomonic for T-cell deficiency;
   b. Mucocutaneous infection with *Candida*;
   c. Systemic infections with filamentous fungi (e.g., *Aspergillus fumigatus*);
   d. Meningitis or systemic infection caused by *Cryptococcus neoformans*.
4. Intracellular bacterial infection is a particular problem in T-cell-deficient patients. These patients are highly susceptible to infection with *M. tuberculosis* or reactivation of latent tuberculosis. They are also susceptible to disseminated infections with poorly pathogenic mycobacteria (e.g., nontuberculous mycobacteria, BCG).
5. Infants with T-cell deficiency are usually lymphopenic and fail to thrive (i.e., fail to maintain normal rates of growth in height and weight).
6. Infants with SCID may develop dermatitis and hepatosplenomegaly due to graft-versus-host disease caused by maternal lymphocytes that have crossed the placenta.
7. Malignancies: T-cell-deficient individuals are prone to develop a range of malignancies where viral infection acts as a co-factor (e.g., Epstein-Barr virus [EBV-] induced non-Hodgkin's lymphoma, Kaposi's sarcoma where human herpes virus 8 is a co-factor). There is also an increase in cutaneous malignancies occurring in an individual exposed to significant amounts of ultraviolet light (basal-cell carcinoma and squamous carcinoma).

Major Categories of Combined Immunodeficiency

SEVERE COMBINED IMMUNODEFICIENCY

SCID comprises a group of inherited diseases characterized by a severe deficit in T-cell development and function with variable defects in B-cell and natural killer or NK cell development. SCID leads to death within the first two years of life, unless patients are rescued by hematopoietic stem cell transplantation (HSCT). These are rare disorders with an estimated frequency between 1 in 50,000 and 1 in 100,000 live births.

Table 5.6 Classification of SCID

Type of SCID	Relative Frequency (%)	Inheritance	Cells Affected	Defective Gene
Reticular dysgenesis	<1	AR	T, B, NK, Leucocytes, platelets	?
T−B−SCID	10	AR	T, B	RAG1/2
	10	AR	T, B	Artemis
T−B+SCID	50	XL	T, NK	IL2R6
	10	AR	T, NK	JAK3
	1	AR	T, NK	IL7RA
	<1	AR	T	CD45
	<1	AR	T	CD36,CD3E
T−B−NK−SCID	20	AR	T, B, NK	ADA
AR, antosomal recessive; XL, X-linked

Classification of SCID

The classification of SCID, based on immunological and genetic criteria, is summarized in Table 5.6.

SCID: Clinical Features

These patients typically present in the first year of life with failure to thrive and recurrent infections caused by bacterial, viral, and fungal pathogens. Infections typically affect the respiratory and gastrointestinal systems. The infections may be caused by common pathogens (adenovirus, respiratory syncytial virus, parainfluenza virus), as well as by opportunistic organisms of low-grade virulence (*Candida, Pneumocystis carinii,* cytomegalovirus). Live vaccines such as BCG can lead to disseminated life-threatening infections. The persistent infections developing in SCID patients rapidly lead to malnutrition, growth impairment, and early death. Because of the patient's inability to reject allogeneic cells, graft-versus-host disease (GvHD) can be caused by transplacentally acquired maternal lymphocytes or by allogeneic cells following blood transfusion. GvHD manifests as skin rashes or hepatosplenomegaly and lymphadenopathy.

The absence of tonsils or other lymphatic tissue may be evident and radiographic studies may reveal thymic-hypoplasia. Lymphopenia (absolute lymphocyte count $<3 \times 10^9$/L in the first year of life) is a characteristic feature seen in over 80 percent of patients with SCID. (Therefore, SCID needs to be excluded in any infant with unexplained lymphopenia.)

Immunological and Molecular Classification of SCID

SCID can be classified in two groups based on the blood lymphocyte phenotype.

■ Patients lacking T cells with normal or increased B cells: T−B+ SCID
■ Patients lacking T and B cells: T−B−SCID

Defects in one of four functionally related genes causes T−B+SCID. X-linked SCID, which is the commonest form, is due to a mutation of the gene encoding the IL-2 receptor γ chain, which is the signal-transducing chain common to the receptors for six cytokines (IL-2, IL-4, IL-7, IL-9, IL-15, and IL-21). The absence of responses to these cytokines causes defects in a broad range of T- and B-cell functions. IL-7 is required for early stages of T-cell development. Lack of response to this cytokine results in T lymphopenia. IL-15 is required for NK-cell development and its lack results in the failure of NK-cell development. Signal transduction through the aforementioned cytokine receptors involves the interaction of the common γ chain with the tyrosine kinase JAK3. This explains why mutations of the *JAK3* gene result in an autosomal recessive form of SCID, with a phenotype similar to X-linked SCID. Mutations of the α chain of IL-2 or IL-7 receptors result in two rare forms of SCID.

T- and B-cell receptors consist of invariant signal-transducing elements combined with elements that make up the variable regions, which contribute to the antigen-binding portion of the receptor. The gene recombination required for generating these receptors requires the function of the product of recombination activating genes 1 and 2 and a number of proteins that are required for DNA repair (DNA-PKcs, KU70, KU80, XRLC4, and DNA-IV). In mice, mutations in any one of these genes produces analogues of SCID.

In humans, T–B–SCID is most common (50 percent of total) caused by mutations of the recombinase-activating genes, *RAG1* or *RAG2*. RAG1 and RAG2 are enzymes responsible for introducing double-stranded DNA breaks, which initiate V(D)J gene rearrangements, required for generating T- and B-cell receptors for antigen. Without normal RAG1 and RAG2 function, T- and B-cell development is arrested early in ontogeny, producing T–B–SCID.

Hypomorphic mutations of *RAG1* or *RAG2* result in a leaky form of SCID called Omenn's syndrome. In Omenn's syndrome, a few T- and B-cell clones may be generated but the full T- and B-cell repertoire fails to develop. The few T- and B-cell clones that leak through may undergo secondary expansion. As a result, patients with Omenn's syndrome may not be markedly lymphopenic but the lymphocyte repertoire is oligoclonal and severe immunodeficiency is the outcome.

T- and B-cell antigen receptors are assembled from the recombination of variable region V(D)J and constant region genes. A protein called ARTEMIS is required for DNA repair, including the repair of DNA breaks generated during V(D)J recombination. Mutation of the gene encoding ARTEMIS results in a rare form of T–B–SCID. These patients also exhibit increased sensitivity to ionizing radiation.

About 15 percent of SCID cases are caused by deficiency of adenosine deaminase (ADA), an enzyme required for the salvage of nucleotides within lymphoid cells. The lack of ADA causes the accumulation of toxic metabolites of adenosine (deoxyadenosine and deoxy-ATP) within lymphoid cells, resulting in their demise. ADA deficiency results in profound lymphopenia affecting T cells, B cells, and NK cells. Rarely, mutations of ADA causing milder forms of enzyme deficiency lead to a milder form of combined immunodeficiency presenting at a later stage in life. Purine nucleoside phosphorylase (PNP) is an enzyme required for purine salvage within lymphocytes, and PNP deficiency causes a milder phenotype of SCID than seen in ADA deficiency. SCID due to PNP deficiency not treated with HSCT is fatal in childhood.

Mutations in proteins required for normal functioning and signal transduction through the T-cell receptor (TCR) cause rare forms of SCID. Mutations of the tyrosine phosphatase, CD45, which helps to initiate signaling by the TCR, results in T–B+ SCID in humans. Mutation of components of CD3-complex (CD3 γ, ε, and δ) result in a SCID phenotype. During signal transduction via TCRs, the protein tyrosine kinases Lck and ZAP70 are required for phosphorylation of ITAMs on the intracytoplasmic segment of the TCR. Deficiency of either of these kinases results in rare forms of SCID.

TCRs of CD8 cells recognize antigenic peptides that are complexed to MHC class I antigens, and TCR of CD4 cells recognize antigen bound to MHC class II on the surface of antigen-presenting cells. Cell-surface expression of MHC class I molecules fails if either of the two transporters of antigenic peptides (TAP1 or TAP2) is lacking. TAP1 and TAP2 help to transfer peptides from the cytosol into the endoplasmic reticulum, for subsequent loading onto newly synthesized MHC class I molecules. In the absence of peptide loading, MHC class I molecules are degraded before reaching the cell surface. In the absence of MHC class I antigen expression, CD8 cell function is deficient, and these cells are not generated within the thymus. The resulting immunodeficiency is milder than SCID and often presents in later life. Paradoxically, viral infections are not a problem in these patients. Some MHC class I deficient patients develop progressive bronchiectasis, while others develop vasculitis affecting the face and upper respiratory tract. It has been postulated that vasculitis seen in these patients may be due to self-destruction of vascular endothelial cells by the unrestrained cytotoxicity of NK cells.

In contrast, MHC class II deficiency results in a profound failure of CD4 cell functions. Lack of thymic CD4$^+$ CD8$^-$ cell selection for survival results in peripheral CD4 lymphopenia. Because CD4 function is required for normal cell-mediated immunity, as well as antibody production, MHC class II deficiency results in a severe form of SCID with a fatal outcome. MHC class II deficiency is due to a mutation in one of four transcription factors (RFXAP, CIITA, RFX5, RFXANK), which regulate MHC class II expression.

TREATMENT OF SCID
Hematopoietic Stem Cell Transplantation

Untreated SCID is invariably fatal in early infancy. Once a diagnosis of SCID is confirmed, irrespective of the molecular diagnosis, HSCT from a human leucocyte antigen (HLA-) identical or haplo-identical family donor is the treatment of choice. Treatment of SCID with HSCT before 3.5 months of age results in good immune reconstitution and 95 percent survive long term. Delay in treatment, or the occurrence of infection, impairs outcome. Infection and GvHD are the main complications following HSCT. North American and European data indicate that long-term survival after transplants from HLA-matched unrelated donors was close to 60 percent. Review of European data between 1968 and 1999 indicates the progressive improvement of outcome, which is mainly because of better prevention of GvHD and the treatment of infection. Analysis of the outcome of European and U.S. bone marrow transplant programs for the treatment of SCID is ongoing and will be regularly reported.

Gene Therapy for SCID

Long-term immune reconstitution has been achieved in patients with SCID caused by the common γ-chain deficiency or ADA deficiency, using gene therapy.

This was achieved by ex vivo gene transfer to hematopoietic stem cells isolated from the patient's bone marrow. These gene-reconstituted stem cells were retransfused into the patient. To date, gene therapy has been restricted to patients without an HLA-matched family donor.

Several cases of leukemia have occurred among γ-chain-deficient patients who received gene therapy. In these cases, the retroviral vector had integrated close to the LMO2 proto-oncogene in the leukemia clone, leading to aberrant transcription and expression of LMO2. Because of this setback, clinical trials of gene therapy for SCID are being carefully evaluated, and more experience is required before the definitive role of gene therapy in SCID is established.

DiGeorge's Syndrome (Thymic Aplasia)

DiGeorge's syndrome (DGS) is secondary to a hemizygous deletion of the short arm of chromosome 22 (DEL 22q. 11.2). This chromosomal defect causes a complex inherited syndrome characterized by cardiac malformations, thymic hypoplasia, palatopharyngeal abnormalities with associated velopharyngeal dysfunction, hypoparathyroidism, and facial dysmorphism. The 22q deletion has an incidence of approximately 1 in 2,500 live births. The associated clinical phenotype is highly variable. About 20 percent of individuals with 22q deletion have thymic aplasia, resulting in T lymphopenia and impaired CMI. In most such cases, the degree of T lymphopenia is modest (partial DGS) and almost complete restitution of the T-cell repertoire and function occurs by two years of age. Therefore, infections characteristic of T-cell deficiency are rare in these individuals. A minority of infected individuals

(<1 percent) exhibit profound T lymphopenia, associated with opportunistic infections and a poor outlook unless rescued with fetal thymic transplant.

The cardiac, velopharyngeal, thymic, and parathyroid abnormalities are due to the defective development of third and fourth pharyngeal arches during ontogeny.

The 22q. 11.2 region contains the *TBX1* gene, which belongs to the T-BOX family of genes that incorporate proteins that regulate embryonic development. Patients with mutations in the *TBX1* genes also develop the clinical features seen in 22q. 11.2 deletion syndrome, suggesting that haplo-insufficiency of the *TBX1* gene may be responsible for the clinical features seen in those with a deletion of the 22q. 11.2 region.

PHAGOCYTE DEFICIENCIES

Neutrophils are the principal circulating phagocyte. During inflammation, neutrophils become activated and migrate into the tissues where they ingest, kill, and digest invading bacteria and fungi. Neutrophil function can be deficient because of a reduction in the number of circulating neutrophils (neutropenia) or due to inherited defects in neutrophil function, which are rare disorders.

Neutropenia

Neutropenia is defined as a decrease in the blood neutrophil count below $1.5 \times 10^9/$L. In some racial groups (e.g., Africans), the normal neutrophil count is somewhat lower (up to $1.2 \times 10^9/$L). While mild neutropnia may be asymptomatic, severe neutropenia (counts $< 0.5 \times 10^9/$L) is invariably associated with the risk of life-threatening

Table 5.7 Causes of Neutropenia

Category of Neutropenia	Condition	Defective Gene
Primary (due to rare gene defects)	Autosomal recessive congenital neutropenia	Homozygous mutations of mitochondrial HS-1 associated protein X1 (HAX1)
	Autosomal dominant congenital neutropenia	In 60% heterozygous mutations of neutrophil elastase gene (ELA-2)
	Cyclical neutropenia	ELA-2
	Shwachman Diamond syndrome	Shwachman Bodian Diamond syndrome gene (SBDS)

Category of Neutropenia	Mechanism of Neutropenia	Cause
Secondary	Reduced neutrophil production in bone marrow	Secondary to viral infection
		Drugs (idiosyncratic) or immune mediated Chemotherapy Radiotherapy Bone marrow failure (leukemia, myelodysplasia, aplasia)
	Reduced neutrophil migration out of bone marrow	WHIM syndrome secondary to mutation of CXCR4 receptor
	Increased peripheral destruction of neutrophils	Autoimmune neutropenia Hypersplenism

microbal sepsis caused by a broad range of endogenous Gram-positive bacteria (*S. aureus*) and Gram-negative bacteria (*E. coli*, *Pseudomonas* spp., *Klebsiella* spp.) as well as fungi (*Candida*). Neutrophils are particularly important for maintaining the integrity of mucous membranes. Hence, oral ulceration and perianal inflammation can be features of severe neutropenia. Causes of neutropenia are summarized in Table 5.7.

Defects in Leucocyte Migration

To reach the sites of inflammation, neutrophils need to migrate across the endothelium into sites of inflammation. For this process to be initiated, sialyl Lewis^X, which is expressed on the surface of leucocytes, needs to interact with E selectin, which is expressed on the luminal surface of the endothelial cells. Leucocytes, which are transiently arrested by the previous interaction, need to bind tightly to the endothelial surface by a second set of interactions. This is between the protein lymphocyte function-associated antigen-1(LFA-1) LFA-1 expressed on the leucocyte surface and its ligand intercellular adhesion molecule-1 expressed on the luminal surface of activated endothelial cells. Leucocyte emigration into the tissues follows these adhesion events. LFA-1 is one of a set of three cell-surface heterodimers composed of a common β chain (CD18) with three separate α chains called CD11a, b, and c. CD18-CD11a heterodimers form LFA-1, CD18/CD11b

Table 5.8 Defects in Phagocyte Function

Phagocyte Deficiencies (excluding congenital neutropenias)	Defective Gene/Pathogenesis	Clinical Features
Chronic granulomatous disease	Mutations in components of the phagocyte oxidase (see text for details)	Pyogenic and fungal infections; lymph node and visceral abscesses; chronic granulomata (see text for details)
Leucocyte adhesin deficiency type 1	Mutation of gene encoding CD18, which is a component of leucocyte adhesins (see text for details)	Delayed umbilical cord separating, omphalitis, pyoderma, periodontitis, leucocytosis
Leucocyte adhesin deficiency type 2	Mutation of gene encoding GDP-fucose transporter (see text for details)	As above plus mental retardation
Rac 2 deficiency	Mutation in *RAC2* leading to impaired actin polymerization/cytoskeletal function	Poor wound healing, leucocytosis
Mendelian susceptibility to mycobacterial infection	Defects in the production or response to IFN-g : Mutated genes include *IL12B*, *IL12RB* *IFNGR1*, *IFNGR2*, *STAT-1*, *TYK2*. Intact response to IFN-γ is essential for control of intracellular bacterial infection. Some *NEMO* mutations cause X-linked susceptibility to mycobacterial infection. See text for full explanation.	Recurrent disseminated infections with poorly pathogenic mycobacteria (NTM or BCG) and systemic infections with non-typhi *Salmonella* species
Hyper-IgE syndrome	Mutations in *STAT-3* leading to a functionally defective form of *STAT 3*. Autosomal dominant inheritance.	Complex phenotype characterized by recurrent abscesses, pneumonia with pneumatocoele formation, elevated serum IgE, dermatosis, dysmorphic features, delayed shedding of decidual teeth, bone abnormalities, selective impairment of anticapsular antibody responses, and impaired acute-phase response following infection. Spectrum of infecting organisms include *S. aureus*, *H. infuenzae*, *S. pneumoniae*, and filamentous fungi.

heterodimers form complement receptor 3, and CD18 combined to CD11c forms complement receptor 4. LFA-1 is required for leucocyte adhesion to endothelial cells while CR3 and CR4 act as receptors for activated complement, aiding ingestion of opsonized microorganisms. Mutation of the gene encoding CD18 (resulting in the lack of expression of LFA-1, CR3, and CR4) results in an inherited primary immunodeficiency called leucocyte adhesin deficiency type 1(LAD1). Mutations of the enzyme GDP-fucosyl transferase prevents post-transcriptional fucosylation of proteins. Such individuals cannot synthesize sialyl Lewis^X. This condition is called leucocyte adhesion deficiency type 2. Leucocytes of the patient with LAD1 and 2 exhibit impaired ability to adhere to endothelial walls and therefore cannot migrate into infected sites.

These patients typically present in early childhood with recurrent pyogenic infection of skin, respiratory, and gastrointestinal tracts as well as mucous membranes. Poor wound healing and delayed umbilical cord separation are typical. Because of impaired neutrophil migration, these patients develop a leucocytosis and pus fails to form at sites of infection. These inherited disorders are typically associated with severe gingivitis and periodontal disease, again indicating the particular importance of normal neutrophil function for maintenance of the health of the dental crevice. Outcome in both conditions is poor, with early death. BMT is curative in LAD1, and oral fucose supplementation is beneficial in LAD2.

Defects in Bacterial Killing

The best example of an immunodeficiency characterized by failure of phagocyte-mediated bacterial killing is chronic granulomatous disease (CGD). In normal neutrophils (and monocytes), bacterial phagocytosis results in the activation of the nicotinamide adenine dinucleotide phosphate (NADPH) oxidase complex, which produces superoxide and generates a milieu within the phagosome that activate the proteolytic enzymes, cathepsin, and elastase. The activity of the proteolytic enzymes is bactericidal. The NADPH oxidase complex comprises two membrane-associated proteins, p91phox and p22phox (also called the α and β units of cytochrome B558, respectively), complexed with three cytosolic cofactors, p47phox, p40phox, and p67phox. Mutations have been identified in four out of five components (p91phox, p22phox, p47phox, p67phox), resulting in defective NADPH oxidase activity, leading to impairment of bacterial killing by phagocytic cells. The result is a clinical syndrome, called CGD, characterized by failure of bacterial degradation in vivo, resulting in the persistence of tissue inflammation with granuloma formation in a variety of organs. CGD due to p91phox deficiency is X-linked, while the other variants of CGD are inherited in an autosomal recessive manner.

In CGD, the bacterial killing mechanisms that depend on the phagocyte oxidase system are inoperative, but the nonoxidative killing mechanisms are still intact. Therefore, patients with CGD are not troubled by the broad range of microbes that a neutropenic patient would be susceptible to. Instead, CGD patients get infections with a restricted range of microorganisms, which are only susceptible to the bactericidal mechanisms initiated by NADPH oxidase activation. The spectrum of microorganisms that causes infections in CGD include S. aureus, Gram-negative bacteria (Burkholderia cepacea, Salmonella, Serratia), and fungi (Aspergillus spp.). Characteristic sites of infection include subcutaneous tissue, lymph nodes, lungs, and liver. Oral and perioral ulceration are common.

The formation of chronic granulomata in various tissues is a typical feature of

CGD. In critical locations, chronic granuloma formation may cause pathology. Granulomatous obstruction of the gastrointestinal or genitourinary tract may be a consequence. Hepatosplenomegaly may occur due to granulomatous infiltration of these organs. A granulomatous colitis, resembling Crohn's disease, occurs in about 15 percent of CGD patients, highlighting the importance of normal phagocyte function for preventing harmful inflammation in the large intestine.

Diagnosis of CGD is based on the ability of stimulated neutrophils from these patients to oxidize dyes to give a colored product or a fluorescent product, detectable by flow cytometry. Prophylactic treatment with IFN-γ substantially reduces the incidence of bacterial and fungal infections in CGD patients, for reasons that are not fully understood.

The cytosolic GTPase Rac2 is required for the normal actin polymerization and optimal function of the phagocyte oxidase system. Rac2 deficiency results in impaired neutrophil mobility and poor superoxide responses to some stimuli. A single affected patient identified to date had a clinical presentation similar to that seen in LAD.

Defects in Killing of Intracellular Bacteria by Activated Macrophages

Some bacterial species (*Mycobacteria, Listeria, Salmonella*) are resistant to the killing mechanisms operating within phagocytic cells and therefore can survive and multiply within monocytes and macrophages. Effective immunity against these organisms depends on T-cell- (and NK-cell-) dependent macrophage activation. Studies in gene-disrupted mouse and human immunodeficiencies have identified that IL-12- and IL-23-dependent interferon gamma (IFN-γ) production is critically important for immunity against intracellular bacterial pathogens. This process is initiated by the stimulation of Toll receptors on the surface of antigen-presenting cells by bacterial ligands such as mycobacterial lipoarabinomannan. This results in the secretion of IL-12 and IL-23 and TNF-α by the antigen-presenting cells. Binding of IL-12 and IL-23 to their respective receptors, expressed on the surface of activated T cells and NK cells, induces these cells to secrete a further cytokine IFN-γ. IFN-γ acting in concert with TNF-α activates macrophages, which are then capable of killing intracellular pathogens (e.g., *Mycobacteria* and *Salmonella*). Individuals with impaired T-cell-mediated immunity (e.g., SCID or HIV infection) are highly susceptible to mycobacterial infections, including infections caused by poorly pathogenic mycobacterial species (nontuberculous mycobacteria and BCG). However, disseminated life-threatening infections by these organisms may also occur in the absence of a recognized primary or secondary immunodeficiency. Genetic analysis of affected kindred to date have identified mutations in seven different genes that participate in the production or response to IFN-γ. These patients are classified under the heading Mendelian susceptibility to mycobacterial disease (MSMD) (OMIM 209950). The genetic lesions responsible for MSMD affect the integrity of the IL-12/23-dependent IFN-γ pathway.

Thus, mutations have been identified in

- The P40 subunit shared by IL-12 and IL-23 (also called IL12B);
- The β chain shared by the IL-12 and IL-23 receptors;
- The TYK2 kinase required for signaling via the IL-12 receptor;

- The α and β chains of the IFN-γ receptor (IFN-γR1 and IFN-γ2);
- The STAT-1 signal transducing molecule, which is required for signaling through the IFN-γ receptor;
- The seventh defect responsible for increased susceptibility to mycobacterial infection is that NFκB essential modulator gene, which is required for NFκB activation, which is critical for signal transduction via the Toll, IL-1, and TNF-α receptors.

The severity of the clinical phenotype of MSMD depends on the genotype. Complete IFN-γR1 or R2 deficiencies lead to the abrogation of responses to IFN-γ. Such patients present in early childhood with disseminated NTM or BCG infections, resulting in a high mortality, despite chemotherapy. Mycobacterial lesions in such patients are multibacillary and associated with poor granuloma formation. In contrast, partial IFN-γR1 deficiency, complete IL-12B deficiency, and IL-12/23 receptor deficiency predispose to mycobacterial infections, presenting at a later age and with a favorable outcome, following chemotherapy. Lesions in these latter patients are paucibacillary and are associated with an intact granulomatous response. Patients with partial or complete STAT-1 deficiency, which impairs the signaling via the IFN-γR results in susceptibility to mycobacteria of low-grade virulence. Complete STAT-1 deficiency also impairs signaling via type I interferon receptors, which predisposes to life-threatening herpes viral infections occurring in childhood. The commonest infections that affect patients with defects in the IL-12/23 are extraintestinal or septicemic, relapsing infections with non-typhoidal *Salmonella* species.

As could be predicted, patients with IL-12/23 defects or partial IFN-γR defects respond to treatment with IFN-γ but those with complete IFN-γ defects are refractory to this therapy.

COMPLEX IMMUNODEFICIENCIES DUE TO MISCELLANEOUS DEFECTS

Wiskott-Aldrich Syndrome

Patients with Wiskott-Aldrich syndrome typically develop eczema; purpura due to thrombocytopenia with small-sized, defective platelets; and a variable immunodeficiency. Antibody production to bacterial capsular polysaccharides is deficient. Patients therefore commonly develop recurrent sinopulmonary infections. T-cell and NK-cell function is deficient and progressive T lymphopenia develops with time. Hence, patients can develop opportunistic infections. Risk of malignancy (especially leukemias or EBV-induced lymphomas) is increased in these patients.

The defective gene, which is on the X chromosome, encodes for the Wiskott-Aldrich syndrome protein, which regulates actin polymerization, and therefore cytoskeletal change is required for normal platelet and lymphocyte function.

DNA Repair Defects Associated with Immunodeficiency

ATAXIA TELANGIECTASIA

Ataxia telangiectasia (AT) is a condition characterized by cerebellar ataxia, oculocutaneous telangiectasia, growth retardation, and a variable immunodeficiency. AT patients show increased sensitivity to ionized radiation and radiomimetic drugs. Increased susceptibility to leukemias and lymphomas is also a feature of this syndrome. Patients often fail to produce antibodies to bacterial capsular polysaccharides and therefore develop sinopulmonary infections. Chromosomal translocations, involving immunoglobulin heavy-chain and TCR loci, are often detected in the T cells of AT patients.

The function of the protein encoded by the affected gene (called ataxia telangiectasia mutated, or ATM) is to detect double-strand breaks in DNA, initiating their repair. Mutated ATM results in defective control of the cell cycle. This explains the radiation sensitivity, abnormal immune cell development and function, and the cytogenetic abnormalities seen in AT.

OTHER DNA REPAIR DEFECTS ASSOCIATED IMMUNODEFICIENCY

Nijmegen breakage syndrome, which is phenotypically similar to AT, is due to a mutation of the *NBS1* gene that encodes a protein that acts as a substrate for ATM. DNA-ligase I defect, which also results in defective DNA repair, manifests with growth retardation and immunodeficiency. The product of the *MRE11A* gene is another component of the DNA damage sensing machinery. Mutation of the *MRE11A* gene results in a condition similar to AT.

IMMUNODEFICIENCIES RESULTING IN DEFECTIVE HOMEOSTASIS OF THE IMMUNE SYSTEM

Defects in the Cytolytic Pathway

The homeostasis of immune responses requires prevention of excessive lymphocyte activation (Table 5.9). The mechanism by which such regulation occurs includes activation-induced cell death of T lymphocytes, which requires the activation of apoptotic pathways. Defects in critical components of these pathways result in susceptibility to hemophagocytic lymphohistiocytosis (HLH), which is usually triggered by an intercurrent viral infection caused by viruses such as EBV or cytomegalovirus. HLH is characterized by massive infiltration of organs, such as the liver, spleen, bone marrow, and central nervous system, by activated CD8$^+$ lymphocytes and macrophages, as well as a massive overproduction of IFN-γ and TNF-α. Severe pancytopenia is typical of this syndrome and is caused in part by phagocytosis of blood cells by activated macrophages and in part is secondary to the infiltration of bone marrow by activated macrophages (histiocytes).

A number of genetic defects that affect the efficiency of T-cell- and NK-cell-mediated cytolysis can predispose to the development of HLH. Cytolysis by T cells and NK cells is initiated by the secretion of contents of cytolytic granules at the immunological synapse between the T cells and the target cells. The process involves the translocation of perforin-containing lytic granules onto the target cell interphase, followed by fusion of these granules with the plasma membrane of the T cell, with release of perforin onto the surface of the target cell. Perforin punches holes in the target cell membrane, causing cytolosis.

Mutation of the perforin (*PRF1*) gene, which encodes for perforin, is one of the genetic defects that predisposes to familial HLH. Perforin-supported cytolysis (by CD-8 cells and NK cells) may damp down immune responses triggered by viral infections by aiding the elimination of antigen-presenting cells or by promoting activation-induced death of T cells.

Table 5.9 Disorders of Homeostasis of Immune Function

Syndromes with Autoimmunity	Gene Defect/Pathogenesis	Chief Clinical Findings
Autoimmune lymphoproliferative syndrome (ALPS)	Defects of components in the apoptosis pathway in lymphocytes: mutations in genes encoding CD95(*TNFRSF6*), CD05 ligand (*TNFSF6*), caspase 10, caspase 8, or NRAS	Lymphadenopathy, hepatosplenomegaly, hypergammaglobulinemia, deficient lymphocyte apoptosis, autoimmune diseases, increased CD4⁻, CD8⁻, T cells
Autoimmune polyendocrinopathy, candidiasis, ectodermal dysplasia syndrome	Mutation in autoimmune regulator gene (*AIRE*) encoding protein required for expression of ectopic antigens in the thymic epithelial cells. This is required for induction of tolerance to autoantigens	Multiple endocrine autoimmunity; chronic mucocutaneous candidiasis
Immune dysregulation, polyendocrinopathy, enteropathy, X-linked (IPEX)	Mutation of *FOXP3* gene whose product is expressed by and is required for function of T-regulatory cells; also mutations in the IL2R gene can cause a similar syndrome.	Childhood onset autoimmune endocrinopathy, enteropathy, eczema
Defects in cytolytic pathways		
Familial hemophagocytic lymphohistiocytosis (HLH)	Defective T-cell- and NK-cell-mediated cytotoxicity due to mutations in genes encoding perforin (*PRF1*), or MUNC protein (*MUNK13-4*) needed for fusion of intracellular vesicles.	Viral infection triggers hemophagocytosis
X-linked lymphoproliferative disorder (XLP)	*SAP* or *XIAP* (see text for explanation of function)	Clinical manifestations precipitated by EBV infection: hepatitis, hemophagocytosis, aplastic anemia, hypogammaglobulinemia, lymphomas
Chediak-Higashi syndrome	Mutation in *LYST* gene. Impaired lysosomal function and defect in sorting cytolytic proteins into secretory granules; poor NK-cell- and T-cell-mediated cytolysis.	Partial albinism, recurrent pyogenic infections, eventually 85% develop accelerated phase with syndrome resembling HLH
Griscelli syndrome (type II)	Deficiency of the RAB27A GTPase required for secretory vesicle function. Exocytosis of cytolytic granules deficient leading to poor NK-cell- and T-cell-mediated cytolysis.	Partial albinism, recurrent pyogenic infections, eventually 85% develop accelerated phase as in Chediak Higashi syndrome.
Disorders of homeostasis of inflammation (autoinflammatory syndromes)		
Syndrome	Gene defect/pathogenesis	Chief clinical findings
Familial Mediterranean fever	*MEFV*: leads to deficiency of pyrin	Periodic fever, amyloidosis

(continued)

Table 5.9 *(continued)*

Syndromes with Autoimmunity	Gene Defect/Pathogenesis	Chief Clinical Findings
Hyper-IgD syndrome	Partial mevalonate kinase deficiency; mechanism of disease uncertain	Periodic fever
TNF-receptor-associated periodic fever	*TNFRSF1*: results in decreased availability of soluble TNF receptor for mopping up TNF	Periodic fever, amyloidosis
Familial cold autoinflammatory syndrome	*CIAS1:* defect in cryopyrin required for leucocyte apoptosis, NFκB signaling and IL-1 processing	Cold-induced urticaria, fever
Neonatal-onset multisystem inflammatory disease (NOMID)	*CIAS1:* as above	Neonatal-onset rash, fever, chronic meningitis, arthropathy
Muckle-Wells syndrome	*CIAS1:* as above	Urticaria, deafness, amyloidosis

Studies of rare immunodeficiency syndromes, all of which are characterized by an increased tendency to develop HLH have identified a number of components required for the normal expression of cytolytic capacity by T cells and NK cells. The intracellular migration and docking of lytic granules requires the function of the small Rab GTPase, RAB27, which is mutated in the Griscelli syndrome characterized by partial albinism, immunodeficiency, and susceptibility to developing HLH. Defective cytolytic granule exocytosis is also characteristic of patients with mutations of the gene encoding the protein MUNK13-4 (*UNC13D*). The tSNARE syntexin 11, which is present in the trans-Golgi network, is also involved in intracellular vesicle trafficking. Mutation of these two genes is responsible for a further form of familial HLH.

Lysosomal trafficking regulator is deficient in individuals with a mutation in the *CHS1* gene. This causes a defect in sorting of cytolytic proteins into secretory granules. This is the underlying defect in the condition called Chediak-Higashi syndrome, which is another condition characterized by susceptibility to HLH.

Immunodeficiencies Characterized by Increased Susceptibility to EBV Infections

XLP is a rare inherited immunodeficiency characterized by life-threatening pathological processes triggered by EBV infections. The manifestations of this condition include fulminant infectious mononucleosis, virally induced HLH, hypogammaglobulinemia, and the propensity to develop malignant lymphomas. Mutation in the gene *SH2D1A* encoding the signaling lymphocyte activation molecule (SLAM) associated protein (SAP) are responsible for more than 60 percent of cases of XLP. SH2D1A−/−mice lack NK T cells and this defect could be corrected by reconstitution of SH2D1A expression within bone marrow cells derived from SH2D1A −/− mice. Patients with XLP also lack NK T cells. Therefore, it is possible that NK T-cell function is essential for controlling EBV infection as well as homeostasis of T-cell responses to this virus. Further support for this theory comes from the recent observation that XLP can also be caused by a mutation in the gene (*BIRC4*) that encodes for the protein X-linked inhibitor of apoptosis (XIAP). XIAP−/− patients also have reduced numbers of NK T cells.

The pathological manifestations of the XLP cannot be completely attributed to the reduced NK- and T-cell function seen in this condition. The SAP, which acts as a signaling adaptor molecule within lymphoid cells, and XIAP, which regulates apoptosis, help in the homeostasis of immune responses in complex ways. Therefore, mechanisms underlying the pathogenesis of XLP are likely to be complicated.

Immunodeficiencies Characterized by Increased Liability to Develop Autoimmunity

Immune responses to self-antigens are prevented by:

1. The elimination of self-reactive B and T cells in the thymus and bone marrow (central tolerance).
2. Inhibition of self-reactive T and B cells that escape central tolerance induction, by the action of regulatory T cells found in the periphery. These T-regulatory cells, which are CD25+ and CD4+, are required for peripheral tolerance and the active suppression of autoimmunity.

IMMUNE DYSREGULATION POLYENDOCRINOPATHY AND ENTEROPATHY, X-LINKED SYNDROME

The product of the *FOXP3* gene (belonging to the forkhead family) is required for the generation and the function of CD4+ CD25+ T-regulatory cells. Mice that are *FOXP3*−/− lack these cells and develop a syndrome characterized by lymphoproliferation and autoimmunity. Expression of ectopic *FOXP3* confers suppressive function on CD4+ and CD25+ T cells. Human males with mutations of the *FOXP3* gene (which is located on the X chromosome) develop a syndrome characterized by neonatal endocrinopathies (including type I diabetes) enteropathy, eczema, immune thrombocytopenia, and cachexia. In these patients, pancreatic islet cell and intestinal mucosal damage are secondary to infiltration of the tissues with mononuclear cells and plasma cells, signifying an autoimmune pathogenesis. This condition is called the immune dysregulation polyendocrinopathy and enteropathy, X-linked (IPEX) syndrome. This condition provides evidence supporting current concepts on the role of T-regulatory cells in preventing autoimmunity.

Recently, mutations in the IL2R gene encoding for the α chain of the IL-2 receptor have been described in patients with the clinical phenotype of the IPEX syndrome. CD4 T cells of these patients fail to produce the immunosuppressive cytokine IL-10.

AUTOIMMUNE LYMPHOPROLIFERATIVE SYNDROME

During lymphocyte development, autoreactive cells are culled by undergoing apoptotic death. During the life span of mature lymphocytes, activation and effector function is followed by activation-induced cell death by apoptosis. Apoptosis thus maintains homeostasis in the immune system by minimizing autoimmune reactions to self-antigens, as well as limiting the total size of the peripheral lymphocyte pool. Antigen-mediated activation of T cells induces them to express a surface receptor FAS (CD95) as well as its ligand, the FAS-ligand. FAS/FAS-ligand interaction activates a biochemical pathway culminating in cell death by apoptosis. Mice that are FAS$-/-$(lpr) or FAS-ligand$-/-$ (gld) develop autoimmunity and develop expansion of their their lymphocyte pool.

ALPS is a rare disease caused by defective cellular apoptosis. Failure of lymphocytes to undergo apoptosis results in impaired homeostasis of the lymphoid population. Patients develop lymphocytosis, hyperplasia of lymphoid organs (spleen, lymph nodes), hypergammaglobulinemia, and autoimmunity (autoimmune cytopenias, Guillain-Barré syndrome). Peripheral blood and peripheral lymphoid tissues characteristically contain an increased population of TCR̃ $\tilde{\alpha}$ β positive CD4$^-$ and CD8$^-$ cells (double negative T cells). Mutations in the FAS-mediated pathway of apoptosis are responsible for most cases. These include mutations of FAS, FAS-ligand, and caspase 10. Caspase 8 deficiency causes impaired CD95-mediated apoptosis as well as a defect in T-, B-, and NK-cell function, manifesting as an immunodeficiency. Recently, an activating mutation in the NRAS gene encoding a GTP-binding protein with a broad spectrum of signaling functions has been found in other patients with ALPS. Defective, IL-2 withdrawal induced, apoptosis of lymphocytes is a characteristic abnormality in these patients.

Autoinflammatory Syndromes

The responses of acute inflammation and fever are protective responses triggered by infection or tissue damage, acting through the innate immune system. The study of a collection of disorders termed *familial periodic fever syndromes* has contributed to our understanding of the physiological processes underlying the homeostasis of inflammation and fever. These inherited disorders are characterized by recurrent episodes of fever and systemic inflammation. These conditions are not associated with autoantibody production or self-reactive T-cell responses. They are collectively called *autoinflammatory syndromes*. Unraveling the pathophysiology of these disorders has given rise to the concept that these conditions are due to an innate immune system that is either oversensitive and prone to activation by minor stimuli or is poorly regulated.

The cleavage of pro-IL-1b to its active product IL-1 by the action of caspase-1 (interleukin converting-enzyme) is a key event in the generation of an acute inflammatory response. Activated caspase-1, intern, is generated from pro-caspase-1 by the action of activated forms of two cytosolic proteins called pyrin and cryopyrin, acting via adaptor proteins. The best-characterized adaptor protein is called ASC (apoptosis-associated speclike protein with a caspase recruitment domain). As summarized in Table 5.9, mutations of components of this system (also called an inflammasome) give rise to most autoinflammatory syndromes characterized to date. The net effect of all these mutations is to impair homoeostasis of the pro-inflammatory cytokine IL-1, NFκB activation, and cellular apoptosis. Impaired cellular apoptosis leads to the persistence of activated leucocytes that would otherwise undergo apoptosis, leading to the resolution of inflammation. Collectively, these abnormalities permit the inappropriate amplification and persistence of inflammatory responses leading to the clinical features of the autoinflammatory syndromes.

INHERITED DEFICIENCY OF THE COMPLEMENT SYSTEM

Activation of the complement system underlies one of the main effector pathways contributing to antibody-mediated immunity. The normal function of the complement system includes defending the body against pyogenic bacterial infection and helping to eliminate immune complexes and damaged cells (Table 5.10).

The key event in complement activation is the proteolytic cleavage of C3 to C3a and C3b. Three pathways can lead to C3 cleavage, namely, classical, alternative, and mannose-binding lectin (MBL) pathways. C3 cleavage leads on to the activation of the terminal complement pathway, causing the generation of the membrane attack complex (MAC), which assembles a lipophilic complex capable of lysing plasma membranes of susceptible cells.

The inability to generate sufficient CD3b results in increased susceptibility to pyogenic sepsis, especially infections caused by encapsulated bacteria. C3 deficiency may be due to complement utilization (e.g., in systemic lupus erythematosus [SLE] or the presence of a C3 nephritic factor) or rarely autosomal recessive C3 deficiency. Factor I deficiency also leads to profound CD3 deficiency due to uncontrolled progression of C3 cleavage. Hereditary C2 deficiency and less commonly inherited C4

deficiency may also be associated with the risk of pneumococcal sepsis.

Protection from Neisserial infection requires the ability to generate the MAC, which lyses these bacteria. Patients with inherited homozygous deficiency of C5, C6, C7, C8, and C9 are susceptible to recurrent meningococcal infections. In Japanese populations, an inherited terminal complement component deficiency leads to about a 5,000-fold increase in the risk of Neisserial sepsis. Primary or secondary CD3 deficiency, which in turn reduces the ability to generate MAC, also results in increased susceptibility to meningococcal infection. Complement deficiency is not a risk factor in sporadic cases of meningococcal disease seen in the population at large.

MBL is a serum collectin that can bind to mannose residues on microbial cell walls. Upon binding of MBL to pathogens, two serine proteases found in serum (MBL-lectin associated serine proteases 1 and 2) become activated. These serine proteases in turn activate the classical pathway at C2 and C4. MBL deficiency may arise because of one of three point mutations in the gene encoding for this protein. Polymorphisms in the promoter region of the gene also influence serum levels of MBL. Low serum levels of MBL may result in an increased incidence of pyogenic infections in young children below two years of age. MBL deficiency is also overrepresented in patients with pneumococcal or meningococcal sepsis. However, the clinical significance of this finding has been disputed. This is because large, long-term prospective studies of adults in Scandinavia have failed to identify increased morbidity due to infectious diseases in MBL-deficient individuals. Therefore, except in young children who have not yet acquired a wide repertoire of protective antibodies, MBL deficiency on

Table 5.10 Complement Deficiency

Deficient Component	Physiological Consequence	Clinical Manifestations
C3 deficiency; factor I deficiency; secondary C3 deficiency due to utilization (e.g., SLE; C3 nephritic factor)	Inability to generate C3b and therefore failure to generate "membrane attack complex"	Recurrent pyogenic sepsis (especially by encapsulated bacteria)
Deficiency of C1q, C1r, C1s, C4, or C2	Failure to generate classical pathway C3-convertase; defective scavenging of apoptotic cells and immune complexes	SLE
Deficiency of properdin or factor D	Failure to generate alternative pathway C3-convertase; failure to opsonize encapsulated bacteria when anticapsular antibody is limiting	Recurrent encapsulated bacterial sepsis
Deficiency of factor H or factor I	Failure to regulate C3 activation	Hemolytic uremic syndrome, membrano proliferative glomerulonephritis
C1 inhibitor deficiency	Failure to regulate C1 activation and kinin generation	Angioedema
CD59	Failure to protect cell surfaces from endogenous C3b	Hemolysis

SLE, systemic lupus erythematosus

its own does not appear to be a significant risk factor for bacterial sepsis.

Complement Deficiency and Autoimmunity

Under physiological conditions, activation of the classical complement pathway helps in the clearance of the circulating immune complexes by the resident macrophages of the reticuloendothelial system. The surface of apoptotic cells activates the classical complement pathway, leading to their efficient clearance by phagocytic cells expressing complement receptors, preventing the generation of autoimmune responses to cellular components.

Deficiency of components required for generating the classical partly C3-convertase may result in impairment of the process described earlier for eliminating immune complexes and "safe" disposal of apoptotic cells. This would explain the increased incidence of SLE-like disorders in patients with inherited C1q, C1r, C1s, C4, C2, C3, factor I, or factor H deficiency.

Factor H Deficiency

Complete or partial factor H deficiency is associated with the occurrence of the hemolytic-uremic syndrome, although the precise underlying pathogenic mechanisms are unknown.

Cell-Surface-Based Inactivators of Complement

CD59 and CD55 are cell-surface molecules anchored by glycosylphosphatidylinositol.

These two proteins inactivate any C3 convertase molecules deposited on cell surfaces. Somatic mutation of the enzyme (PIGA: phosphatidylinositol glycan class A), needed to generate phosphatidylinositol anchors for cell-surface proteins, including CD55 and CD59, in erythroid precursors, results in a condition called paroxysmal nocturnal hemoglobinuria, which is due to the increased susceptibility of red cells to complement-mediated hemolysis. Isolated CD59 deficiency also results in hemolytic anemia.

C1 Inhibitor Deficiency

C1 inhibitor is a serine-protease inhibitor that inactivates the serine esterases generated by complement activation (C1r and C1s), kallikrein of the kinin system, and activated factors XI and XII of the clotting cascade. In the absence of C1 inhibitor, C1 activation results in the depletion of the serum C4 level. (This is useful from a diagnostic point of view.) C1-inhibitor deficiency also results in the inability to inactivate bradykinin, resulting from the unregulated activity of kallikrein. Production of bradykinin in the tissues results in increased vascular permeability, manifesting as attacks of angioedema. Angioedema of the respiratory tract can lead to death from asphyxia. Angioedema of the intestinal tissues results in recurrent episodes of severe abdominal pain due to partial intestinal obstruction, which can mimic an acute abdominal emergency.

C1-inhibitor deficiency arises from a heterozygous mutation of *C1INH* gene, which acts in an autosomal dominant manner. The single normal gene cannot maintain the synthesis of physiologically sufficient quantities of C1 inhibitor. In 85 percent of C1-inhibitor-deficient individuals, the

mutation prevents transcription of the defective gene. In 15 percent of affected individuals, the gene mutation abolishes the activity of the secreted protein. Rarely, autoantibodies to C1 inhibitor can lead to acquired C1-inhibitor deficiency.

DEFECTS IN INNATE IMMUNITY

Defects in the complement pathway resulting in immunodeficiency are summarized in the previous section. Recent work has identified defects in pathways involved in the recognition and response to pathogen-associated molecular patterns. Some of these defects are outlined next.

Defective NFκB activation caused by X-linked hypomorphic mutations of the essential modulator gene (*NEMO*) compromises signaling mechanisms downstream of Toll, IL-1, and TNF-α receptors. These patients are susceptible to infections caused by a range of microorganisms, including mycobacteria, Gram-positive and Gram-negative bacteria, fungi, and viruses.

UNC93B is a protein of the endoplasmic reticulum involved in Toll-receptor activation. Mutations in UNC93B impair the production of IFN-α and IFN-β in response to HSV and other viruses. Affected patients present with *Herpes simplex* viral encephalitis. Recently, heterozygous dominant-negative mutations in the gene encoding toll receptor 3 (TLR3) have been identified in patients with *Herpes simplex* encephalitis. TLR3 is expressed in the central nervous system where it helps to initiate IFN-α and IFN-β responses to viral duble-stranded DNA.

Interleukin-receptor-associated kinase-4 mediates signaling downstream of Toll receptors and members of the IL-1 receptor superfamily. IRAK-4-deficient individuals present during childhood with recurrent, severe, pyogenic sepsis. They are particularly susceptible to recurrent pneumococcal infections.

The signal-transducing molecule STAT-1 is required for signaling via receptors to IFN-γ as well as IFN-α and IFN-β. IFN-γ-receptor-mediated signaling involves the dimerization of phosphorylated STAT-1 molecules. Signaling via IFN-α and IFN-β receptors involves the formation of a complex between STAT-1, STAT-2, and a third protein called interferon-stimulated-gene factor 3-γ. Complete (homozygous) defects of the signal-transducing molecules STAT-1 results in defective responses to IFN-γ, IFN-α, and IFN-β eater leading to the susceptibility to disseminated mycobacterial infections as well as fatal *Herpes simplex* viral infection. Partial STAT-1 deficiency, which interferes with STAT-1 dimerization required for signal transduction via IFN-γ receptors, leads to increased susceptibility to mycobacterial infections. In these patients, the cellular responses to IFN-α and INF-β is intact, thus preserving antiviral immunity.

The WHIM syndrome is a condition characterized by severe warts, hypogammaglobulinemia, and neutropenia. This is the first example of an immunodeficiency caused by aberrant chemokine-receptor function. WHIM syndrome is caused by a mutation in the gene encoding the CXCR 4 chemokine receptor. The mutant form of this receptor shows enhanced responsiveness to its ligand.

The hyper-IgE syndrome (HIES) is a complex clinical entity characterized by recurrent bacterial (*S. aureus*, Gram-negative bacteria) and fungal infections of skin, lymph nodes, lungs, bones, and joints. These patients have elevated serum IgE levels, eosinophilia, dermatitis, facial dysmorphic features, delayed shedding of primary dentition, osteopenia, and impaired acute-phase responses during infections. Most patients have an autosomal dominant inheritance while others are sporadic cases. Patients with classical HIES have heterozygous mutations in the gene encoding the signal-tranducing protein STAT-3. These mutations mainly involve the DNA-binding domain or the SRC homology 2 domain of the protein and are permissive of protein expression. These mutant proteins severely impair the DNA binding of the phosphorylated STAT-3 dimer in response to IFN-α and responses to the cytokines IL-10 and IL-6. Reduced response to IL-6 would explain the defective acute-phase response, and the defective response to IL-10 explains the overproduction of IgE. STAT-3 is essential for the generation of T_H17 cells and for IL-12 signaling, which are required for the secretion of the bactericidal peptides called β-defensins by epithelial cells of the skin and lungs. This may in part explain the increased incidence of severe sepsis.

CONCLUSIONS

Studies in genetically manipulated animals have helped in the development of mechanistic models of antimicrobial immunity. Gene knockout mice have been invaluable for the elucidation of the phenotypic consequences of single-gene defects. Collectively, these animal studies have highlighted candidate genes that should be investigated in patients with increased susceptibility to microbial infection. Comparison of the phenotype of a mouse carrying a defined genetic defect with the clinical and immunological phenotype of patients has been helpful in identifying candidate genes that might be affected in the human patient.

Studies in humans with PID have been complementary. For example, human studies have highlighted that (1) defects in more than one gene can give rise to a similar primary immunodeficiency syndrome; (2) the same genetic mutation can give rise to a variable phenotype, depending on the modulating effect of genetic and environmental influences; and (3) defects in components of innate and adaptive immunity that are required for homeostasis of the immune response may result in autoimmunity or autoinflammatory syndromes rather than increased susceptibility to infection, thus extending the clinical spectrum of "primary immunodeficiency diseases."

In the past decade, we have realized that defects in some components of the innate and adaptive immunity may result in susceptibility to a narrow range of microbial pathogens. This indicates that some immune mechanisms have evolved to deal with specific pathogens but are redundant for immunity against other microorganisms. Such knowledge may lead to the development of novel treatment strategies targeted against specific microbes.

In this review, we have highlighted how defects in individual components of the immune system can lead to the susceptibility to different categories of pathogens. Such analyses help us to understand which components of immunity are nonredundant for protection against different microorganisms. This knowledge also helps us to be guided by the pattern of microbial infections in an individual patient in devising a rational approach to the investigation of patients with suspected immunodeficiency.

The past two decades have seen the development of novel treatment modalities for PIDs. These include the use of Ig replacement therapy (for antibody deficiency), bone marrow transplantation (for SCID), and gene therapy (for the treatment of X-linked SCID and SCID due to ADA deficiency). In X-linked SCID and in ADA-deficiency gene, corrected bone marrow cells have a selective advantage over unmodified stem cells, contributing to successful engraftment by gene-reconstituted cells. The correction of genetic defects in conditions where the expression of the normal molecule does not provide a selective survival advantage will be more difficult and will require the development of more effective genetic vectors. The elucidation of molecular defects underlying PIDs helps in the development of better methods of diagnosing these disorders and genetic counseling of affected families. The contribution of new genetic techniques for elucidating molecular defects underlying PIDs have been described elsewhere (see references list at end of chapter).

BIBLIOGRAPHY

COMPREHENSIVE REVIEWS (PRIMARY IMMUNODEFICIENCY DISEASES)

Primary immunodeficiency diseases. Report of an IUIS Scientific Committee. International Union of Immunological Societies. *Clin Exp Immunol.* 1999;118 (suppl 1):1–28.

Fischer A. Human primary immunodeficiency diseases: a perspective. *Nat Immunol.* 2004;5(1):23–30.

Geha, RS, Notarangelo, LD, et al. Primary immunodeficiency diseases: an update from the International Union of Immunological Societies Primary Immunodeficiency Diseases Classification Committee. *J Allergy Clin Immunol.* 2007;120(4):776–794.

Ochs, HD, Smith, CIE, et al. *Primary Immunodeficiency Diseases: A Molecular and*

Genetic Approach. New York: Oxford University Press; 2007.

SELECTED REVIEWS (MOLECULAR MECHANISMS UNDERLYING PRIMARY IMMUNODEFICIENCIES)

Brydges S, Kastner DL. The systemic autoinflammatory diseases: inborn errors of the innate immune system. *Curr Top Microbiol Immunol.* 2006;305:127–160.

Doffinger R, Patel SY, Kumararatne, DS. Host genetic factors and mycobacterial infections: lessons from single gene disorders affecting innate and adaptive immunity. *Microbes Infect.* 2006;8(4):1141–1150.

Durandy A, Taubenheim N, Peron S, Fischer A. Pathophysiology of B-cell intrinsic immunoglobulin class switch recombination deficiencies. *Adv Immunol.* 2007;94:275–306.

Fischer A, Le Deist F, Hacein-Bey-Abina S, et al. Severe combined immunodeficiency. A model disease for molecular immunology and therapy. *Immunol Rev.* 2005;203:98–109.

Gennery AR. Primary immunodeficiency syndromes associated with defective DNA double-strand break repair. *Br Med Bull.* 2006.

Jouanguy E, Zhang SY, et al. Human primary immunodeficiencies of type I interferons. *Biochimie.* 2007; 89(6–7): 878–883.

Ku CL, Yang K, et al. Inherited disorders of human Toll-like receptor signaling: immunological implications. *Immunol Rev.* 2005;203:10–20.

Marodi L, Notarangelo, LD. Immunological and genetic bases of new primary immunodeficiencies. *Nat Rev Immunol.* 2007;7(11):851–861.

Segal AW. How superoxide production by neutrophil leukocytes kills microbes. *Novartis Found Symp.* 2006;279:92–98; discussion 98–100, 216–219.

Smith TF, Johnston, RB Jr. Functions of the spleen in host defense against infection. *Am J Pediatr Hematol Oncol.* 1979;1(4):355–362.

REFERENCES (DIAGNOSIS AND MANAGEMENT OF IMMUNODEFICIENCIES)

Bonilla FA, Bernstein IL, et al. Practice parameter for the diagnosis and management of primary immunodeficiency. *Ann Allergy Asthma Immunol.* 2005;94(5 Suppl 1):S1–63.

Cavazzana-Calvo M, Fischer, A. Gene therapy for severe combined immunodeficiency: are we there yet? *J Clin Invest.* 2007;117(6):1456–1465.

de Vries E. Patient-centred screening for primary immunodeficiency: a multi-stage diagnostic protocol designed for non-immunologists. *Clin Exp Immunol.* 2006;145(2):204–214.

Ochs HD, Smith CIE, et al. Primary immunodeficiency diseases : a molecular and genetic approach. New York: Oxford University Press; 2007.

Wood P, Stanworth S, et al. Recognition, clinical diagnosis and management of patients with primary antibody deficiencies: a systematic review. *Clin Exp Immunol.* 2007;149(3): 410–423.

REVIEWS (SCIENTIFIC APPROACH TO UNRAVELING THE PATHOGENESIS OF PRIMARY IMMUNODEFICIENCY DISEASES)

Casanova JL, Abel L. Primary immunodeficiencies: a field in its infancy. *Science.* 2007;317(5838):617–619.

Fischer A. Primary immunodeficiency diseases: an experimental model for molecular medicine. *Lancet.* 2001; 357(9271): 1863–1869.

6. Autoimmunity

Haoyang Zhuang, Ph.D., Matthew Kosboth, M.D., Jennifer A. Sipos, M.D., Minoru Satoh, M.D., Ph.D., Lijun Yang, M.D., and Westley H. Reeves, M.D.

DEFINITIONS AND TYPES OF AUTOIMMUNITY

Autoimmunity versus Autoimmune Disease

The classic studies of Paul Ehrlich in the early twentieth century laid the foundation for our current notions of the concept of autoimmunity. Ehrlich used the term *autoimmunity* to signify an immune response against self and introduced the phrase *horror autotoxicus*, suggesting that there are mechanisms to protect against autoimmunity. Over the years, autoimmunity has been recognized as not uncommon and not necessarily detrimental. Thus, an important distinction must be drawn between autoimmunity, which may be asymptomatic, and autoimmune disease, which occurs when autoimmunity leads to an inflammatory response, resulting in tissue injury. An autoimmune response does not necessarily imply the existence of autoimmune disease.

T-Cell versus B-Cell-Mediated Autoimmune Disease

Autoimmune disease may be mediated primarily by T cells, as in multiple sclerosis or the animal model experimental autoimmune encephalomyelitis (EAE). In that case, disease can be transmitted from one animal to another by transferring antigen-specific T lymphocytes. Alternatively, autoimmune disease may be caused by B cells that produce autoantibodies, as in the case of systemic lupus erythematosus (SLE). Autoantibodies bind to self-antigens (proteins, nucleic acids, or other molecules from one's own body, also known as autoantigens) and can damage cells either by binding directly to a cell surface or extracellular matrix antigen or through the formation of immune complexes (see the section "Mechanisms of Autoimmune Tissue Injury and Examples"). Autoantibody-mediated autoimmune diseases sometimes can be transmitted transplacentally, as in the case of neonatal Graves' disease or congenital complete heart block and neonatal lupus. IgG antibodies/autoantibodies can cross the placenta, whereas IgM cannot. Thus, neonatal autoimmune diseases are invariably caused by IgG, not IgM, autoantibodies. In view of the half-life of IgG (twenty-one to twenty-eight days), nearly all maternal IgG disappears from the circulation of the baby by six to twelve months postpartum. Thus, in most cases, neonatal autoimmune disease is transient. One exception is congenital complete heart block, which is thought to be mediated by the transplacental passage of anti-Ro or anti-La autoantibodies that cross-react with cardiac antigens, causing permanent inflammation-mediated damage to the cardiac conduction system.

Systemic versus Organ-Specific Autoimmune Disease

Autoimmune disease also can be classified as systemic or organ specific. Systemic autoimmune diseases, such as SLE, involve multiple organs or tissues, whereas organ-specific autoimmune diseases involve a single organ or tissue, such as the thyroid gland in autoimmune thyroiditis or the islets of Langerhans in type I diabetes (TID). Some of the more common systemic and organ-specific autoimmune diseases are listed in Table 6.1.

MECHANISMS OF AUTOIMMUNE TISSUE INJURY AND EXAMPLES

Tissue damage in autoimmune diseases can occur through several mechanisms, which are analogous to three of the classical types of hypersensitivity reactions: type II (caused by autoantibodies reactive with cell surface or matrix antigens), type III (caused by immune complexes), and type IV (delayed-type hypersensitivity, mediated by T cells).

Type II Autoimmune Reactions

Type II hypersensitivity reactions are caused by antibodies against altered self-proteins, such as penicillin–protein conjugates. In the case of autoimmunity, antibodies generated against cell surface antigens/extracellular matrix proteins may be cytotoxic (type IIA) or they may have agonistic/antagonistic properties (type IIB). Autoantibodies to cell surface antigens may initiate cell destruction by complement-mediated lysis (cell destruction), phagocytosis, or antibody-dependent cell-mediated cytotoxicity (ADCC).

Examples include autoimmune hemolytic anemia (AIHA), and autoimmune thrombocytopenia (Table 6.1). Some autoantibodies bind to surface receptors, either activating (e.g., anti-TSH receptor autoantibodies in Graves' disease) or inhibiting (e.g., anti-acetylcholine antibodies in myasthenia gravis) their function.

Type IIA Autoimmune Reaction: Autoimmune Hemolytic Anemia

AIHA is an example of type IIA autoimmunity. In this disorder, a self-antigen on the surface of erythrocytes elicits an autoantibody response, resulting in the binding of autoantibody to the erythrocyte surface followed by destruction of the antibody-coated erythrocytes by the reticuloendothelial system of the spleen and liver. The mechanism of hemolysis depends on the type of autoantibodies. Autoimmune hemolysis is classified into two groups on the basis of thermal reactivity of the autoantibodies. Warm autoantibodies react optimally at temperatures of 35°C–40°C, whereas cold agglutinins and other cold-reactive autoantibodies react maximally at 4°C. Warm autoantibodies are typically polyclonal IgG but may also be IgM or IgA. Most are IgG1 subclass antibodies reactive with Rh antigens. These antibodies are detected by the direct antiglobulin (Coombs) test (Figure 6.1A). Erythrophagocytosis mediated by Fc receptors on Kupffer cells in the liver and macrophages in the splenic marginal zone is generally the major mechanism of erythrocyte destruction in patients with warm autoantibodies.

In contrast, AIHA induced by cold agglutinins is complement mediated. These autoantibodies are of the IgM class and cannot interact with Fc receptors

Table 6.1 Some Human Autoimmune Diseases

Disease	Organ(s) Involved	Prevalence per 100,000[a]	Female: Male Ratio	Autoantibodies
Systemic autoimmune diseases				
Systemic lupus erythematosus	Joints, skin, nervous system, kidneys, blood cells, heart, lungs	24	9:1	anti dsDNA[b] anti Sm [b] anti ribosomal P [b] anti RNA helicase*
Rheumatoid arthritis	Joints, blood vessels, lungs	860	3:1	anti citrullinated peptides [b] Rheumatoid factor
Sjögren's syndrome	Exocrine glands (salivary and lacrimal glands), kidneys, nerves	14	9:1	anti Ro60 (SS-A) anti Ro52 anti La (SS-B)
Scleroderma	Skin, blood vessels, GI tract, lungs, kidneys	4	4:1	anti topoisomerase I [b] anti fibrillarin (U3 RNP) [b] anti RNA polymerase I [b] anti RNA polymerase III [b]
Polymyositis	Muscles, lungs	5	2:1	tRNA synthetases (histidyl, alanyl, threonyl, glycyl, etc.) [b] Signal recognition particle [b]
Organ-specific autoimmune diseases				
Hashimoto's thyroiditis	Thyroid	982	9:1	Thyroid peroxidase Thyroglobulin
Graves' disease	Thyroid	1152	9:1	Thyroid-stimulating hormone receptor
Addison's disease	Adrenal glands	5	9:1	2I-hydroxylase
Type I diabetes	Pancreatic islet cells	192	1:1	Glutamic acid dehydrogenase, insulin, other islet cell antigens
Pemphigus vulgaris	Skin	N/A	N/A	Desmoglein 3
Bullous pemphigoid	Skin	N/A	N/A	230 kDa hemidesmosomal antigen
Vitiligo	Skin melanocytes	400	1:1	Unknown melanocyte antigens
Goodpasture's syndrome	Kidneys, lungs	0.05	1:1	Type VII collagen
Myasthenia gravis	Nervous system	5	2:1	Acetylcholine receptor
Multiple sclerosis	Nervous system	58	2:1	Unknown myelin antigens
Pernicious anemia	Gastric parietal cells	151	2:1	Parietal cell antigens, intrinsic factor
Primary biliary cirrhosis	Bile ducts	N/A	N/A	Dihydrolipoamide acyltransferase and other antigens [b]
Autoimmune hepatitis	Liver	0.4	9:1	Smooth muscle antigens (F-actin)

(continued)

Table 6.1 (continued)

Disease	Organ(s) Involved	Prevalence per 100,000[a]	Female: male ratio	Autoantibodies
Thrombocytopenic purpura	Platelets	N/A	3:1	Antiplatelet antibodies against GPIIbIIIa and/or the GPIbα complex
Autoimmune hemolytic anemia	Erythrocytes	N/A	~1.5:1	Rh, I, i, and other antigens

N/A, not available.
[a] USA, 1996 estimate; [b] disease-specific autoantibodies.

because there are no Fc receptors capable of binding the μ heavy chain. Idiopathic cold agglutinin disease generally is associated with an IgM paraprotein against the "I" antigen, an erythrocyte surface protein. Unlike IgG, which must be cross-linked, pentavalent IgM fixes complement efficiently without cross-linking. After binding to the erythrocyte's surface at low temperature, IgM cold agglutinins activate C1, C4, C2, and C3b. With rewarming, the antibody can dissociate, but C3b remains fixed irreversibly, which can lead

A Direct Coombs Test Indirect Coombs Test

Patient's red blood cells / Patient's serum / Agglutination / Anti-IgG antibodies / ABO and Rh compatible RBCs

B

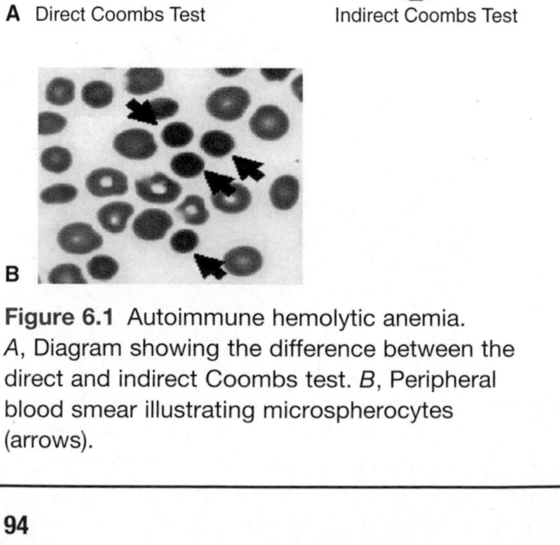

Figure 6.1 Autoimmune hemolytic anemia. *A*, Diagram showing the difference between the direct and indirect Coombs test. *B*, Peripheral blood smear illustrating microspherocytes (arrows).

to recruitment of the terminal complement components (C5–C9, membrane attack complex) and intravascular hemolysis or C3b receptor-mediated phagocytosis by reticuloendothelial cells.

Case 1. Autoimmune Hemolytic Anemia, a Type II Autoimmune Reaction

A twenty-eight-year-old woman with a four-year history of SLE presented for a scheduled follow-up in clinic. Because she avoids the sun and started taking hydroxychloroquine four years ago, her rash and arthritis had improved, but over the past six months, she had become progressively more fatigued and began to notice dark urine. Review of medications, alcohol intake, recreational drug use, and sick contacts was unrevealing. On physical exam, she was mildly tachycardic at 105, with a two out of six systolic ejection murmur at the left sternal border, dullness to percussion over Traubes' space (the normally resonant gastric bubble), and a palpable spleen tip.

Her hemoglobin was 9.5 g/dl (normal 12–16 g/dl), mean cell volume (MCV, a measure of erythrocyte size) was normal at 88 cu μm, and platelets were 75,000/μl (normal 140–400,000/μl). Urinalysis revealed no blood but was remarkable for urobilinogen of 8 mg/dl (normal <2 mg/dl). Hepatic panel was notable for a total bilirubin of 2 mg/dl (normal <1.5 mg/dl) with indirect bilirubin of 1.5 mg/dl (normal <0.8 mg/dl) and direct bilirubin 0.5 mg/dl (normal <0.7 mg/dl). Lactate dehydrogenase was elevated at 350 IU/L (normal <250 IU/L), and corrected reticulocyte count (immature erythrocytes) was 3 percent (normal <1 percent).

Direct Coombs test was positive (Figure 6.1A). Haptoglobin (a scavenger of free hemoglobin) was reduced to <5 mmol/L (normal 10–30 mmol/L). Parvovirus B19, thyroid-stimulating hormone (TSH), vitamin B_{12} level, folate level, iron profile, and ferritin were unremarkable. A review of her blood smear showed numerous spherocytes (spherical erythrocytes instead of the usual biconcave disc shape, the result of damage to the red cell membrane as it passes through the spleen; Figure 6.1B) and confirmed thrombocytopenia (low numbers of platelets). An ultrasound of her abdomen revealed a normal liver but an enlarged spleen.

On the basis of these clinical findings, the diagnoses of AIHA and thrombocytopenia were made. She was treated with prednisone (a corticosteroid) at a dose of 60 mg/day. Initially, her platelet count improved to 120,000. However, after three months of treatment, her anemia did not improve. She gained twenty pounds and noted easy bruising, fatigue, and difficulty sleeping as well as "feeling on edge all the time." Since she had not improved and was experiencing side effects of prednisone, she was given a pneumococcal pneumonia vaccination before surgery to remove her spleen. After splenectomy,

her anemia, thrombocytopenia, and some of her fatigue resolved. After tapering the prednisone dose, she "felt normal." Two years later, her symptoms recurred and laboratory tests confirmed evidence of active hemolytic anemia. A liver-spleen scan indicated the presence of an accessory spleen (present in 10–30 percent of normal population), which was removed. She is currently symptom free.

COMMENT

AIHA in patients with SLE is usually due to the presence of warm-reactive autoantibodies against the Rh antigen. As the autoantibody-coated erythrocytes pass through the spleen, phagocytes bearing Fc receptors remove some of the immunoglobulin on the cell surface along with some of the cell membrane, which subsequently reseals, causing the erythrocyte to take the form of a spherocyte. Eventually, the erythrocyte is unable to be repaired and is removed from the circulation. If this occurs faster than new erythrocytes can be produced (normal life span of an erythrocyte is about 120 days) then anemia develops. The elevated indirect bilirubin (a measure of bilirubin before the liver has a chance to process it) is a result of the increased breakdown of hemoglobin.

AIHA can occur in a variety of circumstances, including neoplastic diseases (most often lymphomas), connective tissue diseases (such as SLE), and infections (viral, bacterial, or mycoplasma). Or it may be drug induced (classically penicillin). The initial treatment is to diagnose and treat the underlying cause or remove offending agents. If this is not possible, corticosteroids such as prednisone are often used. If patients do not respond, then consideration is given to the use of cytotoxic drugs (e.g., azathioprine or vincristine) or splenectomy.

Type IIB Hypersensitivity: Graves' Disease

Graves' disease is an organ-specific autoimmune disease of the thyroid mediated by stimulatory (agonistic) autoantibodies. Autoantibodies to the thyroid-stimulating hormone receptor (TSHR) cause hyperthyroidism in patients with Graves' disease. The pathogenicity of anti-TSHR autoantibodies is demonstrated by the occurrence of neonatal Graves' disease after passive transplacental transfer of IgG thyroid-stimulating autoantibodies from a mother with Graves' disease to the fetus. The anti-TSHR autoantibodies in Graves' disease inhibit binding of TSH to its receptor by binding to a conformational epitope (the part of the antigen recognized by an antibody) of the extracellular domain of the TSHR. Although the autoantibodies appear to interact with TSHR somewhat differently than the natural ligand, they nevertheless stimulate TSHR signaling, causing increased production of thyroid hormone.

Type IIB Hypersensitivity: Myasthenia Gravis

Myasthenia gravis is an autoimmune disease caused by inhibitory (antagonistic) autoantibodies that bind and block the acetylcholine receptor (AChR), causing muscular weakness and fatigue. The AChR is found at postsynaptic membranes of neuromuscular junctions and binds acetylcholine released from a nerve ending, transiently opening a calcium channel. The signal is terminated by acetylcholine esterase, an enzyme located in the basal lamina between the nerve ending and the postsynaptic membrane. As in mothers with Graves' disease, transplacental passage of IgG autoantibodies from mothers with myasthenia gravis can cause transient neonatal myasthenia gravis. Anti-AChR autoantibodies cause disease by downregulating expression of the receptor and by complement-mediated lysis of the cells bearing the AChR. Intermolecular crosslinking of AChR by the autoantibodies may lead to antigenic modulation.

Type III Autoimmune Reactions (Immune Complex Disease)

Autoantibodies also cause disease by forming networks of autoantibodies bound to their antigens (immune complexes). The antigen-antibody complexes can deposit in tissues, causing inflammatory lesions. Studies of serum sickness led to the first description of an immune complex disease. Serum sickness is manifested by fever, glomerulonephritis, vasculitis, urticaria, and arthritis, appearing seven to twenty-one days after primary immunization or two to four days after secondary immunization with a foreign protein. Two consequences of immune complex formation are complement fixation and binding to Fc or complement receptors on phagocytes. Clearance is facilitated by the binding of immune complexes to C3b receptors (CR1) on erythrocytes, which retain the complexes in the circulation until their removal by the reticuloendothelial cells of the spleen or liver.

Immune complex formation is a normal process that removes foreign antigens from the circulation. Removal of immune complexes by phagocytes bearing Fc or complement receptors prevents their deposition at other sites. The efficiency of uptake of immune complexes by either Fc receptors or CR1 is proportional to the number of IgG molecules associated with the complex.

Immune complexes can activate either the classical or the alternative complement pathway. The classical pathway plays a major role in maintaining immune complexes in a soluble form, preventing their deposition in tissues. C3b bound to the solubilized immune complexes promotes their clearance by the erythrocyte complement receptor CR1. If the rate of immune complex formation exceeds the ability to clear these complexes via Fc receptors and CR1, the immune complexes can deposit within tissues, leading to inflammation. This efficient immune complex transport and removal by Fc and complement receptors can be overwhelmed, however, leading to tissue deposition and immune complex disease. This situation may result from overproduction of immune complexes, blockade of phagocytosis by the reticuloendothelial system, or complement depletion resulting in inefficient solubilization of immune complexes.

SLE is the prototype of human immune complex disease. Tissue damage in lupus is mainly caused by immune complexes containing autoantibodies to soluble antigens. These autoantibodies include antibodies against RNA-protein complexes (e.g., anti-Sm, RNP, Ro/SS-A, and La/SS-B antibodies) and DNA-protein complexes (e.g., anti-double-stranded DNA, antihistone, antichromatin antibodies). The target antigens are found mainly in the cell nucleus, although in some cases (e.g., antiribosomal antibodies), they may be cytoplasmic. Immune complexes containing these autoantibodies, especially anti-dsDNA antibodies, are selectively enriched in the renal glomeruli (capillary tufts that produce urine as an ultrafiltrate of blood) of patients with lupus nephritis and are thought to play a critical role in establishing the inflammatory response. Immune complex deposition in the kidney leads to proliferative glomerulonephritis and effacement of the normal glomerular architecture (Figure 6.2). As is the case in serum sickness, active lupus nephritis is frequently associated with hypocomplementemia (Figure 6.2). In addition to the kidneys (glomeruli), immunoglobulin and complement deposits are found in the blood vessels (vasculitis), skin (rashes), nervous system, and other locations. Preformed immune complexes may become trapped in the glomerular filter, or immune complexes may develop in situ because of the interaction of cationic antigens (e.g., histones) with heparan sulfate glycosaminoglycan in the glomerular basement membrane. The association of lupus with deficiencies of the early classical complement components, especially C2 and C4, is consistent with the role of complement pathways in solubilizing immune complexes (see the section "Pathogenesis of Autoimmune Disease").

Case 2. Systemic Lupus Erythematosus, a Type III Autoimmune Reaction

A fifteen-year-old girl developed myalgias (muscle pain), painful and swollen joints, and low-grade fevers and was found to have a positive antinuclear antibodies (ANA) test. Kidney function was normal. She was given a diagnosis of SLE and treated with hydroxychloroquine (an antimalarial), azathioprine (a nucleoside analog), and

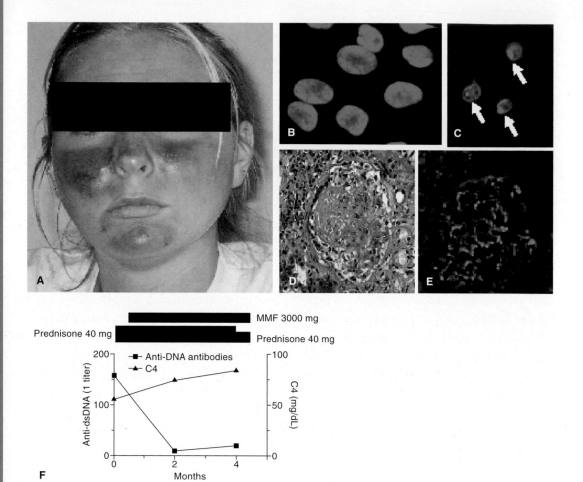

Figure 6.2 Systemic lupus erythematosus. *A,* Acute cutaneous lupus (malar or butterfly rash); *B,* fluorescent antinuclear antibody test (HEp-2 cells were stained with patient serum followed by fluorescein isothiocyanate-labeled goat antihuman IgG antibodies); *C, Crithidia luciliae* kinetoplast staining assay for anti-double-stranded DNA autoantibodies (Crithidia organisms were stained with patient serum followed by fluorescein isothiocyanate-labeled goat anti-human IgG antibodies). Kinetoplasts are indicated by arrows; *D,* hematoxylin and eosin staining of a renal glomerulus illustrating proliferative nephritis and crescent formation; *E,* direct immunofluorescence of a renal glomerulus in lupus nephritis stained for IgG; *F,* classic inverse relationship between anti-dsDNA antibody titer (broken line) and complement (C3, solid line) levels. Bars above the graph depict the doses of prednisone and mofetil mycophenolate (MMF) over the same period.

10 mg/day of prednisone (a corticosteroid). Three years later, she developed alopecia (hair loss) and a red, ulcerating rash of the legs. A skin biopsy was reported to be "consistent with lupus." The skin lesions resolved when the dose of prednisone was increased. For the next five years, her lupus remained well controlled with hydroxychloroquine and intermittent low-dose prednisone until she moved to another state and was unable to continue her health insurance. Several months after stopping all of her medications, vasculitic skin lesions recurred on the legs, and she developed a rash on the face (Figure 6.2A). Laboratory testing revealed that her creatinine (a measure of renal function) was now abnormally elevated at 3.4 mg/dl (normal 1.0 mg/dl),

her albumin was low, and her urine tested positive for protein (proteinuria, >300 mg/dl) and blood (hematuria). Microscopic examination revealed seven erythrocytes per high-power field. Fluorescent antinuclear antibody testing was positive at a titer of 1:640 homogeneous pattern and anti-dsDNA antibodies were detected at a titer of 1:160 using the *Crithidia luciliae* kinetoplast staining assay (Figure 6.2B, 6.2C). Complement components C3 and C4 were low (56 and 11 mg/dl, respectively). She was treated with a high dose of methylprednisolone (another corticosteroid) intravenously followed by prednisone. A renal biopsy was performed and showed proliferative lupus nephritis (Figure 6.2D). Immunofluorescence showed staining of the glomerular basement membrane for IgG (Figure 6.2E) as well as IgM and C3. She was treated with mycophenolate mofetil (MMF, 1,500 mg twice a day), and after four months, her proteinuria and hematuria resolved, the creatinine returned to near baseline (1.1 mg/dL), C3 increased to 85 mg/dl, and anti-dsDNA antibodies decreased to 1:20 (Figure 6.2F).

COMMENT

SLE is the prototype of human immune complex disease. For reasons that are unclear, autoantibodies against dsDNA are involved in the formation of immune complexes that appear to be particularly prone to become trapped in the renal glomeruli, where they can cause inflammation (glomerulonephritis). The levels of anti-dsDNA often are low during periods of disease quiescence. In this case, a flare of disease activity was precipitated by stopping medications that keep the autoimmune response in check (prednisone and hydroxychloroquine), leading to the production of high levels of anti-dsDNA antibodies that could be detected by staining the kinetoplast (a circular DNA molecule) of *Crithidia luciliae* organisms. These autoantibodies formed immune complexes, resulting in the consumption of classical complement components C3 and C4 (the classic inverse relationship between anti-DNA and complement levels, as illustrated in Figure 6.2F). Because the immune complexes were inadequately cleared, they deposited in the renal glomeruli, resulting in the patient's new onset of hematuria and proteinuria and the decline in her renal function (increased creatinine). With reinstitution of appropriate therapy, the anti-DNA levels declined, C3 and C4 levels recovered, and renal immune complex deposition diminished, resulting in an improvement of renal function.

Type IV Autoimmune Reactions (T-Cell Mediated)

Type IV hypersensitivity reactions are mediated by T cells that recognize peptides presented on the surface of antigen-presenting cells in the context of class II major histocompatibility complex (MHC) molecules and that produce the cytokines interferon γ (IFN-γ), interleukin 3 (IL-3), tumor necrosis factor (TNF) α, TNF-β, and granulocyte-macrophage colony-stimulating factor (GM-CSF). These cells constitute a subset of helper T cells termed T_H1 cells. Elaboration of "T_H1 cytokines" leads to macrophage recruitment and activation, enhanced expression of adhesion molecules, and increased production of monocytes by the bone marrow. Delayed-type hypersensitivity in response to the intradermal injection of certain antigens, such as tuberculin (used for tuberculosis skin testing), is a classic example of a type IV hypersensitivity reaction. In the case of autoimmunity, self-antigens (instead of foreign antigens) plus MHC molecules are recognized by the antigen receptors of the TH1 cells. Examples of type IV autoimmune reactions include insulin-dependent diabetes mellitus (pancreatic antigens, such as glutamic acid dehydrogenase, insulin, and other islet cell antigens are recognized), multiple sclerosis (unidentified components of myelin are recognized), experimental antoimmune encephalomyelitis (an animal model of multiple sclerosis in which myelin basic protein (MBP) is recognized), and Hashimoto's thyroiditis (thyroid antigens such as thyroid peroxidase and thyroglobulin are recognized).

Case 3. Hashimoto's Thyroiditis: A Type IV Autoimmune Disease

A thirty-one-year-old woman was seen in the clinic because she had a sensation that something was stuck in her throat. Her older sister had a similar problem. She also noted feeling tired and had gained weight since giving birth to a child five years earlier. Her hair and skin seemed to be getting drier. On examination, her thyroid gland was mildly enlarged on palpation (Figure 6.3A, 6.3B) and ultrasound revealed multiple small nodules and a pseudonodule indicated by the arrow (Figure 6.3C). A needle biopsy of the thyroid revealed a diffuse interstitial lymphocytic infiltrate with formation of lymphoid follicles (Figure 6.3D). Residual thyroid follicles were small, and some contained inspissated colloid.

Complete blood count was notable for mild anemia (hemoglobin 11.3 g/dl). Her T4 level was low (1.9 μg/dl), TSH level was elevated at 25 mIU/L, and serum antithyroid peroxidase and anti-thyroglobulin autoantibodies were detected. Antithyroid-stimulating hormone receptor antibody was negative. She was given a diagnosis of autoimmune (Hashimoto's) thyroiditis on the basis of the low T4 level, elevated TSH, and the autoantibody profile and was treated with thyroid replacement. Her TSH levels normalized and the anemia resolved and she noted a gradual decrease in her fatigue. Her skin and hair dryness improved.

COMMENT

Pathologically Hashimoto's thyroiditis represents an infiltration of the thyroid gland with T and B lymphocytes, which often organize to form germinal centers (Figure 6.3D). The lymphocytic infiltration may be visualized on positron emission tomography scanning as shown in Figure 6.3E. Patients with Hashimoto's thyroiditis may exhibit a focal or diffusely increased 2-[^{18}F]fluoro-2-deoxy-D-glucose (FDG) uptake, which correlates with the T-/B-cell infiltration. The B cells make antibodies against thyroid antigens, as seen in this patient, whereas the T cells produce cytokines that stimulate the B cells and induce the thyroid cells to undergo apoptosis (programmed death). Eventually, the thyroid is destroyed and is unable to secrete thyroid hormone, resulting in hypothyroidism. The diffusely micronodular appearance on ultrasound (Figure 6.3C) is due to disruption of the normal microarchitecture of

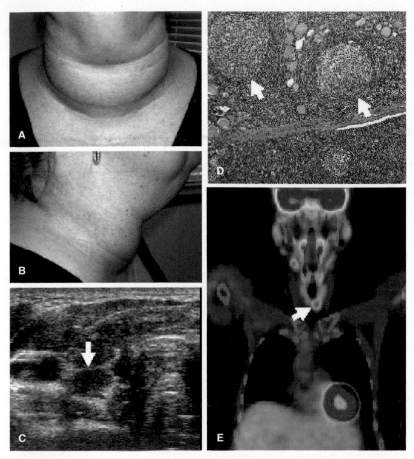

Figure 6.3 Autoimmune (Hashimoto's) thyroiditis. *A*, *B*, Appearance of goiter (diffusely enlarged thyroid gland); *C*, ultrasound image showing a transverse view of the right lobe of the thyroid. The gland is diffusely hypoechoic with multiple small nodules and a pseudonodule. The arrow indicates a pseudonodule (arrow) separated from the remainder of the gland by a fibrous septum. *D*, hematoxylin and eosin staining of the thyroid biopsy illustrating a diffuse lymphocytic infiltrate and the formation of well-organized ectopic lymphoid follicles (arrows). *E*, positron emission tomography image showing focally increased 2-[^{18}F]fluoro-2-deoxy-D-glucose (FDG) uptake in the thyroid gland, correlating with lymphocytic infiltration.

the thyroid gland. The small nodules seen on ultrasound ("pseudonodules") represent germinal centers and areas of focal infiltration in the gland, such as shown in Figure 6.3D.

There may be overlap with Graves' disease, which is manifested by agonistic (activating) antibodies reactive with the TSHR (see "Type II Autoimmune Reactions"). Initially, this antibody may activate the thyroid into *over*secretion of thyroid hormone (seen as increased levels of T4), leading to hyperthyroidism. Eventually, this too may cause destruction of the thyroid gland, resulting in a hypothyroid state.

The cause of Hashimoto's thyroiditis is unknown. There are familial linkages (as seen in this patient). Other conditions that may predispose to Hashimoto's are physical stress, radiation, viral infections, increased iodine, medications (most notably amiodarone, lithium, and interferon-α), other autoimmune diseases (most notably Sjögren's syndrome), female gender, and pregnancy.

Epidemiology of Autoimmune Disease

There are nearly 100 different forms of auto-immune disease, making these disorders a major cause of chronic illness, affecting up to 3 percent of the general population. Nearly any organ can be affected by either systemic or organ-specific autoimmune disease (Table 6.1). Women make up nearly 75 percent of all individuals afflicted by autoimmune disease, making these disorders one of the ten leading causes of death in women less than sixty-five years old. However, the female-to-male ratio varies widely among different diseases, being as high as 9:1 in SLE, Sjögren's syndrome, and autoimmune thyroiditis and as low as 1:1 in TID, Goodpasture's syndrome, and vitiligo (Table 6.1). The mean age of onset also varies widely, with some disorders typically occurring early in childhood (e.g., TID, juvenile rheumatoid arthritis), others in the childbearing years (ages 15–45, e.g., SLE), and still others in later life (e.g., Sjögren's syndrome). There may be striking ethnic/racial predispositions to autoimmune disease. For example, SLE is about three times more prevalent in individuals of African, Asian, or Latin ancestry than in individuals of European ancestry, whereas Sjögren's syndrome and multiple sclerosis are more prevalent in those of European ancestry. The racial/ethnic differences are likely to reflect differences in the frequencies of disease susceptibility genes. The costs of these disorders to society are enormous. Rheumatoid arthritis (RA) affects

2.1 million Americans (1.5 million women and 600,000 men) at an annual cost of about $6,000 per patient (direct medical costs and indirect costs such as absence from work). Lupus affects 500,000 Americans at an estimated annual cost of $13,000 per patient, a total $6.5 billion per year.

ANIMAL MODELS OF AUTOIMMUNE DISEASE

The difficulty in carrying out randomized, well-controlled research in patients complicates studies of the pathogenesis and treatment of human autoimmune disease. Often the simplest course is to first study the disease in an appropriate animal model. However, because animal models of disease rarely are identical to the human disorder, the suitability of a particular model in any given situation must be considered carefully before undertaking animal studies. The list of animal models of autoimmune disease is extensive, and only some of the more commonly studied models can be reviewed here (see also Table 6.2).

SLE (NZB X NZW F1, MRL, BXSB, TMPD)

Numerous mouse strains have been studied over the years as animal models of SLE. Some strains develop lupus spontaneously, such as NZB X NZW (F1) (NZB/W) hybrid mice, MRL mice, and BXSB male mice. Other models, such as tetramethyl-pentadecane (TMPD, pristane) induced lupus, are inducible with chemicals. The spontaneous models afford hope that if the genetic defect(s) responsible for lupus-like disease in these mice can be identified, similar defects will be found in human lupus. However, the inducible TMPD

Table 6.2 Key Features of Selected Animal Models of Autoimmune Disease

Animal Model	Disease	Susceptible Strains	Similarities to Human Disease	Differences from Disease
(NZB X NZW)F1	SLE	N/A	Glomerulonephritis, ANA, anti-dsDNA, female > male	Autoantibody profile, no vasculitis
MRL *lpr/lpr*	SLE (RA)	N/A	Lymphadenopathy, glomerulonephritis, erosive arthritis, vasculitis, female > male	FAS deficiency causes mainly hematological autoimmunity in humans
BXSB male	SLE	N/A	Glomerulonephritis	Only male is affected, limited autoantibody profile
TMPD-induced lupus	SLE (RA)	BALB/c, C57BL/6, SJL, DBA/1, DBA/2, 129Sv, and most others	Glomerulonephritis, erosive arthritis, pulmonary vasculitis, ANA, anti-dsDNA, anti-Sm/RNP, female > male, increased interferon α/β	Not genetically mediated (but influenced by the genetic background)
Collagen-induced arthritis	RA	DBA/1 and others	Chronic, erosive inflammation of peripheral joints	Induced by immunization. In mice, males have a greater susceptibility. Primarily affect ankles rather than knees
TTP deficiency	RA	129Sv	Erosive, polyarticular symmetrical arthritis	Patchy alopecia, dermatitis, conjunctivitis, and "kangaroo" hunched posture
K/BxN	RA	BALB/c and others	Erosive, polyarticular symmetrical arthritis	Induced by autoantibodies; no RF or anti-CCP antibodies
EAE	MS	SJL and others	Relapsing-remitting or chronic-progressive, highly variable neurological disorder	Inducible instead of developing spontaneously, might require adjuvants
NOD	TID	N/A	Insulin-dependent diabetes	Autoimmune sialadenitis, autoimmune thyroiditis, autoimmune peripheral polyneuropathy, SLE-like disease, and prostatitis

MS, multiple sclerosis; N/A, not applicable; RA, rheumatoid arthritis; SLE, systemic lupus erythematosus; TID, type I diabetes; TMPD, tetramethylpentadecane; TTP, tristetrapolin; EAE, experimental autoimmune encephalomyelitis.

model more closely mimics the abnormalities in interferon (IFN) α and β production seen in most lupus patients.

NZB/W F1 MODEL

The NZB/W model was the first murine model of lupus nephritis. New Zealand Black (NZB) mice develop AIHA and the female New Zealand White (NZW) mice develop mesangial glomerulonephritis late in life. In contrast, the F1 hybrid (NZB/W) develops early-onset severe (proliferative, immune complex-mediated) glomerulonephritis along with ANA, antichromatin, and anti-dsDNA antibodies. However, these mice lack other classic clinical and serological manifestations of SLE, such as arthritis, inflammatory skin rashes, serositis, and anti-Sm autoantibodies. Extensive genetic analysis of this strain has revealed three major susceptibility intervals on chromosomes 1, 4, and 7. Each of these intervals appears to contain multiple disease-susceptibility genes and several candidate genes have been identified. NZB/W mice have been used widely for preclinical studies of various therapeutic interventions for lupus nephritis.

MRL MODEL

MRL mice, an inbred strain derived from several other strains, develop ANAs and late-onset glomerulonephritis reminiscent of SLE. A spontaneously occurring mutation led to impressive lymphoproliferation (*lpr* mutation), severe, early-onset nephritis closely resembling proliferative lupus nephritis, the development of erosive arthritis (more characteristic of RA than SLE), salivary gland inflammation (reminiscent of Sjögren's syndrome), vasculitis, and skin disease resembling cutaneous lupus. Both MRL and MRL *lpr/lpr* mice develop a host of autoantibodies characteristic of SLE, including anti-Sm and anti-dsDNA as well as severe hypergammaglobulinemia. These autoantibodies develop earlier in the presence of the *lpr* mutation, which generally accelerates the onset of lupus-like disease in this strain. The abnormalities caused by the *lpr* mutation are due to an ETn retrotransposon insertion into the *Fas* gene, which encodes an important protein mediator of apoptosis. Defective apoptosis of lymphocytes leads to the accumulation of $CD3^+CD4^-CD8^-$ ("double negative") T cells, accounting for the massive lymphoproliferation seen in MRL *lpr/lpr* mice.

BXSB MODEL

This strain was created by crossing male SB/Le and female C57BL/6J mice. Male, but not female, BXSB mice develop severe glomerulonephritis, lymphadenopathy, splenomegaly, AIHA, and anti-dsDNA autoantibodies. Thus, the sex predilection is an important difference from human lupus and most other murine lupus models. A mutant gene located on the Y chromosome, designated *Yaa* (Y chromosome-linked autoimmune acceleration), causes accelerated lupus-like disease in male BXSB mice. A recent study showed that the *Yaa* mutation results from translocation of a 4-megabase portion of the X chromosome to the Y chromosome, leading to increased expression of several genes that are normally X linked, including TLR7.

TMPD-INDUCED LUPUS

Intraperitoneal injection of pristane (2, 6, 10, 14 tetramethylpentadecane, TMPD) can induce a lupus-like syndrome in non-autoimmune-prone mice characterized by proliferative glomerulonephritis, erosive arthritis, pulmonary vasculitis, and a variety of lupus autoantibodies, including anti-dsDNA and anti-Sm. All or nearly all immunocompetent mouse strains are susceptible to lupus induced by this hydrocarbon oil. This inducible model of lupus is, at least so far, unique in reproducing the increased levels of IFN-α and IFN-β seen in the majority of lupus patients. The disease is largely abrogated in type I interferon receptor-deficient mice.

Rheumatoid Arthritis (Collagen-Induced Arthritis, TTP Deficiency, K/BxN Model)

RA is a systemic autoimmune disease characterized by prominent joint involvement. Arthritis is typically associated with erosion of cartilage and subchondral bone, formation of an inflammatory tissue, consisting of activated macrophages, T cells, fibroblasts, and other immune cells (pannus). This can ultimately result in joint destruction and significant joint deformities. In addition to the joints, RA can cause vasculitis, splenomegaly, and leukopenia (Felty's syndrome), interstitial lung disease, and other abnormalities. Rheumatoid factor (an autoantibody against the Fc portion of immunoglobulin) and antibodies against citrulline-modified proteins or peptides (usually detected as antibodies against an artificially produced cyclic citrullinated peptide, or CCP) are typical serological findings in RA, although not all patients exhibit these abnormalities. Several animal models of RA exist, but they do not precisely reproduce the clinical and laboratory abnormalities.

COLLAGEN-INDUCED ARTHRITIS (CIA)

Immunization of susceptible rodent strains with type II collagen (CII) leads to the development of a severe polyarticular arthritis resembling human RA. Although induced by heterologous CII, immunization leads to a response against autologous CII. CIA can be induced in susceptible strains of mice, rats, and primates. Histologically, both RA and CIA are characterized by an intense synovitis accompanied by erosion of cartilage and subchondral bone by a pannuslike tissue. Unlike human RA, CIA is monophasic. In addition, there are important serological differences. In general, rheumatoid factor is not produced in CIA and antibodies against CCP are absent.

TTP DEFICIENCY

Tristetraprolin (TTP) is a transcription factor that can bind to and destabilize mRNAs encoding TNF-α and granulocyte-macrophage colony-stimulating factor (GM-CSF). Mice deficient in TTP develop a complex syndrome characterized by cachexia, polyarticular arthritis, dermatitis, autoimmunity, and myeloid hyperplasia accompanied by extramedullary hematopoiesis (erythrocyte production outside of the bone marrow). TTP knockout mice exhibit exuberant inflammatory pannus and bony erosions. These mice also produce high titers of anti-DNA, and ANAs; however, rheumatoid factors are absent.

K/BxN MODEL

Although RA has been considered primarily a type IV autoimmune reaction for many years, the finding that autoantibodies against glucose 6-phosphate isomerase (GPI) can transfer RA-like joint disease to normal mice has rekindled interest in the possibility that antibody-mediated autoimmune mechanisms (type II or type III) could play a role in the pathogenesis of

RA. K/BxN T-cell-receptor transgenic mice express a transgenic T-cell receptor specific for a peptide of the ubiquitously expressed self-protein GPI. Arthritis in this model is initiated by antibodies against GPI. The resulting synovitis is chronic, erosive, and associated with pannus formation. Paradoxically, although the GPI antigen is ubiquitous, autoimmunity is focused on the joints. It appears that the GPI protein, not a cross-reactive synovial antigen, is the target of the pathogenic antibodies. Although the histological appearance of the affected joints is reminiscent of RA, there is no evidence that RA in humans can be caused by antibodies against GPI. The classic serological abnormalities, rheumatoid factor, and anti-CCP antibodies are not seen, and anti-TNF-α antibodies have little effect in this model.

Multiple Sclerosis (Experimental Autoimmune Encephalomyelitis)

Multiple sclerosis (MS) is a chronic autoimmune disease affecting the central nervous system, including the brain and spinal cord. The disease affects about 350,000 Americans and about 1.1 million worldwide. Age of onset is typically twenty to forty years old, women are affected more frequently than men (2:1 ratio), and it is most prevalent in individuals of northern European ancestry. It is thought to be mediated primarily by a T-cell-mediated attack on the myelin sheaths of certain nerve fibers, resulting in inflammation, demyelination, and gliosis (scarring). In addition, autoantibodies against components of myelin such as myelin oligodendrocyte glycoprotein (MOG) may be seen and also may contribute to disease pathogenesis by fixing complement. During the course of disease,

the lesions classically occur at different times and in different locations. Symptoms include sensory loss, paresthesias (numbness, tingling), visual changes due to optic neuritis, tremor, ataxia, weakness, spasticity, and other neurological symptoms. Patients with MS can exhibit either a relapsing-remitting or a progressive course.

EAE is a model of MS induced in susceptible animals by immunization by intact myelin or components of myelin, the sheath that surrounds certain neurons. Like CIA for RA, EAE can be induced in several species, including mice, rats, guinea pigs, rabbits, and primates. Although induced by heterologous antigen(s), the disease is autoimmune. Several proteins have been used to induce EAE, including MBP, proteolipid protein (PLP), and MOG. Different antigens cause somewhat different clinical manifestations. By administering the antigen with complete Freund's adjuvant and pertussis toxin, the blood-brain barrier is disrupted, permitting access by immune cells. The resulting demyelinating disease closely resembles human MS and is thought to be mediated primarily by T cells because disease can be transferred to normal animals by T cells (type IV autoimmune reaction). There is only limited evidence that an immune response to MBP, PLP, or MOG is involved in human disease, and it is hypothesized that other myelin antigens may be the targets of autoreactive T cells in MS.

Type I Diabetes (Nonobese Diabetic Mouse Model)

TID is an autoimmune disease in which the insulin-producing β cells in the pancreatic islets of Langerhans are gradually destroyed by autoreactive T cells over a period of months to years. After about 80 percent of the islet cells are destroyed, insulin deficiency and a severe form of insulin-dependent diabetes marked by ketoacidosis develops. The disease usually affects children and young adults but can occur at any age. Males and females are affected equally. The highest incidence is in Scandinavians (35 per 100,000 per year). Individuals with a genetic susceptibility to the disease are thought to develop autoimmunity in response to an undefined environmental trigger. Most patients with TID produce anti-islet cell autoantibodies reactive with insulin, glutamic acid decarboxylase, ICA-512/IA-2, phogrin, or other antigens. These autoantibodies generally appear before the onset of clinical diabetes and have been used for early diagnosis of the condition.

The nonobese diabetic (NOD) mouse is the most useful model of autoimmune TID. NOD mice spontaneously develop marked infiltration of T cells into the pancreatic islets. The infiltrating T cells selectively destroy the pancreatic β cells. In addition to diabetes, NOD mice spontaneously develop autoimmune responses involving other tissues, including salivary gland, lacrimal gland, thyroid gland, parathyroid gland, adrenal gland, testis, large bowel, and red blood cells. NOD mice also are susceptible to exogenously induced autoimmune diseases, such as experimental autoimmune thyroiditis, colitis-like wasting disease, encephalomyelitis, and SLE. Defects related to several genes, including the MHC class II, CTLA-4, and IL-2, have been associated with the susceptibility to diabetes. T cells play an important role in the development and progression of disease, whereas B cells are not required at the effector stage of TID in NOD mice.

Autoimmune Thyroiditis (Experimental Autoimmune Thyroiditis)

Experimental autoimmune thyroiditis is induced in mice by immunization with murine thyroglobulin plus complete Freund's adjuvant. The mice develop autoantibodies against thyroglobulin and histological changes consistent with those seen in human autoimmune thyroiditis. It is a useful model for studying the pathogenesis of human chronic (Hashimoto's) thyroiditis.

PATHOGENESIS OF AUTOIMMUNE DISEASE

Genetic Predisposition

Genetic, environmental, and random (stochastic) factors all play a role in the pathogenesis of autoimmune diseases. Family members of affected individuals are at higher risk for developing autoimmune disease than the general population. The relative risk to siblings of affected individuals (probands) versus the risk in the general population (λ_s = disease prevalence in siblings of affected individuals ÷ disease prevalence in the general population) is a useful way to estimate the importance of genetic factors. The relative risk is between five- and fiftyfold higher in siblings of affected probands than in unrelated individuals in most autoimmune diseases (Table 6.3). Part of this effect is accounted for by MHC-linked genes.

Twin studies illustrate the importance of these genetic factors. If the concordance rates in monozygotic and dizygotic twins are about the same, the genetic effect is small. For most autoimmune diseases, concordance rates are 15–30 percent for monozygotic twins versus 2–5 percent for

Table 6.3 Twin Studies Illustrating the Importance of Genetic Factors in Autoimmune Disease

Disease	Concordance Rates		Sibling Risk/Population Risk (λ_s)	
	Dizygotic Twins	Monozygotic Twins	Overall	Attributable to MHC
Systemic autoimmune diseases				
Rheumatoid arthritis	4%	12–15%	8	1.6
SLE	2%	24%	20	N/A
Organ-specific autoimmune diseases				
Type 1 diabetes	5%	33%	15	2.4
Multiple sclerosis	3.5%	21–40%	20	2.4
Graves' disease	0%	36%	15	N/A

Compiled from the following references: Vyse TJ, Todd JA. Genetic analysis of autoimmune disease. *Cell*. 1996;85:311–318; Jarvinen P, Aho K. Twin studies in rheumatic diseases. *Semin Arthritis Rheum*. 1994;24(1):19–28; Brix TH, Christensen K, Holm NV, Harvald B, Hegedus L. A population-based study of Graves' disease in Danish twins. *Clin Endocrinol*. 1998;48(4): 397–400; Redondo MJ, Fain PR, Eisenbarth GS. Genetics of type 1A diabetes. *Recent Prog Horm Res*. 2001;56:69–89; Kahana E. Epidemiologic studies of multiple sclerosis: a review. *Biomed Pharmacother*. 2000;54(2):100–102.

dizygotic twins, consistent with a sizeable genetic effect (Table 6.3). Identification of the actual mutations or genetic polymorphisms that confer susceptibility to autoimmune diseases has been complicated by the fact that most autoimmune disorders appear to involve multiple genes, each with only a small effect. Moreover, many autoimmune "diseases" are actually "syndromes" that may arise through a variety of different pathogenic mechanisms and genetic abnormalities. Even in the inbred lupus-prone mouse strain NZB/W, ten or more susceptibility loci are thought to contribute to disease severity in an additive fashion (threshold liability model). Human SLE and other autoimmune diseases also are likely to be highly complex genetically. Interestingly, there may be some overlap genetically between different forms of autoimmune disease, such as SLE and type I diabetes. More than half of the linkages identified in genomewide scan-

ning studies of a variety of systemic and organ-specific autoimmune diseases map nonrandomly into eighteen chromosomal clusters, possibly explaining the occurrence of several autoimmune diseases in a given individual or family. For example, Hashimoto's thyroiditis is associated with a variety of organ-specific (e.g., TID, pernicious anemia, autoimmune hepatitis, and Addison's disease) and systemic (e.g., lupus, RA, and Sjögren's syndrome) autoimmune diseases. Pedigrees with more than one systemic autoimmune disorder are not unusual. Of course, shared environmental influences could also explain familial clustering.

Among candidate genes, the MHC class II molecule is the most comprehensively studied. MHC polymorphisms are associated with development of RA, SLE, MS, TID, and other autoimmune diseases (Table 6.3). RA is a striking example. A shared epitope, consisting of a 5-amino acid sequence motif in the third allelic hypervariable region of the HLA-DRβ1 chain (QKRAA in the *0401 allele, QRRAA in the *0404 and *0101 alleles), is carried by 90 percent of patients with RA and is associated with disease severity. In addition to MHC-linked genes, mutations or genetic polymorphisms involving non-MHC genes also are strong candidates for autoimmune disease susceptibility genes (Table 6.4). These include genetic polymorphisms or deficiency of molecules involved in the response to or clearance of immune complexes (e.g., C1q, C4, FcγRIIa, FcγRIIb, FcγRIIIa, mannose-binding lectin), which are associated with SLE, as well as genes influencing T-cell activation (*PTPN22*, *CTLA-4*), cytokine responses (*STAT-4*, *IRF-5*, *Tyk2*), or programmed cell death (*Fas*, *PDCD1*; Table 6.4).

Many, if not most, systemic and organ-specific autoimmune diseases are thought to be multifactorial, involving multiple genetic defects consistent with the *threshold liability model of multifactorial inheritance*. This model supposes a continuously distributed genetically determined liability to the development of disease. Individuals who develop disease will bear multiple disease susceptibility genes. Because of the normal distribution of genes, first-degree relatives will have much higher risk of developing disease than the general population, second-degree relatives will have a moderate risk, and third-degree relatives will have low risk.

Environmental Triggers of Autoimmune Disease

Environmental factors can trigger autoimmune disease in susceptible hosts, as illustrated by the initiation of disease by sun exposure in a subset of lupus patients. The wavelengths most likely to induce lupus fall in the UV range: UVC (200–290 nm), UVB (290–320 nm), and UVA (320–400 nm). UVB irradiation is mostly absorbed in the upper layers of the epidermis, whereas the longer wavelength UVA is able to reach the dermis. UV exposure can induce apoptosis and release of immune mediators and activation of resident dendritic cells and T cells. Expression of certain self-antigens, such as Ro60/Ro52, on the surface of the apoptotic cells may lead to antibody-mediated inflammatory responses that could play a role in the pathogenesis of skin rashes in lupus.

The importance of environmental factors is further illustrated by the induction of a murine lupus syndrome by the hydrocarbon pristane (see "Animal Models of Autoimmune Disease"), which appears to act, in part, through the induction of type I interferon (IFN-α and IFN-β) production. Many other chemicals and drugs have been implicated as triggers of autoimmunity or autoimmune disease. Procainamide, hydralazine, chlorpromazine, methyldopa, quinidine, minocycline, and nitrofurantoin all have been associated with the induction of ANAs and in some cases antineutrophil cytoplasmic antibodies as well as in the pathogenesis of "drug-induced lupus," most frequently manifested by serositis (inflammation of the pleura or pericardium) and arthritis. Silica is recognized as a precipitating factor for scleroderma, cigarette smoke may aggravate RA, and trichloroethylene is thought to promote lupus in animal models and possibly humans. Other chemical agents implicated in the pathogenesis of autoimmunity include heavy metals such as mercury, gold, and cadmium, pesticides, herbicides, hydrazine, and certain dyes.

Table 6.4 Some Candidate Non-MHC Autoimmune Disease Susceptibility Genes

Gene	Abnormality	Disease Association	Defect
C4	Deficiency	SLE	IC clearance
FcγRIIa	R131	SLE	Inflammatory response to ICs
FcγRIIb	T232	SLE	Inflammatory response to ICs
FcγRIIIa	F176	SLE	Inflammatory response to ICs
CTLA-4	+49G	SLE, TID, Graves' disease, Hashimoto's thyroiditis, Addison's disease, celiac disease	Control of T-cell activation
PTPN22	W620	SLE, RA, TID, RA, JRA, Graves' disease, vitiligo	Control of T-cell activation
STAT4	SNP rs7574865	SLE, RA, TID, autoimmune thyroiditis, myasthenia gravis	Cytokine signaling
IRF-5	SNP rs2004640 T allele	SLE	Cytokine signaling
Tyk2	SNP rs2304256	SLE	Cytokine signaling
PDCD1	SNP rs11568821 (PD-1.3)	SLE	Programmed cell death
Fas	Deficiency	Autoimmune cytopenias	Programmed cell death
Foxp3	Deficiency	Organ-specific autoimmune disease (TID, autoimmune thyroiditis)	Control of T-cell activation (deficiency of T_{reg})

IC, immune complex; JRA, juvenile rheumatoid arthritis; RA, rheumatoid arthritis; SLE, systemic lupus erythematosus; TID, type I diabetes.

Infections also are implicated in the pathogenesis of autoimmune disease. The classic example is rheumatic fever, which is thought to be a consequence of cross-reactivity or "molecular mimicry" between antigens carried by certain strains of streptococci and self-antigens of the heart. Mycoplasma pneumonia can induce the production of cold agglutinins, polyclonal cold-reactive IgM autoantibodies against the erythrocyte I, or i antigens that can cause complement-mediated AIHA (see "Type II Autoimmune Reactions"). A variety of other parasitic (e.g., schistosomiasis, Chagas' disease), bacterial (e.g., *Helicobacter pylori*, staphylococci, salmonella, Lyme borreliosis), mycobacterial (e.g., tuberculosis, leprosy), and viral (e.g., cytomegalovirus, Epstein-Barr virus, hepatitis C, Coxsackie virus, parvovirus B19) infections can be complicated by autoimmunity. Proposed mechanisms include molecular mimicry and the chronic overproduction of cytokines, such as IFN-α. Indeed, therapy with IFN-α can lead to the development of autoimmune diseases such as autoimmune thyroiditis and SLE.

Maintenance of Self-Tolerance

Environmental triggers, such as sunlight, drugs/chemicals, and infectious agents, act on a genetic background that regulates tolerance to self. The immune system has evolved a remarkable ability to distinguish self from nonself. Immune tolerance is achieved by multiple mechanisms, operating both centrally and peripherally. Central tolerance occurs during the development of T and B lymphocytes in the thymus and bone marrow, respectively. This mostly involves the deletion of autoreactive cells before they exit the primary lymphoid organs. In general, lymphocytes exhibiting strong reactivity for ubiquitously expressed self-antigens are deleted in this manner, whereas autoreactive cells of lower affinity for self may escape central tolerance. These cells are held in check by peripheral tolerance mechanisms. Peripheral tolerance is mediated by deletion, anergy, and suppression as well as by "neglect" or "ignorance," acting on autoreactive lymphocytes after they exit the primary organs. In general, lymphocyte activation requires two signals, one delivered by the antigen receptor (T-cell antigen receptor or surface immunoglobulin) and second, a *co-stimulatory* signal. For T-cell activation, this co-stimulatory signal is delivered by the interaction of molecules expressed on the surface of professional antigen-presenting cells or B cells, such as CD80 and CD86, which interact with CD28 (or other receptors) on the T-cell surface. In the case of B cells, the co-stimulatory signal is delivered by CD40 ligand, a surface protein expressed by activated helper T cells that interacts with CD40 on the surface of B lymphocytes. In the absence of a co-stimulatory signal, engagement of the T- or B-cell antigen receptor leads to a state of anergy (the inability of the lymphocyte to respond to its specific antigen).

Many self-antigens are expressed at a very low level that is insufficient to induce T-cell activation. In the case of T cells, which recognize short peptides associated with MHC molecules, the induction of self-tolerance requires the generation of a sufficient amount of self-peptide in antigen-presenting cells to stimulate T-cell deletion or anergy. Self-peptides that are generated inefficiently by the antigen-presenting cells can neither stimulate immunity nor induce tolerance; that is, the immune system remains "ignorant" of them. If these minor self-peptides are produced in larger amounts and exposed to the immune system in the presence of an inducer of co-stimulatory molecules (e.g., adjuvants), they have the capacity to stimulate an immune response. This has been shown experimentally with peptides generated in vitro using proteolytic enzymes or using synthetic self-peptides.

Regulatory T cells (T_{reg}) also play an important role in maintaining peripheral tolerance. Several different subsets of T_{reg} have been reported, but one of the most intensely studied is the $CD4^+CD25^+Foxp3^+$ subset, which represents about 10 percent of total $CD4^+$ cells. These cells regulate T-cell activation by a cell–cell contact-dependent mechanism and through the secretion of inhibitory cytokines such as IL-10 and transforming growth factor-beta (TGFβ). They suppress both naïve and memory T-cell responses and down-regulate the expression of pro-inflammatory cytokines and co-stimulatory molecules on the antigen-presenting cells. These cells are induced in an antigen-specific manner, but the subsequent suppressive effects are not antigen specific. Genetic defects in

Foxp3, a transcription factor that is the key controller of T_{reg} function, lead to organ-specific autoimmune or autoinflammatory diseases. The scurfy mouse has an X-linked defect of the *Foxp3* gene that is lethal in males, which exhibit hyperactivation of $CD4^+$ T cells and overproduction of inflammatory cytokines. *Foxp3* mutations in humans are the cause of the IPEX (immune dysregulation, polyendocrinopathy, enteropathy, X-linked syndrome) syndrome. These individuals develop organ-specific autoimmune diseases, such as TID, autoimmune thyroiditis, and inflammatory bowel disease. Interestingly, however, the development of systemic autoimmune disease is not part of the syndrome in either mice or humans.

Finally, antigen-presenting cells play an important role in the induction of tolerance. Dendritic cells can either initiate T-cell activation and proliferation or promote peripheral tolerance through the deletion of autoreactive T cells, depending on their maturation state. Tolerance is induced when antigens are presented by immature dendritic cells and these cells also play a role in the generation and maintenance of T_{reg}.

TREATMENT OF AUTOIMMUNE DISEASE

Treatment for autoimmune disease is diverse, and in recent years, the options have increased rapidly. Organ-specific autoimmune diseases of endocrine function, such as TID and autoimmune thyroiditis, may be treated with hormone replacement. In contrast, other forms of organ-specific autoimmune disease such as autoimmune thrombocytopenia, AIHA, and multiple sclerosis are treated with immunosuppressive medications, as are the majority of systemic autoimmune diseases. Immunosuppressive medications can be categorized by mode of action.

Anti-inflammatory Agents

Nonsteroidal anti-inflammatory drugs have been used since the 1800s when salicin was extracted from willow bark (1828) and sodium salicylate (1875) and aspirin (1899) were synthesized. A large number of these drugs, which either selectively or nonselectively inhibit the enzyme cyclooxygenase (a synthetic enzyme for prostaglandins), are currently in use to treat inflammatory disease. Although most of their anti-inflammatory properties derive from the inhibition of prostaglandin synthesis, at high doses, there is inhibition of the transcription factor nuclear factor κB (NFκB), a key mediator of inflammatory cytokine production. Corticosteroids have a more potent effect on NFκB and consequently a greater anti-inflammatory effect.

Philip S. Hench discovered the anti-inflammatory properties of cortisone in 1949. Corticosteroids are a mainstay of therapy for many systemic autoimmune diseases, including SLE, RA, and inflammatory myopathies such as polymyositis. Corticosteroid therapy also is used for the treatment of some of the more serious organ-specific autoimmune diseases, such as AIHA, autoimmune thrombocytopenia, multiple sclerosis, and Goodpasture's syndrome. Corticosteroids reduce inflammation by multiple mechanisms of action. One major action is enhanced transcription of an inhibitor of NFκB called IκB. IκB dimerizes with NFκB, inhibiting the production of inflammatory cytokines mediated by this transcriptional pathway. In addition, corticosteroids promote the differentiation of a subset of anti-inflammatory macrophages that produce the cytokine IL-10.

Antimalarial Drugs

Antimalarial drugs have been used for the treatment of SLE and RA since the early 1900s. The precise mechanism of action remains uncertain, but they have been shown to inhibit cytokine (IL-1 and IL-6) production in vitro. The antimalarials pass freely through cell membranes at neutral pH, but in acidic environments, such as endosomes, they become protonated and can no longer diffuse freely. This leads to concentration of the drug within endosomes and the collapse of endosomal pH gradients. It has been proposed that the inhibition of endosomal acidification interferes with antigen processing or, alternatively, that there is an effect on the interaction of microbial substances such as unmethylated CpG DNA or uridine-rich RNA with endosomal toll-like receptors (TLR9 and TLR7/TLR8, respectively). In addition to SLE and RA, antimalarials are used in the treatment of juvenile rheumatoid arthritis, Sjögren's syndrome, and inflammatory myopathies.

Anticytokine Agents

The development of TNF-α inhibitors in the 1990s ushered in a new era of therapy of autoimmune disease using "biologicals" capable of interfering with the interactions between cytokines and their receptors. The initial clinical use of TNF inhibitors such as etanercept (a soluble recombinant TNF receptor II linked to the Fc portion of human IgG1), infliximab (a chimeric human-mouse anti-TNF-α monoclonal antibody), and adalimumab (a fully humanized monoclonal antibody against TNF-α) in RA demonstrated that although multiple cytokines may be involved in disease pathogenesis (in RA, IL-1, and IL-6 in addition to TNF-α), inhibitors of a single cytokine pathway may show therapeutic efficacy. In addition to RA, TNF-α inhibitors are used for treating inflammatory bowel disease, psoriasis, and psoriatic arthritis and are being tested in sarcoidosis, Wegener's granulomatosis, pyoderma gangrenosum, SLE, and Behcet's syndrome.

Anti-TNF therapy is only the tip of the "biological iceberg." Recombinant IL-1 receptor antagonist (anakinra) has been approved for the treatment of RA, and numerous other cytokine antagonists are currently in clinical trials or under development.

Methotrexate

Methotrexate is a folic acid analog used extensively for the treatment of RA. It appears that its ability to inhibit dihydrofolate reductase is not responsible for its efficacy in RA, however. Instead, activity may be related to effects on aminoimidazole-carboxamide ribotide transformylase, leading to the release of adenosine, a potent anti-inflammatory molecule that inhibits neutophil adherence to fibroblasts and endothelial cells. Methotrexate inhibits IL-1 and increases the expression of TH2 cytokines (e.g., IL-4), leading to decreased production of TH1 cytokines (e.g., IFN-γ).

Anti-T-Lymphocyte Therapy

T cells play a key role in the pathogenesis of type IV autoimmune reactions and also are critical for generating the T-cell-dependent autoantibodies mediating type II and type III autoimmune diseases. Consequently, considerable effort has gone into the development of therapeutic agents that selectively or nonselectively target T lymphocytes. Drugs that target primarily T cells include cyclophosphamide, azathioprine, cyclosporin A, tacrolimus, and the biological CTLA4-Ig. Cyclophosphamide is an alkylating agent that substitutes alkyl radicals into DNA and RNA. The drug is inactive by itself but is converted to an active metabolite responsible for its immunosuppressive effects. It is used for the treatment of lupus nephritis and other life-threatening complications of SLE and other systemic autoimmune diseases.

Azathioprine is a purine analog that inhibits the synthesis of adenosine and guanine. Like cyclophosphamide, it is converted to an active metabolite (6-mercaptopurine), which inhibits the division of activated B and T cells. Azathioprine is used in the treatment of RA, SLE, autoimmune hepatitis, inflammatory myopathy, vasculitis, and other autoimmune disorders.

Unlike cyclophosphamide and azathioprine, cyclosporine and tacrolimus (FK506) have immunosuppressive properties that are highly selective for T cells. Both agents interfere with the phosphatase calcineurin, ultimately leading to an inhibition of the activation of the transcription factor NFAT (nuclear factor of activated T cells). Cyclosporine binds to the intracellular protein cyclophilin and tacrolimus to a protein called FK binding protein. The cyclosporine-cyclophilin and tacrolimus-FK binding protein complexes bind to calcineurin, preventing its activation by intracellular calcium, and the activation of NFAT. Although used most frequently to prevent transplant rejection, these agents have been shown to have activity in the treatment of RA, SLE, and certain forms of vasculitis.

The CTLA4 (CD152) molecule is an inhibitory receptor expressed by activated T cells that block the co-stimulatory interaction between CD80 or CD86 on the surface of antigen-presenting cells and CD28 on T cells. It acts by binding CD80/CD86 with greater affinity than CD28. CTLA4 is expressed late in T-cell activation and serves to turn off the activated state. CTLA4-Ig (abatacept) is a recombinant chimera of CTLA4 and the Fc fragment of IgG1. CTLA4-Ig/abatacept is used for the treatment of RA and is active in mouse models of lupus. Clinical trials in SLE patients are in progress.

Anti-B-Lymphocyte Therapy

Rituximab is a cytotoxic chimeric human-mouse monoclonal antibody with a high affinity for CD20, a pan-B-cell surface antigen. It was developed originally for the treatment of B-cell lymphomas. The killing of B cells by rituximab is thought to depend on both the specific recognition of B cells by this monoclonal antibody and natural killer (NK) cell-mediated antibody-dependent cellular cytotoxicity (ADCC) of those cells. There is considerable evidence that the interaction of B-cell-bound monoclonal antibodies with NK cell CD16 (FcγRIIIA) is a critical event leading to ADCC following treatment with rituximab. Rituximab appears to have activity in a variety of autoimmune diseases associated with autoantibody production, including RA, SLE, polymyositis/dermatomyositis, Sjögren's syndrome, and cryoglobulinemic vasculitis.

Intravenous Immunoglobulin

Intravenous immunoglobulin (IVIG) is a preparation of human immunoglobulin pooled from thousands of healthy individuals. It was originally developed for replacement therapy in humoral immunodeficiency syndromes but has more recently become an important therapeutic modality in severe autoimmune disorders, such as thrombocytopenic purpura, AIHA, neuroimmunological diseases such as Guillain-Barré syndrome, SLE, certain forms of vasculitis, and polymyositis/dermatomyositis. The mechanism of action remains unclear, but IVIG may block the function of Fc receptors expressed by phagocytes of the reticuloendothelial system and also induces FcγRIIB (inhibitory Fc receptor) expression on infiltrating macrophages in the K/BxN model of RA. An additional mode of action may involve the presence of anti-idiotypic antibodies that block the antigen combining sites of pathogenic antibodies. The duration of action is limited by the metabolism of serum immunoglobulin, and generally, IVIG is regarded as a temporary measure that is followed by more definitive therapy.

Autologous Hematopoietic Stem Cell Transplantation (HSCT)

The ability to adoptively transfer autoimmune diseases with bone marrow transplantation in a variety of animal models provides strong evidence that these disorders are mediated by cells derived from hematopoietic cells. There is compelling evidence that autoimmune disease results from a loss of B- or T-cell tolerance to certain self-antigens. Hematopoietic stem cells are the earliest progenitor cells of the immune system and give rise to B and T lymphocytes as well as antigen-presenting cells (monocytes, macrophages, and dendritic cells). The rationale for HSCT as a therapy for autoimmune disease is based on the concept that the peripheral expansion of autoreactive T- and B-cell clones is central to the pathogenesis of autoimmunity. If these autoantigen-specific cells can be deleted and the immune system regenerated with "normal" hematopoietic stem cells, there is the potential to effect a "cure" of autoimmune disease. Therapy is based on the mobilization of hematopoietic stem cells using C-CSF or G-CSF plus cyclophosphamide. There is the risk during mobilization of flares caused by G-CSF treatment. The stem cells are depleted of lymphocytes and enriched for CD34$^+$ cells followed by expansion and reinfusion into the same donor after "conditioning." The conditioning regimen involves cyclophosphamide treatment or other immunosuppressive treatments aimed at depleting mature lymphocytes. Phase III clinical trials of the efficacy of autologous HSCT in MS, SLE, RA, and scleroderma are ongoing or planned. Promising preliminary results have been obtained with all of these conditions, but further study is needed.

THE FUTURE

Therapy Directed at Inflammatory Pathways

The pace of changes in the field of autoimmunity is rapid. Recent advances in understanding the importance of key inflammatory pathways involved in specific diseases, such as the TNF-α pathway in RA, inflammatory bowel disease, and other disorders, have been quickly followed by new biological therapies designed to interfere with these pathways.

With recent data increasingly underscoring the importance of type I interferon pathways in the pathogenesis of lupus, it seems reasonable to expect that therapies directed at preventing the excessive production of IFN-α/-β will be tested in the near future. As always, a major challenge in immune therapy will be to treat the key immunological defects selectively, leaving the remainder of the immune system intact to deal with infections. As the important immunological pathways become better defined, it may be feasible to selectively target one part of the pathway while leaving others intact. For instance, type I interferon is produced through several interrelated pathways. If only one of them is found to be abnormal in SLE, it may be feasible to selectively blockade that pathway, leaving the others intact to deal with viral and other types of infections.

Gene Therapy

Although considerable progress has been made in defining the genetics of autoimmune disease, nearly all of the major systemic autoimmune diseases are highly complex, multigene disorders, even in animal models. In comparison with single-gene diseases, such as cystic fibrosis or alpha 1-antitrypsin deficiency, it may prove considerably more difficult to correct genetically complex autoimmune disorders using standard gene therapy approaches. However, there may be reason for cautious optimism because inhibition of a single cytokine (TNF-α) can have a significant beneficial effect in the treatment of a multigenic autoimmune disorder (RA). At least in mice, retroviral transduction of *Foxp3* has been shown to convert naïve T cells into cells that phenotypically and functionally resemble T_{reg}. Whether this approach

will be applicable to the therapy of autoimmune disease remains to be determined.

Cell Therapy

Another promising possibility involves manipulating tolerance through the use of suppressor T cells or immature dendritic cells. Decreasing the numbers of $CD25^+CD4^+Foxp3^+$ cells in mice can induce a variety of organ-specific autoimmune conditions. Conversely, expansion of this subset can be used to induce immune tolerance in transplantation models. There is considerable interest in the potential use of T_{reg} expansion either in vivo or in vitro in the treatment for autoimmune disease. T_{reg} are highly proliferative in vivo, and certain drugs, such as rapamycin, may increase the ratio of T_{reg} to T effector cells. Alternatively, T_{reg} can be expanded in vitro in the presence of high doses of IL-2 and self-antigen followed by reinfusion, an approach that has been used successfully in the treatment of TID in NOD mice.

Whereas mature dendritic cells are highly potent stimulatory antigen-presenting cells, immature dendritic cells are tolerogenic. Dendritic cell therapy is being explored as a means of both promoting immunity (mature DCs) and inducing tolerance (immature DCs). Immune silencing may be made feasible by loading DCs ex vivo with self-antigens followed by treatments that render them tolerogenic (TGF-β, retinoic acid, or rapamycin, for instance). Reinfusion of these cells may be useful for inducing tolerance, though numerous obstacles remain.

Stem Cell Therapy

Although the bulk of evidence suggests that autoimmune diseases arises primarily due to defects in the immune system, therapy directed at repairing the target organs also may be equally important. Thus, there is increasing interest in the possibility of repairing damage at the level of the target organs with stem cell therapy.

MESENCHYMAL STEM CELLS

Found in bone marrow, cord blood, spleen, adipose tissue, and other tissues, mesenchymal stem cells (MSCs) are a well-characterized population of adult stem cells that can give rise to three main cell types, including adiopocytes, chondrocytes, and osteoblasts. However, these cells may be induced experimentally to undergo differentiation into other cell types as well, such as neural cells and myogenic cells. Isolation, amplification, and large-scale in vitro culturing of MSCs has been mastered to a degree appropriate for clinical applications, making MSCs good candidates for use in tissue repair. These cells can be maintained and propagated in culture for long periods, without losing their capacity to form the cell types discussed earlier. Another advantage is that MSCs can take up and retain introduced genes, a property that can be exploited for the delivery of clinically beneficial proteins to targeted locations. MSCs are also amenable to cryopreservation, allowing their future use in "off-the-shelf" therapies. Animal studies seeking to reconstitute or repair damaged cartilage, bone, muscle, heart muscle, and tendon using MSCs have shown great promise, raising the possibility that they might one day be used for repairing tissues damaged by autoimmune attack. Indeed, cell therapy using MSCs can prevent damage to the joints in collagen-induced arthritis and also can ameliorate end-organ damage in EAE and murine lupus.

Interestingly, allogeneic bone marrow–derived MSCs or stromal cells suppress in vitro T- and B-cell proliferation in a non-MHC-dependent manner. The immunosuppressive activity of MSCs has been attributed to effects on the expansion of the $CD25^+CD4^+Foxp3^+$ T_{reg} population.

Current tissue engineering strategies tend to rely on the use of autologous sources of adult stem cells. However, data demonstrating that the transplantation of allogeneic adult mesenchymal stem cells is feasible have the potential to revolutionize this field. With routine access to adult stem cells at the point of care, physicians may be able to incorporate tissue-engineering approaches into the management of autoimmune disease.

HUMAN EMBRYONIC STEM CELLS

Very recent advances in stem cell technology enable the generation of pluripotent human stem cells from human somatic cells using a process known as reprogramming or dedifferentiation. The procedure exploits viral vector-mediated expression of only four genes (namely, *c-myc, oct3/4, sox2, and klf4*) to reprogram mouse and human somatic cells (specifically, skin fibroblasts) into embryonic-like "induced pluripotent stem cells" (iPS cells). These cells appear to be just as plastic as embryonic stem cells, but one drawback to their clinical application in humans is the use of lentiviral or other retroviral vectors to introduce the genes. Although still at an early stage, the use of iPS cells could greatly advance the practicality of regenerative medicine as a therapeutic option. By creating patient-specific, pluripotent human stem cells, cell replacement therapies that avoid human embryo destruction may now be within reach.

ACKNOWLEDGMENTS

We thank Drs. Richard Lottenberg and Neil Harris (University of Florida Division of Hematology-Oncology) for providing the micrograph of spherocytes.

BIBLIOGRAPHY

REVIEWS

Atkinson MA, Eisenbarth GS. Type 1 diabetes: new perspectives on disease pathogenesis and treatment. *Lancet.* 2001;358:221–229.

Drayton DL, Liao S, Mounzer RH, Ruddle NH. Lymphoid organ development: from ontogeny to neogenesis. *Nat Immunol.* 2006;7:344–353.

Feldmann M, Brennan FM, Maini RN. Role of cytokines in rheumatoid arthritis. *Annu Rev Immunol.* 1996;14:397–440.

Goodnow CC, Cyster JG, Hartley SB, et al. Self-tolerance checkpoints in B lymphocyte development. *Adv Immunol.* 1995;59:279–368.

Miyara M, Sakaguchi S. Natural regulatory T cells: mechanisms of suppression. *Trends Mol Med.* 2007;13:108–116.

SUGGESTED READING

Anolik JH, Barnard J, Cappione A, et al. Rituximab improves peripheral B cell abnormalities in human systemic lupus erythematosus. *Arthritis Rheum.* 2004;50:3580–3590.

Boackle SA, Holers VM, Chen X, et al. Cr2, a candidate gene in the murine Sle1c lupus susceptibility locus, encodes a dysfunctional protein. *Immunity.* 2001;15:775–785.

Bruhns P, Samuelsson A, Pollard JW, Ravetch JV. Colony-stimulating factor-1-dependent macrophages are responsible for IVIG protection in antibody-induced autoimmune disease. *Immunity.* 2003;18:573–581.

Clynes R, Dumitru C, Ravetch JV. Uncoupling of immune complex formation and kidney damage in autoimmune glomerulonephritis. *Science.* 1998;279: 1052–1054.

Ehrchen J, Steinmuller L, Barczyk K, et al. Glucocorticoids induce differentiation of a specifically activated, anti-inflammatory subtype of human monocytes. *Blood.* 2007;109:1265–1274.

Jacobson DL, Gange SJ, Rose NR, et al. Epidemiology and estimated population burden of selected autoimmune diseases in the United States. *Clin Immunol Immunopathol.* 1997;84:223–243.

Kouskoff V, Korganow AS, Duchatelle V, Degott C, Benoist C, Mathis D. Organ-specific disease provoked by systemic autoimmunity. *Cell.* 1996;87:811–822.

Kremer JM, Westhovens R, Leon M, et al. 2003. Treatment of rheumatoid arthritis by selective inhibition of T-cell activation with fusion protein CTLA4Ig. *N Engl J Med.* 349:1907–1915.

Nacionales DC, Kelly-Scumpia KM, Lee PY, et al. Deficiency of the type I interferon receptor protects mice from experimental lupus. *Arthritis Rheum.* 2007;56:3770–3783.

Traynor AE, Schroeder J, Rosa RM, et al. Treatment of severe systemic lupus erythematosus with high-dose chemotherapy and haemopoietic stem-cell transplantation: a phase I study. *Lancet.* 2000;356:701–707.

7. Chronic Lymphocytic Leukemia

Nicholas Chiorazzi, M.D., and Manlio Ferrarini, M.D.

INTRODUCTION

Any cell of the immune system (see Chapter 1, Figure 1.1) can undergo malignant transformation giving rise to leukemia, lymphoma, or myeloma. In this chapter, we focus on B-cell-type chronic lymphocytic leukemia (B-CLL), the most common leukemia in the Western Hemisphere. This B-cell lymphoproliferative disorder arises among the aging population, increasing in incidence in a linear fashion after age 50. Therefore, its incidence is likely to increase as the baby boomer generation enters the sixth decade. Because patients with the disease in general have an extended clinical course (three to twenty-five years), B-CLL is categorized as one of a group of indolent leukemias/lymphomas. However, despite progress in therapeutic strategies, B-CLL remains an incurable disease.

An abundance of new information has become available within the past decade, such that B-CLL is now divided into two related conditions, both originating from antigen-selected B lymphocytes but differing in clinical course. Some patients live several decades, often without treatment, and others succumb to the disease in a few years. Here we shall discuss the possible mechanisms causing expansion and conversion of normal B lymphocytes to leukemic clones and determining the differences between the two major B-CLL subtypes. First, we will review normal B-cell development and the aberrant transformation to leukemia.

B-CELL ACTIVATION AND MATURATION

The enormous diversity of the normal B-cell-antibody repertoire initiates in the bone marrow where B lymphocytes rearrange their immunoglobulin (Ig) variable (V) region gene segments coding for the B cell's receptor for antigen (BCR) (Figures 7.1 and 7.2). The diversity in the repertoire continues to grow after binding antigen, when the B cell enters a lymphoid follicle and, with the help of other cells and cytokines, creates a structure called the *germinal center* (GC) where the cell proliferates and accumulates somatic mutations in its BCR-encoding genes (Figure 7.3). These mutations may produce amino acid changes in the binding site of the BCR, which can improve or create new antigen-binding specificity. Enhanced affinity B cells survive, whereas those having BCRs that either do not bind antigen or bind self-antigens die. The GC reaction usually occurs in secondary lymphoid follicles with the help of T lymphocytes. This mutation and selection process can take place in response to bacteria without T-cell help in the marginal zones outside of lymphoid follicles, although in this case, antigenic stimulation does not always induce mutation of IgV_H genes.

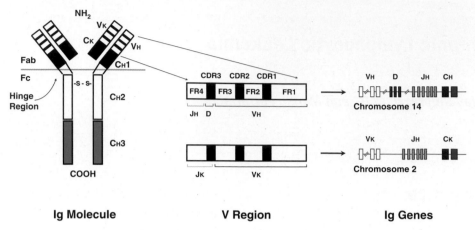

Ig Molecule   **V Region**   **Ig Genes**

Figure 7.1 Ig molecules and their genes. Ig molecules can be divided into two fragments, Fab and Fc, by enzymatic digestion; the former fragment engages antigen and the latter fragment mediates effector functions. The two fragments differ in *IgV* gene composition, with the Fab region, containing the antigen-binding site, being composed predominantly of the Ig variable region gene segments (*IGHV*, *IGHD*, and *IGHJ*) and the Fc region composed completely by an *IGHC* gene.

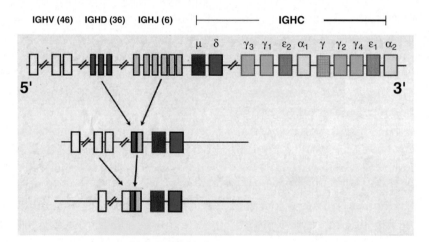

Figure 7.2 *IGHV* gene rearrangements. To code for a complete Ig molecule containing both Fab and Fc regions, several *Ig* genes need to be brought together from distinct locations and joined. This is a multistep process involving first the rearrangement of one of thirty-six *IGHD* gene segments with one of six IGHJ segments. Subsequently this unit is rearranged and combined with one of forty-six *IGHV* genes. In normal B-cell development, the first rearrangement contains the *IGHC* μ gene.

CHARACTERIZING THE HETEROGENEITY OF B-CLL BY MOLECULAR AND CLINICAL SUBTYPES

Based on their mutation status, B-CLL patients can be divided into two groups: those whose B-CLL cells use unmutated IgV_H genes (U-CLL) and those whose B-CLL cells use mutated $Ig\ V_H$ genes (M-CLL). Initially, it was believed that the two types of B-CLL cells could be generated by virgin and memory cells, respectively, although, as we shall discuss, there is now evidence

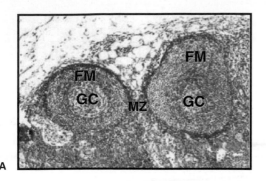

A

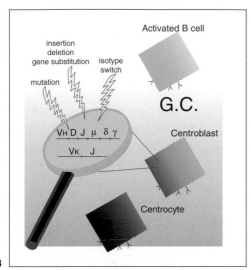

B

Figure 7.3 Germinal center and the germinal center reaction. *A*, Photomicrograph of two adjacent germinal centers within a mesenteric lymph node, with germinal center (GC), follicular mantle (FM), and marginal zone (MZ) areas. *B*, On close inspection of the DNA sequence of the rearranged *IgVHDJH*, one notices somatic changes that arise during the time the activated B cell resides in the GC. These changes involve predominantly point mutations and isotype class switching, although other less frequent events such as nucleotide deletion or insertion can occur. These changes occur at the centroblast stage of B-cell maturation; at the centrocyte stage, rescue from apoptosis is achieved by antigen binding through the BCR and T-cell interaction.

that both B-CLL subtypes derive from (auto)antigen-experienced B cells.

B-CLL cells are monoclonal B-cell expansions as documented by the expression of monotypic (i.e., either κ or λ) surface Ig and the CD19 antigen; this is in line with the presence of monoclonal rearrangements of VDJ genes in the leukemic cells. Most B-CLL cells also express activation markers and, like normal activated B cells, have low levels of surface IgM and IgD. The expression of CD5, usually thought of as a lineage marker, is characteristic of B-CLL cells and should be considered part of their activation status as it can with normal B cells when stimulated through several receptors, including the BCR. The presence of these markers and the degree of activation varies in different B-CLL cases.

B-CLL clones can be further subdivided based on their activation marker expression: in one subgroup, the majority of leukemic cells express two activation markers, that is, CD38 and ZAP-70; and in the other, the majority of the cells lack these markers. The two molecules appear to be involved in the regulation of signals delivered by the BCR. The CD38$^+$ ZAP-70$^+$ B-CLL subset is primarily characterized by the presence of more members of the leukemic clone-bearing markers of activated B cells. These activation marker-defined subgroups also differ in their expression of several other molecules up-regulated by cellular activation.

In comparing these two subsetting schemes – the first based on IgV_H mutation status and the second on activation markers – CD38$^+$ZAP-70$^+$ B-CLL clones generally use unmutated IgV_H genes, whereas CD38$^-$ZAP-70$^-$ B-CLL clones mainly use mutated IgV_H region genes. Although the subdivision into CD38$^+$ZAP-70$^+$ U-CLL and CD38$^-$ZAP-70$^-$ M-CLL is true for the majority of patients, it is not universal since about 25 percent of cases are discordant for the expression of the three markers.

It is interesting to note the correlation between the molecular characterizations of the patients' clones with the patients' clinical course. Of major clinical and investigative importance are the observations that IgV_H gene mutation status and ZAP-70 and CD38 expression have clinical relevance, since cases in whom the majority of the cells express CD38, ZAP-70, and exhibit unmutated IgV_H genes have a more aggressive clinical course (Figure 7.4). Correspondingly, those patients whose clones are in the main CD38$^-$ZAP-70$^-$ and express mutated IgV_H genes generally fare better and have a good prognosis. In those individual cases that are discordant for the expression of these markers, there is nevertheless generally a direct correlation

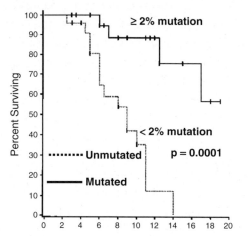

Figure 7.4 *IGHV* mutation status is a robust prognostic marker in B-cell-type chronic lymphocytic leukemia (B-CLL). CLL cases can be divided into two categories based on the presence of somatic mutations in the expressed *IGHV* gene. Those patients whose CLL cells have an IgV_H gene that differs by greater than 2 percent from its germ line counterpart have a much longer survival time than those patients whose cells use an IgV_H gene that differs by less than 2 percent. This distinction has major prognostic value. Reprinted by permission from Damle RN, Wasil T, Fais F, et al. *IgV* gene mutation status and CD38 expression as novel prognostic indicators in chronic lymphocytic leukemia. *Blood*. 1999;94:1840–1847.

between the number of unfavorable markers and clinical outcome.

DEVELOPMENT OF B-CLL FROM NORMAL B LYMPHOCYTES: SIGNALS AND MECHANISMS INITIATING THE GROWTH AND ACCUMULATION OF LEUKEMIC LYMPHOCYTES

The major events in tumorigenesis have traditionally been grouped into inducing and promoting factors. Inducing factors cause transforming mutations, whereas promoting factors sustain the proliferation and survival of cells undergoing or having undergone transforming mutations. It is useful to apply such principles to B-CLL.

Despite active research, to date no genetic aberration (inducing factor), shared by all patients, has been found in B-CLL. The monoclonality of B lymphocytes that develop in this disease implies that such a lesion existed in the cells initiating the clone. Although characteristic DNA abnormalities can occur later in the development of B-CLL clones, these are rarely found in the initial phases of the disease.

In contrast, several stimulatory signals delivered from the microenvironment may represent important promoting factors in the development and evolution of the disease. One of these – antigen stimulation – appears to play a major role in the pathogenesis of B-CLL; this conclusion is based on the existence of remarkable similarities in the structures of BCRs of unrelated patients. This similarity in BCR structure is especially striking for about 25 percent of patients, with some patients' clones using identical IgV_H, D, and J_H genes. Extraordinarily, in some of these cases, these rearranged Ig heavy-chain genes are paired with identical IgV_L genes, yielding antigen-binding sites that are virtually identical at the amino acid level. Given the enormous number of possible combinations of IgV gene segments encoding antibody-binding domains, one would not expect to find B-CLL patients having such structurally similar "stereotypic" BCRs by chance until well over 1 million cases have been screened. Hence, their occurrence is not likely random, making a plausible argument for the importance of antigen stimulation and drive in this disease.

Foreign antigens or autoantigens could prompt normal B lymphocytes to become B-CLL cells by selecting B-cell clones with restricted stereotypic BCRs. The nature of the antigens that select for these highly restricted BCRs (possibly unique to B-CLL) is largely unknown, although currently under investigation. It may be they result from infection due to a specific microbe common among patients, which has been found for gastric lymphomas. Alternative possibilities are that both environmental and autologous antigens may be involved. Indeed, it appears that intermittent and interchangeable encounters with microbial antigens and autoantigens, especially those generated during cell death and oxidative and other forms of stress, are key.

How would the transition from normal B cells to leukemic cells via antigen stimulation occur? Normal B lymphocytes using unmutated IgV genes produce antibodies that are frequently polyreactive, binding carbohydrates, nucleic acids, and phospholipids. Such antibodies provide the first line of defense against microorganisms and promote the clearance of autoantigens and their fragments. B-CLL cells frequently display polyreactive BCRs, thereby making it possible that they derive from normal polyreactive B lymphocytes that have been repeatedly stimulated in

vivo by a combination of nonprotein self- and microbial antigens.

Similarly, such a mechanism could also promote the origin of M-CLL. As already mentioned, IgV_H gene mutations can occur without T-cell help in marginal zones outside of GCs. Because mutations can sometimes favor autoreactivity, such autoreactive B cells would become expanded. However, expansion would stop if IgV gene mutations alter BCR structure in such a way that antigen binding is no longer sufficient to induce B-cell signaling.

With continued expansion leading (or not) to accumulation of $IgVH$ gene mutations as explained by the T-cell-dependent versus T-cell-independent models mentioned earlier, it becomes increasingly likely that a cell develops a genetic abnormality as in an initial inducing lesion that would lead to relatively unrestrained expansion. Such a cell is primed for leukemic transformation.

A hypothesis such as this implies that it might be possible to detect clonal expansions in healthy subjects. In fact, small numbers of apparently clonal B cells with B-CLL cell characteristics do exist in the blood of about 3.5 percent of disease-free individuals. An even higher proportion of such clones have been found in the blood of first-degree relatives of patients with B-CLL (as often as 12 percent). Although such studies of the BCRs of B lymphocyte expansions in normal disease-free individuals are limited, they further support this hypothesis in that these expansions are not only monoclonal but also use some of the same genes commonly encoding the BCRs of B-CLL clones.

In addition to antigen stimulation, B-CLL cells also receive receptor-mediated signals as well as soluble factors, such as cytokines and chemokines, from other lymphoid and nonlymphoid cells. In particular, it is thought that in vivo B-CLL cell interactions with stromal cells and "nurselike" cells can rescue normally (ex vivo) apoptosis-prone B-CLL cells from death. The natural ligand of CD38, CD31, is displayed on stromal and nurselike cells as well as on endothelial cells and might be involved in setting up these rescue signals. Such contact-derived and soluble signals can go on to up-regulate anti-apoptotic genes, such as *Bcl-2*, *survivin*, and *Mcl-1*, which could rescue B-CLL cells from apoptosis and facilitate their growth.

CORRELATIONS BETWEEN THE CELLULAR AND MOLECULAR FEATURES OF THE DISEASE WITH THE CLINICAL COURSE OF B-CLL

How might features of the repertoire of IgV_H genes used by B cells in B-CLL, the mutation status of these genes, and expression of molecules related to cellular activation and BCR signal transduction (CD38 and ZAP-70) be relevant to the clinical course of B-CLL? The disease manifests differently in different patients, depending on the utilization of mutated or unmutated IgV_H genes and the expression of ZAP-70 and CD38 by the leukemic cells (Figure 7.5). One explanation is that activation via the BCR following recognition of (self-)antigens activates the cells in vivo, accompanied by expression of CD38 and ZAP-70. Because the majority of U-CLL clones contain a self-reacting BCR, while most M-CLL clones do not, it is not unexpected that more activation markers are found on U-CLL cells. In addition, B-CLL clones from patients in different prognostic subsets differ in signaling capacity, with an intact BCR signal transduction pathway found most fre-

quently among patients exhibiting unfavorable prognostic markers. Thus, continuous (auto)antigenic stimulation would likely represent a major factor for U-CLL cases and much less likely for M-CLL.

Similarly, there is a rough correspondence between the clinical course of patients and the development of chromosomal abnormalities in their clones. Recurrent chromosomal lesions typically found in B-CLL patients include deletions at 13q14.3, 11q22–23, 17p13, and 6q21, and amplifications of all or portions of chromosome 12. Deletion at 13q14.3 is found in greater than half of B-CLL cases over time and is linked to loss of two micro-RNAs that can regulate *Bcl-2* expression. However, this particular chromosomal abnormality is not especially dangerous because patients exhibiting this deletion on one allele and no other DNA lesions in their clones have a clinical course that is benign and comparable to normal age-stratified individuals. In contrast, deletions at 11q22–23, 17p13, and 6q21 are generally associated with more aggressive disease, perhaps because these deletions may affect important genes such as *p53* (17p13 deletion), and *ataxia telangiectasia mutated* (*ATM*; 11q22–23 deletion). Longitudinal studies, albeit on a relatively limited number of patients, demonstrated that these ominous cytogenetic abnormalities accumulate progressively in the course of the disease and more frequently in patients with U-CLL.

These considerations are in line with the results of in vivo labeling experiments that involve incorporation of nonradioactive deuterium into newly synthesized DNA of dividing cells. These studies have shown B-CLL clones to be dynamic, having measurable birth rates from about 0.1 to >1.0 percent of the clone/day. Although only a minority of cells in a B-CLL clone can

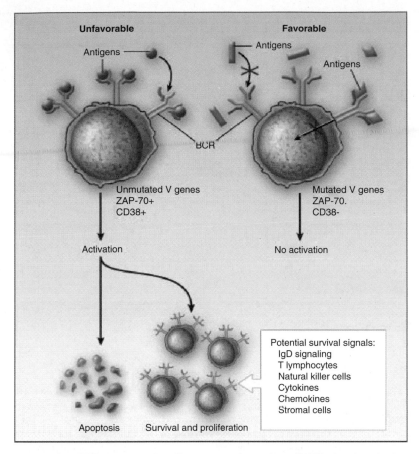

Figure 7.5 Differences in B cell's receptor for antigen (BCR) signaling in the two subgroups of B-cell–type chronic lymphocytic leukemia (B-CLL). B-CLL clones from patients with unmutated IgV_H genes (U-CLL) frequently differ from those from mutated $IgVH$ (M-CLL) patients in the ability to transduce an activation signal through the BCR. In the case of U-CLL, patients that are more likely to have an unfavorable clinical course, BCR-mediated signals deliver an apoptotic signal unless influenced by other survival signals. In the case of M-CLL patients who are more likely to have a more favorable clinical course, BCR-mediated signals are ineffective either because the BCR has been altered and no longer binds available (auto)antigens or because after antigen binding the BCR is incapable of signaling due to anergy. Reprinted with permission from Chiorazzi N, Rai KR, Ferrarini M. Chronic lymphocytic leukemia. *N Engl J Med*. 2005;352:804–815.

be shown to divide using this approach, estimates of the leukemic cell burden of a typical B-CLL patient are of the order of about 10^{12} cells, and therefore about 10^9 to 10^{10} new leukemic cells would be generated daily. Such rates of cell division are sufficient to permit more dangerous clonal variants to emerge and to influence clinical course and outcome over time.

SUMMARY REMARKS ON THE DEVELOPMENT, GROWTH, AND EVOLUTION OF B-CLL

On the basis of the foregoing information, we propose a model for the development of B-CLL (Figure 7.6). B-CLL cells are able to avoid apoptosis and even to proliferate by receiving growth and stimulatory

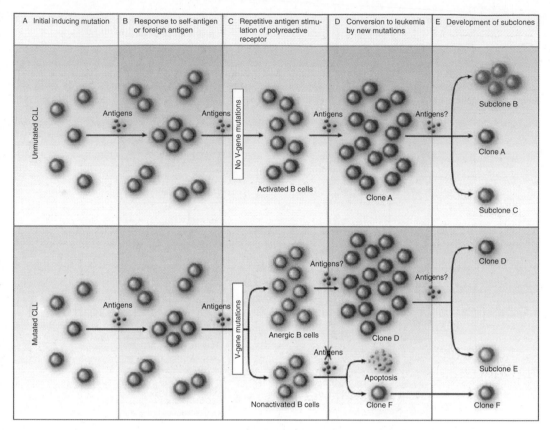

Figure 7.6 Model to explain the development and evolution of B-CLL. See text for description. Reprinted with permission from Chiorazzi N, Rai KR, Ferrarini M. Chronic lymphocytic leukemia. *N Engl J Med*. 2005;352:804–815.

signals from the environment delivered through their BCR or other receptors; these signals likely involve autologous and foreign antigens, cytokines, and chemokines, as well as yet-to-be-defined ligands on accessory and stromal cells. The cell's BCR mediates major growth effects in cases for which the receptor is polyreactive, binding autoantigens and foreign antigens, while maintaining its capacity to transmit stimulatory signals to the cell nucleus. Both self-reactivity and intact BCR signal-transducing capacity are more frequently found in U-CLL; hence, the more active clonal expansion and clinical aggressiveness of patients with such clones.

Because in vitro observations demonstrate the absence of lesions in the major apoptotic pathways, our model posits the absence of an intrinsic cell death defect in the majority of the leukemic clones. We do not rule out the possibility that developing genetic alterations in the evolving clone can tip the balance between pro- and anti-apoptotic molecules in such a way as to favor B-CLL cell survival. However, the influence of external signals appears to dominate based on current knowledge. This is in line with the in vivo labeling studies indicating the dynamic nature of CLL clones.

ANIMAL MODELS OF B-CLL

While an enormous amount of new information has been gleaned by directly studying human B-CLL cells, animal models are now contributing to our understanding of the human disease. For example, New Zealand Black (NZB) mice spontaneously develop, with age, an expansion of IgM^+CD5^+ B cells that resembles B-CLL. However, because frank leukemia occurs randomly in only a minor subset of animals, this model has been used sparingly.

In recent years, however, a variety of transgenic mouse models have been developed that lead to diseased phenotypes resembling human B-CLL more closely and reproducibly. We focus on three models that have been especially helpful.

Transgenic mice expressing the *TCL1* gene in murine B cells develop a polyclonal expansion of B lymphocytes early in life that becomes progressively more restricted until a monoclonal population emerges after about one year in most animals. The genetic and phenotypic features of this murine leukemia resemble those of the aggressive, treatment-resistant cases of human U-CLL. Although it is of interest that *TCL1* is an activator of the PI3K-Akt oncogenic signaling pathway, a pathway not infrequently active in human CLL, the extent to which overexpression of this gene leads to human B-CLL remain to be elucidated, as an overexpression of *TCL1* in human B-CLL patients is not uniform.

Another mouse model that develops features resembling human B-CLL involves the overexpression of two genes: *BCL-2* and *TRAF2* (TNF-receptor-associated factor 2). This double transgenic animal is especially intriguing because of the already mentioned recent work showing that the deletion at 13q14, often seen in human B-CLL, involves the loss of micro-RNAs 15a and 16-1, which affects expression of *BCL2*. As with the *TCL1* transgenic mice, these animals develop $CD5^+$ B-cell clones,

eventually with massive splenomegaly and leukemia.

In the third transgenic model, overexpression of *APRIL* (*a pro*liferation *i*nducing *li*gand) in murine T cells leads indirectly to B-cell proliferation and survival because of signaling through its receptors BCMA and TACI. Unlike the previous two transgenic animals, however, expansions of $CD5^+$ B cells occur in only 40 percent of animals, with these B cells locating predominantly in the spleen and rarely passing into the blood. Nevertheless, as *APRIL*'s action involves the TRAFs and leads to NFκB activation, this model may prove helpful in linking signals from soluble ligands and surface receptors to the NF,κB pathway, a pathway known to be constitutively active in some B-CLL clones.

Finally, transfer of human B-CLL cells into immune-deficient mice may bypass the ex vivo apoptosis tendency of B-CLL cells, enabling their survival and amplification in vivo. Such an approach may also make it possible to define and test new therapeutics to treat this currently incurable disorder.

CLINICAL IMPLICATIONS AND THE DEVELOPMENT OF NOVEL THERAPEUTICS

Currently used clinical staging systems defined by Rai and by Binet help clinicians to monitor disease progression and decide when to treat patients. Because of difficulties distinguishing patients with poor prognosis at the onset of disease using these staging systems, the generally used practice is to wait to start therapy until the patient's clinical course becomes evident ("wait and watch" mode). However, the molecular and cellular markers that reflect intrinsic properties of leukemic cells present at the disease onset can help to distinguish patients that will follow worse clinical courses, regardless of their Rai and Binet risk categories at diagnosis. Although determination of *IgVH* gene mutation status is not yet routinely available, measurement of CD38 and ZAP-70 has become more widely available. Thus, although the wait-and-watch mode is still being followed in current clinical practice, it may be substituted for by new more aggressive strategies in the future. The new prognostic markers indicate that 30–50 percent of the patients have features portending a poor outcome, and therefore an early start of therapy may be justified in such poor-prognosis groups. This strategy is plausible, considering that continued proliferation and expansion of the neoplastic clone facilitates accumulation of ominous cytogenetic abnormalities. However, before any recommended guidelines can be proposed, clinical trials must test the use of early intervention in patients in poor-prognosis groups.

New knowledge about the biology of B-CLL can provide clues for novel therapeutic targets. For example, since B-CLL cells must interact with the stroma in bone marrow or other peripheral lymphoid tissues to survive, furthering our knowledge of these interactions may generate new objectives for innovative therapies. Another compelling set of options may derive from specific inhibition of the BCR or CD38 signaling pathways or other pathways in which ZAP-70 is crucial. Likewise, the possibility of using cell-cycle-specific drugs is worth being explored in clinical trials, given the documented active turnover of B-CLL cells. Finally, because up to 20 percent of patients with the worst prognostic markers have stereotypic antigen receptors, these common structures may be feasible as vulnerable points of attack. As the antigens that engage these receptors become more precisely defined, it may be possible to use these to develop an arsenal of specific therapies.

BIBLIOGRAPHY

REVIEWS

Chiorazzi N, Ferrarini M. B cell chronic lymphocytic leukemia: lessons learned from studies of the B cell antigen receptor. *Annu Rev Immunol.* 2003;21:841–894.

Chiorazzi N, Rai KR, Ferrarini M. Chronic lymphocyrtic leukemia. *N Engl J Med.* 2005;352:804–815.

Ferrarini M, Chiorazzi N. Recent advances in the molecular biology and immunobiology of chronic lymphocytic leukemia. *Semin Hematol.* 2004;41:207–223.

Stevenson F, Caligaris-Cappio F. Chronic lymphocytic leukemia: revelations from the B-cell receptor. *Blood.* 2004; 103(12):4389–4395.

SUGGESTED READING

Bichi R, Shinton SA, Martin ES, et al. Human chronic lymphocytic leukemia modeled in mouse by targeted TCL1 expression. *Proc Natl Acad Sci USA.* 2002;99:6955–6960.

Binet JL, Auquier A, Dighiero G, et al. A new prognostic classification of chronic lymphocytic leukemia derived from a multivariate survival analysis. *Cancer.* 1981;48:198–206.

Burger JA, Kipps TJ. Chemokine receptors and stromal cells in the homing and homeostasis of chronic lymphocytic leukemia B cells. *Leuk Lymphoma.* 2002;43:461–466.

Calin GA, Dumitru CD, Shimizu M, et al. Frequent deletions and down-regulation of micro-RNA genes *miR15* and *miR16* at 13q14 in chronic lymphocytic leukemia. *Proc Natl Acad Sci USA.* 2002;99:15524–15529.

Dameshek W. Chronic lymphocytic leukemia – an accumulative disease of immunologically incompetent lymphocytes. *Blood.* 1967;29(suppl):566–584.

Damle RN, Wasil T, Fais F, et al. Ig V gene mutation status and CD38 expression as novel prognostic indicators in chronic lymphocytic leukemia. *Blood.* 1999;94:1840–1847.

Deaglio S, Capobianco A, Bergui L, et al. CD38 is a signaling molecule in B-cell chronic lymphocytic leukemia cells. *Blood.* 2003;102:2146–2155.

Dohner H, Stilgenbauer S, Benner A, et al. Genomic aberrations and survival in chronic lymphocytic leukemia. *N Engl J Med.* 2000;343:1910–1916.

Fais F, Ghiotto F, Hashimoto S, et al. Chronic lymphocytic leukemia B cells express restricted sets of mutated and unmutated antigen receptors. *J Clin Invest.* 1998;102:1515–1525.

Ghia P, Caligaris-Cappio F. The indispensable role of microenvironment in the natural history of low-grade B-cell neoplasms. *Adv Cancer Res.* 2000;79: 157–173.

Ghia P, Prato G, Scielzo C, et al. Monoclonal CD5+ and CD5- B-lymphocyte expansions are frequent in the peripheral blood of the elderly. *Blood.* 2004;103:2337–2342.

Hamblin TJ, Davis Z, Gardiner A, Oscier DG, Stevenson FK. Unmutated Ig VH genes are associated with a more aggressive form of chronic lymphocytic leukemia. *Blood.* 1999;94:1848–1854.

Messmer BT, Messmer D, Allen SL, et al. *In vivo* measurements document the dynamic cellular kinetics of chronic lymphocytic leukemia B cells. *J Clin Invest.* 2005;115:755–764.

Pekarsky Y, Zanesi N, Aqelian RI, Croce CM. Animal models of chronic lymphocytic leukemia. *J Cell Biochem.* 2006;100: 1109–1118.

Rai KR, Sawitsky A, Cronkite EP, Chanana AD, Levy RN, Pasternack BS. Clinical staging of chronic lymphocytic leukemia. *Blood.* 1975;46:219–234.

Rassenti LZ, Hunynh L, Toy TL, et al. ZAP-70 compared with immunoglobulin heavy-chain gene mutation status as a predictor of disease progression in chronic lymphocytic leukemia. *N Engl J Med.* 2004;351:893–901.

Rawstron AC, Yuille MR, Fuller J, et al. Inherited predisposition to CLL is detectable as subclinical monoclonal B-lymphocyte expansion. *Blood.* 2002;100:2289–2890.

Wiestner A, Rosenwald A, Barry TS, et al. ZAP-70 expression identifies a chronic lymphocytic leukemia subtype with unmutated immunoglobulin genes, inferior clinical outcome, and distinct gene expression profile. *Blood.* 2003;101:4944–4951.

Zupo S, Isnardi L, Megna M, et al. CD38 expression distinguishes two groups of B-cell chronic lymphocytic leukemias with different responses to anti-IgM antibodies and propensity to apoptosis. *Blood.* 1996;88:1365–1374.

8. Immunology of HIV Infections

Anders G. Vahlne, M.D., Ph.D.

INTRODUCTION

An estimated 33 million people globally are infected with the AIDS virus (HIV-1). Most of the infected individuals are poor, live in developing countries, and have little access to health care. Although initiatives are under way to bring proper medications to these individuals via a large infusion of money, this will benefit only approximately 2.5 million individuals and prevent 12 million new cases, as pointed out in a 2007 *New York Times* editorial. The remainder of these infected individuals will continue to increase the number of newly infected individuals. In this context, the medications decrease the viral load in treated individuals, but medications are expensive and would not reach many of the infected individuals living in developing countries.

Thus, many researchers are focusing on studies of the immunological concepts involved in the disease, not only to understand in greater detail why some individuals remain uninfected (they are not immune since some "resistant" women later acquire human immunodeficiency virus, or HIV), despite repeated exposure to infected individuals, but also to explore various vaccine candidates and concepts that might prevent the disease before exposure to the virus – candidates that would be cheap to make and inexpensive to deliver.

IMMUNOLOGICAL AND BIOLOGICAL PARAMETERS OF DISEASE

The pattern of disease progression has now been well documented. Following infection with the virus, the virus hones to and infects cells with CD4 receptors. During the early phase, individuals may experience a flu-like illness with mild fever, cough, and occasional chills. The symptoms subside, and the individual may be asymptomatic for many years. In reality, the disease is progressing, and it is a long battle between the immune response with production of new $CD4^+$ cells and the dying (apoptotic) HIV-infected CD4 cells. Eventually, the host immune system deteriorates, and the individual succumbs to the complications secondary to loss of the cellular immune system (see Figures 8.1 and 8.2). The pattern and complications are quite similar to those seen in primary immunodeficiency diseases (see Chapter 5). However, it has been a well-known observation that some individuals, especially sex workers with repeated exposure to the virus, are relatively resistant to HIV acquisition.

One of the earliest markers in the progression of HIV-1 infection was the presence of NEF in the viral strain. NEF is a 27–34 D myrisolated protein unique to primate lente viruses. A functional NEF protein is important for the development of high viremia and AIDS in simian immunodeficiency virus (SIV) in infected rhesus

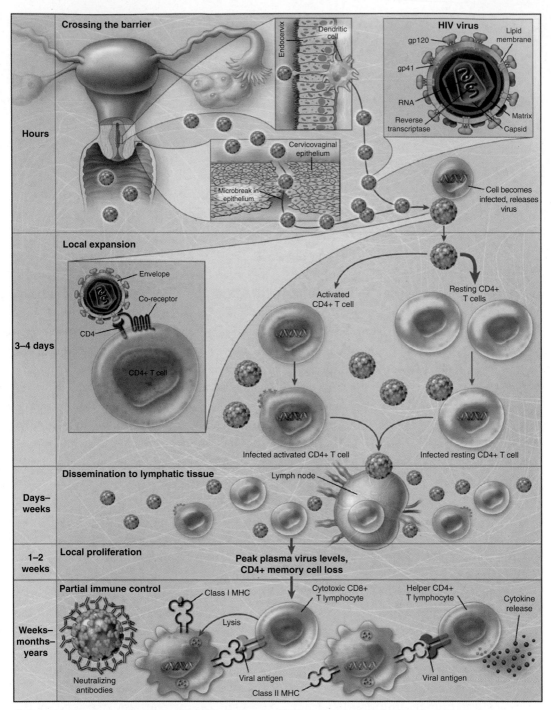

Figure 8.1 Early events in the vaginal transmission of HIV, modeled after studies of simian immunodeficiency virus infection in nonhuman primates. The binding of the HIV gp120 envelope protein to CD4 T cells results in conformation change in the envelope, interaction with the co-receptor, and fusion of the viral and cell membranes, thus giving the HIV genome access to the interior of the cell. The infected cells are carried first to draining lymph nodes and then spread systemically. HIV-specific immune responses, including increases in CD8[+] T cells and eventually neutralizing antibodies, only partially control infection. As a result, in the absence of effective vaccination or therapy, a slow and continued depletion of CD4[+] T cells ensues and there is a progression to AIDS. Reprinted by permission from Macmillan Publishers: Haase AT. Perils at mucosal front lines for HIV and SIV and their hosts. *Nat Rev Immunol.* 2005;5:783–792.

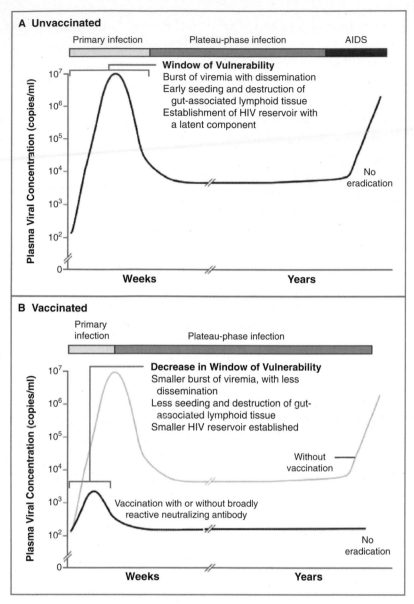

Figure 8.2 Panel *A* shows the course of infection in unvaccinated persons. The primary stage of HIV infection (yellow) starts with a burst of viremia, dissemination of the virus, early seeding and destruction of gut-associated lymphoid tissue, and establishment of a viral reservoir with a latent component. HIV levels in plasma then decline to a set point that lasts from months to years. Eventually, in the absence of effective therapy, the virus escapes immune control and AIDS results (red). Panel *B* shows the hypothetical course of infection in vaccinated persons. A T-cell vaccine might decrease the burst of viremia and dissemination that occurs in primary infection (yellow), preserving gut-associated lymphoid tissue, diminishing the viral reservoir, decreasing virus levels at the set point, and increasing the length of time that viral levels are controlled (blue).

macaques. An important observation first noted in the macaques and later in humans was that animals infected with NEF-deleted virus were resistant to subsequent challenge with pathogenic wild-type viruses. This was followed by the observation in humans that some individuals with long-term non-progressive HIV-1 infection (persons who showed no clinical or immunological signs of immunodeficiency despite being HIV seropositive for over a decade) turned out to be infected with viruses carrying deletion in their NEF gene.

More recently, a large body of evidence has appeared that shows that NEF has many important effects on many cells of the immune system. Both exogenous and endogenous NEF down-regulates HLA-ABC molecules critical for the initiation of cytotoxic T lymphocyte (CTL) responses, thus impairing antigen presentation to HIV-specific CD8[+] lymphocytes. NEF and gp120 also are able to down-regulate major histocompatibility complex class I (MHC-I) in dendritic cells (DCs) and introduction of exogenous NEF leads to up-regulation of MHC-II molecules, thereby favoring CD4[+] T-cell activation. This step increases the "pool" of lymphocytes permissive to infection. However, endogenous NEF does not modulate MHC-II surface expression; rather it induces a loss of co-stimulation. These results underscore the pleiotrophic action of NEF. On one hand, exogenous NEF triggers ABC-mediated bystander T-cell activation, ensuring viral spread, while endogenous NEF induces a loss of co-stimulation, favoring immune evasion.

Another area of interest has been the observation that NEF-pulsed DC produces a wide variety of cytokines and chemokines typical of mature DC. This up-regulation of cytokine production might promote bystander stimulation of T cells that cluster around DC and could enhance HIV-1 replication in CD4[+] T cells.

In summary, the selective effects of the NEF protein may markedly enhance viral pathogenesis and progression to disease. It does this by hijacking DC functional activity and favoring HIV replication via bystander activation of CD4+ cells and the escape of HIV-1 from immune surveillance by blocking CD8+ cells' functional competence. Thus, efforts directed toward blocking NEF influence in viral replication may have long-term beneficial effects on therapeutic management of the disease.

Approximately 5–10 percent of sex workers in Kenya remained HIV uninfected despite engaging in unprotected sex with many male clients and the frequent acquisition of other sexually transmitted infections. Because of the pioneering work of Plummer and associates, the scientific reasons for this extraordinary resistance to the virus in these women are beginning to unfold.

Turning first to examination of CD4[+] T-cell immune responses in seronegative sex workers compared with HIV-positive women, CD4[+] T cells that produced interferon gamma (IFN-γ) in response to HIV p24 were detected in exposed seronegative sex worker (ESN) women, albeit at a much lower level than in HIV-positive women. However, ESN women had a 4.5-fold stronger CD4[+] proliferation response to the p24 peptide compared with the HIV-positive group. These data suggest that CD4[+] T cells in ESN women recognize HIV and have an enhanced ability to proliferate to the p24 protein.

Perhaps more important has been the examination of the CD8[+] cells in these ESN individuals. Because IFN-γ production correlates with cytotoxic functions, the CD8[+] T lymphocyte IFN-γ response to HIV p24 peptide in ESN women was compared with HIV-positive individuals. Approximately 40 percent of ESN women had a CD8$^+$ IFN-γ-positive response, and this was five times lower in magnitude than that of HIV-positive women. The breadth of the response was very narrow and focused primarily on one peptide that is similar to KK10 protective peptide when compared with the HIV-positive group. In HIV-positive women, lower CD4$^+$ counts influenced the number of CD8$^+$ cells producing IFN-γ, which may undermine the ability to control HIV. These results indicate ESP women have an HIV-1 p24 peptide-specific CD8$^+$ IFN-γ response, providing evidence to the specificity needed for an effective HIV vaccine.

Further studies of these women centered around the known polymorphisms of the IL-4 gene and resistance to infection. Using microsatellite genotyping methods coupled with the genomic sequencing, three polymorphisms in the interferon regulatory factor (*IRF-1*) located at 619a, 179, and 6516 of the gene, showed association with resistance to HIV infection. Peripheral blood mononuclear cells from these patients showed significantly lower-based *IRF-1* expression and reduced responsiveness to IFN-γ stimulation. This study added *IRF-1*, a transcriptional immunoregulatory gene, to the list of genetic correlates of altered susceptibility to HIV-1.

One of the key cells in the immune surveillance system is the native DC, which is well equipped for activation of both the innate and adaptive immune response. It has been demonstrated that some DC-tropic viruses such as influenza virus leave DC function intact while other viruses such as HIV and cytomegalovirus have evolved strategies to impair DC functions, thereby enhancing the virus's ability to persist and escape immune surveillance.

DC interaction with HIV is relevant to the pathogenesis of AIDS because they are present in the mucosa and skin of humans and are believed to be the first HIV-1 targets following sexual transmission of the virus. Both myeloid DC and plasmacytoid DC possess the receptors for HIV entry; that is, CD4, CXR4, and CCR5 can be infected but with a lower efficacy than CD4$^+$ cells or macrophages. The long-term result of this infection is that DC remains a reservoir for the production and persistence of the HIV-1 virus, and the virus induces several functional impairments and variations in the DC population. Thus, the number of both myeloid DC (MDC) and peripheral DC (PDC) are significantly decreased in HIV-positive progressors, while remaining unaltered in HIV-positive long-term nonprogression. The destruction of these cells may be a consequence of direct lytic infection or as targets for specific CTL or through a block in DC development from peripheral CD34$^+$ stem cells. More recent evidence supports the notion that both midi and pad show impaired functional capacity in HIV-positive patients. Since both DC subsets participate in the initiation of innate and adaptive immune responses, infection, depletion, and dysfunction of DCs may contribute to the immunosuppression seen in HIV disease. Therefore, DCs play a dual role in HIV infection: they trigger both innate and adaptic immune responses to control the infection, but they also represent a viral reservoir for infection of permissive CD4$^+$ T cells.

Although the story of the African sex workers who seem to be immune to HIV infection has captured the imagination of many researchers, there is another model of natural immunity that needs examination in more detail. Most babies born to HIV-infected mothers also escape infection even after potential intrauterine exposure and, more important, exposure to virus-contaminating blood and secretions during labor and delivery. Finally, breast-fed infants ingest hundreds of liters of virus-infected breast milk. Many factors such as CD4 cell counts and viral load in the secretions must be considered. One should add that, like the sex worker model, it is a "real"-world situation of viral encounter opening a window to the "in vivo" infection moment. Although interesting, there are, however, several drawbacks to the model; notably, the newborn is immunologically immature compared with later in life. However, their capacity to produce CC cytokines is greater compared with their mothers whether she is HIV infected or not (see Figure 8.3). This is consistent with the expected skewing toward a stronger innate response rather than the adaptive response.

The initially unexpected finding of HIV-specific CD4$^+$ and CD8$^+$ T-cell responses among uninfected sex workers paved the way to the fact that natural protective immunity may exist. It has been difficult to repeat these studies in infants because of

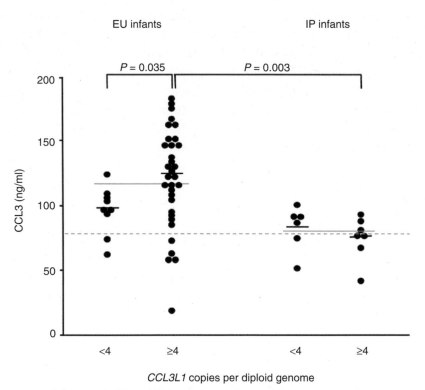

CCL3L1 copies per diploid genome

Figure 8.3 CCL3 production by cord blood cells. CCL3 concentrations in mitogen-induced mononuclear cell cultures of umbilical cord blood from exposed and uninfected (EU) and intrapartum-infected (IP) infants are stratified on the basis of low numbers (less than 4) or high numbers (4 or more) of CCL3L1 copies per diploid genome. Small, black horizontal lines, median values; solid gray lines across low and high groups, median values for each total group; gray dashed line, median value for uninfected controls. Reprinted by permission from Macmillan Publishers: Tiemessen CT, Kuhn L. CC chemokines and protective immunity: insights gained from mother-to-child transmission of HIV. *Nat Immunol.* 2007;8:219–222.

small blood volumes. Nevertheless, some studies, using IL-2 production as a marker following stimulation with envelope peptides, have shown that none of the children with apparent HIV-specific T-cell response developed HIV infections despite exposure to HIV through breast-feeding.

However, this observation does not completely explain why some babies are infected with HIV and others are not. In a landmark study, Gonzalez and colleagues (2005) showed that segmental duplication occurred in the gene CCL3L1-like chemokine. CCL3L1 as well as CCL3 are ligands for CCR5 and are associated with lower susceptibility to HIV. Moreover, a study of maternal-infant HIV transmission has shown that a phenotype of deficient mitogen-induced CCL3 production is associated with a greater risk of HIV infection during labor and delivery. Thus the maternal-infant model has demonstrated that the protein encoded for one or both of the functional genes (*CCL3* or *CCL3L1*) is involved, suggesting that the abundance of this protein may be important in HIV-protective immunity. Functional capacity, not just gene copies (four or more in some cases) of these proteins, is important. This suggests that the "susceptibility phenotype" lives at the level of induction of gene expression (see Figure 8.3) of *CCL3* and *CCL3L1*, resulting in qualitative differences in protein production.

Turning to their use as vaccine candidates, Tiemessen and colleagues (2007) suggest that, if CCL3 is a crucial molecule in protection against HIV by virtue of its adjuvant ability, it may be useful as a vaccine adjuvant. In this manner, one does not have to rely on the host's ability to produce it (production may be deficient in certain populations; see Figure 8.4).

Innate immunity has been mostly neglected in favor of HIV-specific

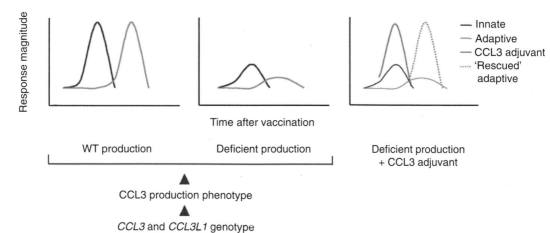

Figure 8.4 Possible influence of *CCL3* and *CCL3L1* genotype on the development of adaptive immunity to HIV vaccines and restoration of loss of function in people with deficient production through the provision of CCL3 as adjuvant. *CCL3* and *CCL3L1* genotypes determine the production phenotype as wild type (WT) or deficient (red arrowheads). *Left*, wild-type production of CCL3 as the critical component of a rapid innate immune response (red line) that "instructs" the effective development of subsequent adaptive immunity (green line). *Middle*, deficient production of CCL3 "translates" into an ineffective adaptive immune response. *Right*, provision of CCL3 as an adjuvant (blue line) compensates for deficient host production and restores the development of adaptive immunity to wild-type capability (dashed green line). Reprinted by permission from Macmillan Publishers: Tiemessen CT, Kuhn L. CC chemokines and protective immunity: insights gained from mother-to-child transmission of HIV. *Nat Immunol*. 2007; 8:219–222.

immunity in HIV vaccine studies. CCL3 production should be considered a correlate of protective immunity. A desired response would be sufficient production of CCL3 at the site of HIV and vaccine encounter. It is imperative to delineate the precise functions of CCL3 in the immune response to HIV, aside from its noncytolytic inhibitory effect on HIV, as the ability of CCL3 to drive the development of adaptive immunity might be the crucial factor in overall protection. Many important questions arise, given the findings outlined here. How should HIV vaccines be designed? How can people who would be poor responders to vaccines (deficient CCL3 producers) be identified? How can the genetically encoded loss of function be overcome, and how can molecules be identified that can compensate for this? Innate immunity must become a more integral component of studies of HIV vaccines, as understanding the interaction between innate and adaptive immunity may hold the key to understanding what constitutes protective immunity to HIV. Studies of uninfected infants born to HIV-infected mothers offer a unique human experimental model for extending the understanding of such phenomena.

ANIMAL MODELS OF HIV INFECTION

Although many questions concerned with HIV biology were first learned in cultured cell lines infected with HIV or SIV, it became obvious that these cultured lines did not truly mimic the wild-type infections seen in animal models. A number of small rodent models, such as the SCID mouse, were developed and were helpful but somewhat artificial and did not really mimic human disease.

In fact, a significant obstacle in HIV vaccine research has been the difficulty in developing an appropriate animal model with many of the features of human HIV infection. The only animals susceptible to experimental infections with HIV are chimpanzees, *Pantroglodytes*, and pigtail macaques, *Macaca nemestrina*. These animals maintain low levels of persistent virus but do not develop clinical manifestations of AIDS. In contrast, Asian monkeys, especially rhesus monkeys from India, are highly susceptible to SIVmac infection and progressively develop an immunodeficiency syndrome that is similar to human AIDS. Plasma viral levels during acute and chronic SIVmac251 infection in these animals parallel those observed in humans, with some animals containing virus spontaneously and progressing to disease slowly as in HIV-1 infected human long-term nonprogressors. In contrast, others maintain high viral loads and behave like human rapid progresses. As in HIV-1 infected humans, the cellular immune response to SIVmac during acute and chronic disease differs significantly, and evidence of immune escape has been well documented. This is particularly true of the mucosal immune system, especially the many $CD4^+$ CCR-5+ T cells in the gut-associated lymphoid tissue, the major site of viral replication and of $CD4^+$ T-cell depletion in SIV-infected macaques. This also mimics the human disease and thus the SIV macaque model is currently considered the most appropriate animal model for studies on potential protective immune responses against HIV.

A second animal model of HIV vaccine research is based on the use of SIV/HIV hybrid viruses that were engineered to carry the *env* gene from HIV into the content of the SIV genome. These viruses do replicate in rhesus macaques and after serial macaque passages do lead to the emergence of highly pathogenic SHIV variants that can wipe out circulating CD4$^+$ T cells within a few weeks and lead to a lethal immunodeficiency syndrome within a year of infection.

However, the problem has been whether these variants, like SHIV 89.6P, are relevant to HIV infections. For example, they exhibit an "X4" cellular tropism and are therefore easier to contain by vaccine-induced immune response than "R5" viruses such as SIV. If we could obtain SHIV strains with R5 tropism, this might be a better model to study.

The real problem with the monkey models is that experiments to evaluate vaccine efficacy requires challenging the vaccinated animals with high doses of virus to get 100 percent infection, that is, 10^3–10^5 TCID50 equivalent to 5×10^7 SIV RNA copies/ml. This is in marked contrast to natural exposure to HIV in humans wherein the doses of 10^3 HIV RNA copies/ml of seminal plasma have been reported. However, these results are quite different in mucosal challenge, wherein reported low doses (10–30 TCID50) with SIV results in the same viral and immunological kinetics of infection as high-dose challenges. Thus, this new type of mucosal challenge might change the results of preclinical vaccine efficacy studies in the future.

VACCINES TO PREVENT HIV INFECTION

Despite the many efforts to develop a safe and effective vaccine against HIV infection, the results to date have been negative or controversial at best. Among the reasons for this state of affairs have been the enormous genetic diversity of the virus and the unique features of the HIV envelope protein. One thing we have learned from studies of HIV pathogenesis, however, has been that a vaccine that induces a strong and specific T-cell immune response in the absence of broadly neutralizing antibodies may blunt initial viremia, even if the infection is not completely prevented. Moreover, they may prevent the mass destruction of CD4$^+$ T cells, thereby helping to control the infection and prolong disease-free survival.

Before we go to the actual vaccine candidates, some knowledge of the structure of the HIV is warranted. HIV, together with the simian, feline, and bovine immunodeficiency viruses (SIV, FIV, and BIV) all belong to the genus lentivirus in the family of *Retroviridae*. These viruses characteristically produce slowly progressive infections, and the replication depends on an active reverse transcriptase enzyme to transform the viral RNA genome into a proviral DNA copy that integrates into the host cell chromosome. This step provides the enormous genetic diversity of HIV isolates in the infected cell, since the reverse transcriptase step is often fraught with errors in replication.

Two types of HIV have been described: HIV-1 and HIV-2, the latter being less virulent, less transmissible, and confined mostly to West Africa. HIV-1 is phylogenetically close to SIVcpz commensural virus in chimpanzees, which probably arose as a specific transmission event from chimps to humans. However, SIVmac is the etiological agent of simian AIDS and has many of the features of HIV AIDS. HIV-1 is further divided into three major groups: M (major), O (outlier), and N (non M or O). Most of the strains responsible for the AIDS epidemic belong to the M group, and this group has been divided into ten different subgroups known as clades (A–K).

The genome of HIV is a single-stranded positive small RNA molecule, approximately 9.5 kbs in length and encodes the typical retrovirus proteins Gag further divided into M (matrix), C (capsid), and N (nucleocapsid); Pol, cleaved into protease, reverse transcriptase, and integrase; and ENV 160 kD glycoprotein, divided into an external gp120 and a trans-membrane gp41 subunit that together form trimeric spikes on the surface of the virion. Furthermore, the HIV genome encodes a variety of nonstructural proteins such as transactivation protein (Tat) splice regulator protein (Rev) and accessory proteins such as Nef, Vpr, and Vpn.

VACCINE CANDIDATES

There have been many attempts to construct a vaccine that is both protective and has a low cost of production; yet, there is still not a promising candidate. Part of the problem is that to be effective the vaccine has to be given early or before exposure to the virus. Ideally a vaccine could prevent the disease entirely or at least shut down the viremie phase (see panel B of Figure 8.4). For the sake of convenience, we have listed the vaccine approaches separately with their promises and caveats.

Live Attenuated Vaccines

The observation that NEF strains could offer protection against challenge with pathogenic SIV infections in rhesus macaques served as the model for the use of this type of attenuated vaccine. However, this mutant's drawback is that it produces a lifelong persistent viral infection in the host. The positive side is that although the attenuated vaccine does not prevent infection with a wild-type SIV infection, it does prevent that infection from going on to produce the disease AIDS. Thus, this approach does not appear feasible now. However, what is being explored is the nature of the protective immune response in these monkeys after infection with the attenuated virus.

Several reports raise the question whether these attenuated vaccines will give the broad protection so eagerly sought. As Anne Piantadosi and colleagues (2007) have pointed out, HIV-1 superinfection (reinfection) does not always protect against other strains. In their studies, they screened a cohort of high-risk Kenyan women by comparing partial *gag* and *envelope* sequences over a five-year period, beginning with the primary infection. Of thirty-seven women screened, seven were found to have superinfections, including cases in which both viruses were from the same HIV-1 subtype A. In five cases, the superinfecting strain was detected in only one of the two genomes examined, suggesting that recombination frequently occurs following HIV-1 superinfection. They conclude that superinfection commonly occurs after the immune response against the initial infection has had time to develop and mature. Supporting this claim was an earlier report by Altfeld et al. in *Nature* in which this superinfection occurred despite broad CD8[+] T-cell responses (twenty-five distinct epitopes) to many HIV viral proteins. They conclude that superinfection can occur in the setting of a strong and broadly directed virus-specific CD8[+] T-cell response.

Yet, other reports by Chakraborty and colleagues indicate that superinfection may not be so high. They studied fourteen HIV seroconcordant couples (i.e., partners were independently infected with different HIV-1 strains) with high risk of re-exposure to the virus. Phylogenetic analyses based on *pol* and *env* global sequences obtained from more than a 100 longitudinal plasma samples over one to four years failed to detect HIV-1 superinfection in this cohort of patients. They conclude that chronic HIV infection seems to confer protection against superinfection with a second HIV-1 strain. Obviously, more work needs to be done to determine what factors are responsible for superinfection in some individuals and protection in others, both at high risk of reinfection.

Inactivated Viral Vaccines

Although the initial results with inactivated vaccine were negative with high doses of formalin treatment (loss of antigenicity of the viral envelope proteins), it was quickly discovered that by using low doses of formalin, the antigenicity of the envelope proteins was preserved. This preparation was capable of inducing viral neutralizing antibodies in both mice and nonhuman primates. This area is presently being actively pursued, but the problem will be overcoming the rapidly changing antigens of the wild-type virus.

A second approach has been to inactivate the domains of two nucleocapsid protein zinc fingers. This has been achieved by treating these complexes with mild oxidation or alkylation procedures, which completely inactivates both HIV-1 and SIV but keeps the envelope glycoprotein spikes intact and functional. Studies in the SIV macaque model revealed that monkeys vaccinated with the inactivated virus were *not* protected against infection with the wild-type virus, but the levels of SIV viremia were low and there was no depletion of CD4+ T cells.

Subunit Vaccines

Most of the research efforts in HIV vaccines have gone into the subunit vaccines involving the gp120 envelope proteins, which also includes the gp41 domain. Both of these proteins do elicit neutralizing antibodies to the homologous vaccine strain but not to heterologous primary isolates in the animal model. Despite these caveats, two large-scale phase III clinical trials of this type of vaccine have been carried out involving 7,500 high-risk individuals. Neither of these trials showed a significant reduction in HIV infection in the vaccinated individuals, even with continuous booster shots during the three-year trial. A number of other trials involving trimeric gp140, a DNA vaccine encoding a V2-deleted gp140 and other combinations, are in various phases, but the results are not known at present.

Cellular Vaccines

A strong and specific T-cell immune response in the absence of broadly neutralizing antibodies may blunt the initial viremia, even if the infection is not completely prevented. Thus, more recent vaccine efforts have been directed toward stimulating the cellular immune response. Particular attention has been paid to those vaccines that induce an HIV-specific CD8+ CTL response whose role in the control of virus load and evolution of disease has been well documented in the macaque model. Although the T-cell vaccines do not prevent the HIV infection, they do help vaccinees who get infected to control viral replication and reduce viral loads, thus resulting in less risk of transmission of the disease to seronegative partners.

Vaccines have been based on this strategy with particular emphasis on the use of naked DNA vaccines and live recombinant vectors, for example, naked DNA vaccines expressing the HIV-1 *gag* gene and either IL-12 or Il-15, which was developed by Wyeth and is presently in several phase I trials in the United States, Brazil, and Thailand. DNA vaccines have been found to be most useful as priming vaccines in prime-boost strategies, using live recombinant vaccines for booster immunization.

While the original recombinant HIV vaccines used vaccinia virus and were well tolerated, safety considerations in immunodeficient hosts has led investigators to substitute the canarypox virus for the vaccinia virus. However, the immunogenicity of the pox-virus-based vaccines in humans has been relatively modest with less than 35 percent of the vaccinees scoring positive for T-cell responses. In contrast, replication-defective adenovirus type 5 (ad5) appears to be one of the most promising live virus vectors for HIV vaccines. Merck has used this complex and showed that 50 percent of the volunteers had significantly long-lasting $CD8^+$ T-cell responses to HIV-1 peptides. A trivalent recombinant ad5-*gag/pol/nef* complex has been engineered and retested in human volunteers. A phase II trial of this candidate is being investigated in 1,200 men and 400 women at high risk of exposure to HIV infection who will be followed for three years. The results of this trial will appear in 2008.

FUTURE DIRECTIONS FOR RESEARCH

The use of antiretroviral combination regimes has made significant advances in the treatment of HIV infections in industrialized countries. However, these treatments are expensive and would only reach a limited number of infected individuals, especially in developing countries where most of the epidemic is occurring.

Thus, the need for a safe, effective, inexpensive vaccine to prevent further spread of the infection becomes an increasingly important goal. Unfortunately, most of the vaccine trials to date have not been successful in this regard, and many investigators have turned their attention to vaccines that, if given early in the infection, may protect individuals from developing AIDS. A number of these vaccines show promise and are in various stages of clinical or nonhuman primate trials. As stated in the 2007 *New England Journal of Medicine* article by Johnson and Fauci, "There is optimism that even a less than perfect vaccine could benefit individual recipients and the at risk community…. However such a vaccine will have to be delivered as part of a comprehensive multifaceted prevention program."

These are, however, to be considered as first-generation vaccines. The ultimate goal will be to produce an effective preventive vaccine. This will require new thinking about vaccine approaches, innovative solutions, and persistence, but the total prevention of this devastating disease is a worthwhile goal.

BIBLIOGRAPHY

REVIEWS

Duerr A, Wasserheit JN, Corey L. HIV vaccines: new frontiers in vaccine development. *Clin Infect Dis*. 2006;43:500–511.

Girard MP, Osmanor SK, Kieny MP. A review of vaccine research and development: the human immunodeficiency virus (HIV). *Vaccine*. 2006;24:4062–4081.

Johnson MJ, Fauci AS. Current concepts: an HIV vaccine – evolving concepts. *New Engl J Med*. 2007;356:2073–2081.

SUGGESTED READING

Altfeld M, Allen TM, Yu XG, et al. HIV-1 superinfection despite broad CD8+ T cell responses containing replication of the primary virus. *Nature*. 2002;420:434–439.

Chakraborty B, Valer L, De Mendoza C, Soriano V, Quiñones-Mateu ME. Failure to detect human immunodeficiency virus type 1 superinfection in 28 HIV-seroconcordant individuals with high risk of reexposure to the virus. *AIDS Res Hum Retroviruses*. 2004;20: 1026–1031.

Devito C, Broliden K, Kaul R, et al. Mucosal and plasma IgA from HIV-1-exposed uninfected individuals inhibit HIV-1 transcytosis across human epithelial cells. *J Immunol*. 2000;165:5170–5176.

Devito C, Hinkula J, Kaul R, et al. Mucosal and plasma IgA from HIV-exposed seronegative individuals neutralize a primary HIV-1 isolate. *AIDS*. 2000;14:1917–1920.

Editorial. *New York Times*. June 1, 2007.

Ellenberger D, Otten R, Li B, et al. Evidence of protection after reported mucosal SHIV challenges to HIV-1 vaccinated rhesus types. AIDS Vaccine Meeting, Montreal Quebec, Canada. Abs. 110; 2005.

Gonzalez E, Kulkarni H, Mangamo A, et al. The influence of CCL3L1 gene-containing segmented duplications M HIV-1/AIDS susceptibility. *Science*. 2005;307:1434–1440.

Heeney JL. Primate models for AIDS vaccine development. *AIDS*. 1996;10(suppl A): S115–S122.

Kaul R, Dong T, Plummer FA, et al. CD8[+] lymphocytes respond to different HIV epitopes in seronegative and infected subjects. *J Clin Invest*. 2001;107(10):1303–1310.

Kaul R, Plummer FA, Kimani J, et al. HIV-1-specific mucosal CD8[+] lymphocyte responses in the cervix of HIV-1-resistant prostitutes in Nairobi. *J Immunol*. 2000;164:1602–1611.

Kaul R, Rowland-Jones SL, Kimani J, et al. Late seroconversion in HIV-resistant Nairobi prostitutes despite pre-existing HIV-specific CD8[+] responses. *J Clin Invest*. 2001;107:341–349.

Piantadosi A, Chohan B, Chohan V, et al. Chronic HIV-1 infection frequently fails to protect against superinfection. *PLoS Pathog*. 2007;3(11):e177.

Quaranta MC, Mattiol B, Giordoni L, Viora M. The immunoregulatory effects of HIV-1 Nef on dendritic cells and the pathogenesis of AIDS. *FASEB J*. 2006;20:2198–2208.

Rowland-Jones S, Pinheiro S, Kaul R. New insights into host factors in HIV-1 pathogenesis. *Cell*. 2001;104: 473–476.

Tiemessen CT, Kuhn L. CC chemokines and protective immunity: insights gained from mother-to-child transmission of HIV. *Nat Immunol*. 2007;8(3):219–222.

9. Immunological Aspects of Allergy and Anaphylaxis

Paul M. Ehrlich, M.D., and Jonathan D. Field, M.D., F.A.A.A.I.

INTRODUCTION

Adverse responses to otherwise innocuous substances we are exposed to constitute the crux of allergic reactions. Reaction to exposure to these substances may vary from a slight rash, easily treated with an antihistamine, leukotriene modifier, or corticosteroid cream, to a multisystemic reaction, with catastrophic consequences or anaphylaxis. All that will be discussed in this chapter have, as a common factor, various aspects of the immune system with inflammatory responses involving these seemingly innocuous substances.

Allergic reactions may be found in up to 20 percent of the general U.S. population, but by the age 6, 40 percent of the children in the United States have some sort of allergic problems. Although most of these children have respiratory problems, such as allergic rhinitis or bronchial asthma, many of those with allergies may also have atopic reactions to foods or medications. As antigens are slowly introduced into an infant's environment or diet, the child's propensity to deal with these new substances may not be developed. In addition, children's airways are small, their gastrointestinal tracts are not developed, and their immune systems are not ready to meet the challenges of these newly introduced proteins called *allergens*. Most responses are Gell and Coombs type I or immediate hypersensitivity reaction. This reaction will be described in the next section.

ALLERGIC HYPERSENSITIVITY

In 1964, Gell and Coombs classified four types of immunologically mediated hypersensitivity states. The majority of disease states encountered in the clinical practice of allergy are related to type I, or *immediate-type hypersensitivity*. In this model, an allergen interacts with preformed IgE on the surface of a mast cell or basophil. This interaction causes cross-linking of the FceRI receptor and release of multiple mediators, including histamine, leukotrienes, and various interleukins. Depending on the relative localization of release, clinical states such as *allergic asthma*, *allergic rhinitis*, or *systemic anaphylaxis* occur. Of the remaining clinical allergy hypersensitivity states, type IV, or *delayed-type hypersensitivity*, is most common. In this type, T-cell antigen receptors on T_H1 or T_H2 lymphocytes bind to tissue antigens, causing clonal expansion of lymphocytes and release of pro-inflammatory lymphokines. Distinct clinical entities such as *contact dermatitis* (e.g., poison ivy) or tuberculin skin test sensitivity in pulmonary tuberculosis may occur relative to the site of the tissue antigen.

Table 9.1 Gell and Coombs Classification of Immune-mediated Allergic Responses

Type	Mechanism	Responses
I	IgE mediated	Anaphylaxis, urticaria
II	Complement-mediated cytotoxicity	Cytopenias
III	Immune complex deposition	Vasculitis/ nephritis
IV	Delayed-type hypersensitivity	Dermatitis or hepatitis

ATOPY

Clinical allergic diseases are predominately type I, or IgE mediated. Approximately 40 percent of people in Western nations are inclined toward an exaggerated IgE response to multiple environmental allergens such as pollen or animal dander. This allergic state, known as *atopy*, is the result of multiple genetic and environmental factors.

Our current understanding of the development of an IgE response favors a T_H2 T-cell induction. When specific inhaled, ingested, or absorbed proteins, or allergens, appropriately stimulate this subset of the T-cell population, a series of cellular reactions occurs that leads to IgE antibody production.

Inhalation of most proteins does not cause IgE-mediated responses, whereas a limited number of small protein allergens can elicit such reactions. Although the mechanism of allergic induction is not completely clear, some general principles have emerged. Allergens presented transmucosally at very low doses induce IgE responses by T_H2 cells. This subset of cells produces the primary cytokines, interleukin-4 (IL-4) and interleukin-13 (IL-13). These interleukins interact with receptors on B lymphocyte cell surfaces, which promote class switching to the IgE antibody subclass. The subsequent class switch produces antigen-specific IgE antibodies with specificity toward common allergens such as pollen, animal dander, food, or venom.

Genetic studies of atopic families have identified regions on chromosome 11q and 5q that affect IgE production. Chromosome 5 contains multiple genes, including those for IL-4, IL-5, and granulocyte-macrophage colony-stimulating factor. Eosinophil survival and mast cell proliferation are just a few pro-allergic effects of these cytokines. Chromosome 11 encodes the beta subunit of the high-affinity IgE receptor. Increased expression of this receptor on mast cells leads to a more vehement response to small numbers of antigens. This increased expression explains how exposure to minute amounts of allergen, such as venom from a stinging insect, can produce systemic anaphylaxis.

Although atopy has a strong genetic component, environmental factors best explain the recent global trend toward increased prevalence of allergic disease. Predictive factors include the following: (1) decreased exposure to infectious disease during early childhood, (2) changes in diet, (3) higher levels of allergen exposure, and (4) increased environmental pollution. Of these factors, variances in exposure to infectious disease appear to have the greatest correlation with atopy. Epidemiological studies point out a negative association between atopic disease in children and a history of measles or hepatitis A virus infection. It is hypothesized that infections such as these tilt the production of cytokines toward interferon gamma (IFN-γ) and the T_H1 cytokines, thereby decreasing production of T_H2 allergic cytokines such as IL-4. This theory's attractiveness may be its ability to explain the global increase in atopy due to decreased infection rates in Westernized regions with aggressive vaccination programs. Current research trials use this theory with protein vaccines that promote T_H1 responses to shift the immune system away from this allergic phenotype. In this chapter, we highlight the common clinical manifestations of atopy and demonstrate how immunological reactivity to key antigens underscores each condition. Although the Gell and Coombs classification is not universally applicable, the fundamental immunological processes apply in most of the common clinical hypersensitivity states discussed next.

SYSTEMIC ANAPHYLAXIS AND ANAPHYLACTOID REACTIONS

Overview

Systemic anaphylaxis represents the clinical manifestation of type I hypersensitivity that occurs when a specific antigen and a homocytotrophic antibody interact. The reaction can be sudden and progress rapidly, often without a clear cause. Death can occur because of vascular collapse or airway obstruction. The term *anaphylaxis* is derived from the Greek *ana*, meaning backward, and *phylaxis*, meaning protection. Poiter and Richet coined the term in 1902 after sea anemone antigen injected into a previously tolerant dog caused a fatal reaction instead of the expected immunological protection, or prophylaxis.

Generally, antigen-specific IgE antibodies on mast cells, or basophils, interact with previously encountered antigens

mediating anaphylaxis. Mast cells are found in large numbers beneath cutaneous and mucosal surfaces and are closely associated with blood vessels and peripheral nerves. Basophils, most closely related to eosinophils, function similarly to mast cells. Basophils are present in the circulation, while mast cells are present only in tissue but in much greater numbers. When either of these cell types is triggered, a biphasic release of mediators occurs. The pathophysiology of anaphylaxis is clinically defined by the physiological effects of the immediate-phase and late-phase mediators on the target organs. By definition, anaphylaxis involves the cardiovascular, respiratory, gastrointestinal, or epidermal system; in most cases, multiple organs are involved.

In the immediate phase, preformed enzymes and toxic mediators such as histamine, tryptase, and heparin are the predominant bioactive substances released. Acting on H_1 and H_2 receptors, histamine promotes multiple effects such as increased vascular permeability, vasodilatation, constriction of bronchial smooth muscle, and increased mucous secretion. Clinically, these reactions lead to

1. Airway and laryngeal edema and bronchospasm with potential for complete asphyxiation;
2. Gastrointestinal tract smooth muscle contraction, causing pain, vomiting, and diarrhea;
3. Blood vessel dilatation with potential for progression to circulatory collapse;
4. Cutaneous vascular permeability, resulting in flushing, urticaria, and angioedema.

Late-phase reactions are characterized by induced production of mediators such as leukotrienes, chemokines, and cytokines, which are not preformed. Therefore, the effects of these mediators are seen later into the course, usually hours after the onset of an anaphylactic reaction. The late-phase effects include activation and recruitment of T_H2 inflammatory cells, including neutrophils and eosinophils, as well as promulgation of the smooth muscle contraction and vasodilatation initiated by the immediate-phase reactants.

Treatment of anaphylaxis is aimed at restoring blood pressure, decreasing tissue edema, and reversing bronchospasm. Subcutaneous or intravenous epinephrine, oral or intravenous antihistamines, and systemic steroids are the mainstay of treatment. Patients should be monitored for at least six to twelve hours because late-phase reactions are possible.

Experimental Models

Animal models have been use to understand various manifestations of anaphylaxis. Circulatory collapse typically occurs in dogs; rabbits may suffer acute pulmonary hypertension; and guinea pigs may experience acute respiratory obstruction. These reactions are classically mediated by the interaction of IgE; the high-affinity IgE receptor found on mast cells, $F_{ce}RI$; and histamine. However, findings from several rodent studies suggest an alternative pathway involving the IgG receptor ($F_{c\gamma}RIII$), macrophages, platelets, and platelet-activating factor (PAF) may be more important in anaphylaxis than previously realized. Strait and colleagues immunized wild-type, IgE-deficient, $F_{ce}RI$-deficient, and mast cell–deficient mice using goat antimouse IgD antibody. This technique induced mastocytosis and a large response to goat antigen (IgG) with increased IgE

and IgG production. After fourteen days, they challenged the mice with antigen (goat IgG) or rat antimouse IgE monoclonal antibody (mAb). The severity of anaphylaxis was gauged by changes in body temperature, physical activity, and mortality. Findings in this experimental model included similar anaphylactic responses regardless of anti-IgE, mAb-induced, or goat IgG antigen challenge. Anti-IgE, mAb-induced anaphylaxis was $F_{ce}RI$ dependent and mediated predominantly by histamine. In contrast, antigen-induced anaphylaxis was $F_{c\gamma}RIII$ and macrophase dependent with PAF as the predominant mediator. This mouse model provides evidence that anaphylaxis may have alternative pathways and mediators contributing to its pathogenesis. Table 9.2 summarizes key substances and their role in anaphylactic reactions.

Representative Agents Causing Anaphylaxis

Multiple substances have been implicated as possible causes of anaphylaxis. The most common substances include drugs, specifically low-molecular-weight compounds. In most cases, the parenteral mode of administration is implicated, although oral, inhaled, and even cutaneous exposure can induce anaphylaxis as well.

Penicillin, the prototypic beta-lactam antibiotic, is the most frequent cause of anaphylaxis in humans. The reaction occurs when the compound is covalently bound to tissue carrier proteins to form drug-protein conjugates known as *haptens*. Ninety-five percent of tissue-bound penicillin is haptenized as benzylpenicilloyl, termed the *major antigenic determinant*. IgE antibodies directed at this hapten appear to be implicated in type I hypersensitivity reactions.

Table 9.2 Mediators of Anaphylaxis

Mediator	Action	Signs/Symptoms
Histamine	Vasodilatation	Pruritis, edema, wheezing, diarrhea, hypotension
Leukotrienes	Bronchoconstriction	Wheezing
Platelet-activating factor	Bronchoconstriction, vasodilatation	Wheezing, hypotension
C3a, C5a	Smooth muscle contraction, vasodilatation	Wheezing, hypotension
Tryptase	Proteolysis	Edema, smooth muscle contraction

Skin testing using a commercially available benzylpenicilloyl polylysine conjugate (Pre-Pen) may be used to predict the likelihood of an immediate-type reaction. Skin testing cannot predict non-IgE-mediated reactions; therefore, a thorough history to determine the necessity for skin testing is important.

Insect venom, another common cause of anaphylaxis, accounts for approximately forty to fifty deaths each year in the United States. The Hymenoptera order, including hornets, wasps, honeybees, and yellow jackets, contains the most common allergenic species. Immunotherapy is 90 to 95 percent effective after five years of therapy.

Foods, including nuts and crustaceans (i.e., shrimp), are frequently the cause of anaphylactic reactions. With exercise-induced anaphylaxis, certain foods that are normally tolerated such as celery, apples, and shrimp can induce anaphylaxis when ingestion is followed by exercise.

In recent years, natural rubber latex has been recognized as a source of anaphylaxis. Exposure can occur through contact or inhalation, and various scenarios of exposure include surgical procedures, dental exams, or sexual intercourse with latex condoms. Health care workers and spina bifida patients are particularly at risk. IgE antibodies to latex antigen *Hev b1* have been demonstrated by immunoassay and are felt to play a pathogenic role in this clinical entity.

Anaphylactic reactions involve an immunological mechanism. However, there are subsets of reactions clinically indistinct from anaphylaxis, which occur in a non-IgE-mediated fashion. In these anaphylactoid reactions, certain substances such as morphine and other agents such as radiocontrast media are common triggers. In contrast to IgE-mediated anaphylaxis, prior exposure is generally not required. In non-IgE anaphylaxis, some patients with selective absence of IgA demonstrate anaphylactic symptoms following transfusion of IgA-containing plasma. Physiological changes such as exercise, emotions, and overheating can provoke symptoms in patients with cholinergic anaphlyactoid reaction. In this rare condition, an increase in core body temperature causes a rise in plasma histamine from mast cells. This disease is an exaggerated form of urticaria, described later in this chapter. In all cases, no single pathogenic mechanism has been defined, but it is likely that direct mast cell activation accounts for most of these disorders; complement activation has also been reported.

ALLERGIC CONJUNCTIVITIS

Overview

The eye, one of the initial exposure interfaces for allergens, is a common site for allergic disorders. Symptoms can range from mild eye itching to chronic cataracts and blindness. These disorders are differentiated by their clinical presentation as well as by the nature of the immunological changes occurring in the conjunctival surface. Ocular allergic inflammation is typically associated with IgE-mediated mast cell activation. Mast cell–derived mediators (e.g., histamine, proteases, leukotrienes, and cytokines) initiate a cascade of events that culminate in the infiltration and migration of inflammatory leukocytes (neutrophils, eosinophils, and lymphocytes) to the ocular tissue. This trafficking of inflammatory cells requires attraction of these cells initiated by chemokines, and directed migration of the inflammatory cells out of the bloodstream to the surface epithelium using adhesion molecules and their receptors. These immunological reactions lead to the common allergic ocular diseases described next.

Clinical Disease States

Allergic eye disease consists of four overlapping conditions, including (1) seasonal and perennial allergic conjunctivitis, (2) vernal conjunctivitis, (3) giant papillary conjunctivitis, and (4) atopic keratoconjunctivitis. Distinct immunological changes occurring at the conjunctival surface give rise to the clinical spectrum seen in ocular allergy.

Seasonal allergic conjunctivitis is the most common form of allergic ocular disease. Changes in the conjunctiva include a visible increase in the type and number of cells provoking allergy symptoms, usually in spring and in fall. The aforementioned cell types, such as mast cells and eosinophils, interact and release a variety of allergic mediators when exposed to seasonal aeroallergens such as tree or grass pollen. Preformed mediators are released in an immediate phase, and newly formed mediators appear approximately eight to twenty-four hours after exposure. These mediators have overlapping biological functions that contribute to the typical ocular itching, redness, and watery discharge associated with allergic eye disease. Inflammatory markers include up-regulation of intercellular adhesion molecules such as ICAM-1. Increased levels of helper T cell 2 subset (T_H2) cytokines, including IL-4, are found in the eye tissues during allergy season. Clinically, the conjunctiva is red, with a clear discharge. The eye is almost uniformly pruritic. Seasonal allergic conjunctivitis is commonly associated with rhinitis, but it may be the predominant symptom of allergy.

Perennial allergic conjunctivitis, in contrast, is associated with a persistent increase in the number of these allergic cell types throughout the year as well as specific IgE (dust, mold, animal dander) found in the tears of affected individuals.

Vernal conjunctivitis is a chronic, bilateral conjunctival inflammatory disease found primarily in young males with history of atopy during spring months. Initial symptom onset is before puberty, and symptoms dissipate by the third decade of life. In severe cases, vernal conjunctivitis can lead to corneal scarring and permanent vision loss. Histopathologically, conjunctival infiltration with basophils, eosinophils, plasma cells, lymphocytes, and macrophages characterizes vernal conjunctivitis. With this cellular milieu, it appears that vernal conjunctivitis is a combined immediate- and delayed-type hypersensitivity reaction.

Giant papillary conjunctivitis is a chronic inflammatory process that leads to the production of giant mucosal ducts, or papillae, on the conjunctival lining of the upper eyelids. The immunopathologic mechanism is complex and is theorized to be a mechanical trauma culminating in a mast cell–mediated delayed-type hypersensitivity.

The major signs and symptoms include itching and a clear or white stringy discharge. A "cobblestone" appearance is typical. It is commonly associated with contact lens use. Foreign bodies and ocular sutures or prosthetics may be causal as well. Treatment typically involves avoidance of the inciting process or use of ocular anti-inflammatory agents such as cromolyn sodium or topical corticosteroids.

Atopic keratoconjunctivitis (AK) is observed in approximately 15 to 40 percent of patients with atopic dermatitis. Whereas allergic conjunctivitis is usually a self-limiting process, AK is chronic and can potentially cause loss of vision. Immunological and immunohistochemical studies reveal mast cells, IgE antibody, eosinophils, and other inflammatory cells in similar quantities to those found in allergic conjunctivitis. The finding of lymphocyte involvement explains the chronic nature of the disease as well as the threat to sight. Additional findings include antibodies to ICAM-1 and HLA-DR throughout the ocular epithelium, suggesting increased antigen presentation. Also, increased level of RANTES, an eosinophil homeostasis chemokine, are observed in immunohistochemical studies of the epithelium. Fibroblast numbers are increased in the connective tissue with an increased level of collagen compared with normal tissue. This infiltration is likely critical to the sight-threatening nature of the disease. Table 9.3 summarizes the histopathological and other laboratory manifestations of ocular disease.

Treatment is aimed at reducing the local inflammation. Ocular mast cell stabilizer drops such as olopatadine are the mainstay of treatment. In addition, treatment of nasal symptoms with nasal anti-inflammatory sprays promotes patency of the nasolacrimal duct. This combination treatment allows the eye to drain excess allergens, therefore diminishing allergic responses in the eye.

Experimental Models

Animal models of ocular allergies have been developed in the past years to establish new therapeutic approaches and assess immunological mechanisms. The current animal models are based on sensitization to and subsequent challenge with small numbers of allergens such as ovalbumin (Ova), ragweed pollen, or cat epithelium. The murine model of allergic conjunctivitis represents the presently preferred species for investigating the immunological basis of the disease.

Magone and colleagues applied such a model to evaluate the role of various cytokines, including IL-4, IFN-γ, and IL-12, in the early and late phases of ocular allergy using knockout (KO) mice and neutralizing antibodies. In this model, multiple mice experimental groups, including (1) ragweed-sensitized wild type, (2) IL-4KO type, (3) IL-12KO type, (4) IFN-γKO type, (5) anti-IL-12/mAb-treated, and (6) anti-IFN-γ mAb-treated mice were challenged with ragweed allergen ten days after immunization. An additional group received recombinant murine IL-12. They

Table 9.3 Histopathological and Laboratory Findings in Allergic Eye Disease

Disease	Histopathology	Laboratory Manifestations
Allergic conjunctivitis	Mast cell/eosinophil infiltration in epithelium and substantia propria; mast cell activation; up-regulation of ICAM-1 on epithelial cells	Increased tear-specific IgE antibody; histamine, tryptase, TNF-α
Vernal keratoconjunctivitis	Increased eosinophils, mast cells in conjunctival epithelium and substantial propria; eosinophil major basic protein deposition in conjunctiva, CD4$^+$ cells; increased collagen; increased ICAM-1 on corneal epithelium	Increased specific IgE/IgG antibody in tears; reduced serum histaminase activity; increased serum levels of nerve growth factor and substance P
Giant papillary conjunctivitis	Giant papillae; mast cells in epithelium; conjunctival thickening	Increased tryptase in tears; no increased histamine in tears
Atopic keratoconjunctivitis	Eosinophils in conjunctival epithelium and substantia propria; increased mast cells, increased collagen; increased CD4/CD8 ratio in conjunctival epithelium	Increased serum eosinophils and IgE; increased specific IgE in tears; decreased cell-mediated immunity; increased conjunctival eosinophils

found the anti-IL-12 antibody-treated and IL-12KO type mice failed to show allergic cellular infiltration into the conjunctiva. IFN-γKO type mice, however, had a significantly stronger immediate-type hypersensitivity reactions and prolonged allergic cellular infiltration after ragweed exposure. Overall, their data provided evidence of IL-12 as an inducer of the late phase of ocular allergy. Additionally, the data suggest IFN-γ as a limiting factor of the late phase and a potential therapeutic cytokine in the prevention of chronic allergic disease. Further research is aimed at preventing initial sensitization to allergens.

ALLERGIC DISEASE OF THE RESPIRATORY TRACT

The nature of the respiratory process involves inhalation of airborne allergens. As a result, the components of the respiratory tract, including the nose, sinuses, and lungs, are disproportionately affected by allergic disease. In clinical practice, the common manifestations include seasonal or perennial allergic rhinitis, allergic sinusitis, and allergic asthma. The former two are often described together as allergic rhinosinusitis. Although clinically distinct, each condition involves similar underlying immunologic processes that will be discussed next.

Allergic Rhinitis

OVERVIEW

The nose has five major functions, including (1) olfaction, (2) aiding speech, (3) airflow to the lungs, (4) humidifying and warming air, and (5) filtering potentially irritating particles from the air. Allergic reactions occurring in the nose can have severe effects on all levels of function, usually divided into primary and consequential, or secondary symptoms. Typical primary symptoms include nasal congestion, runny nose or rhinorrhea, as well as itchy palate and ears. Secondary symptoms include involvement of the middle ears, eustachian tubes, and sinuses, inducing symptoms such as headache, ear pain, and decreased hearing. Multiple central nervous system complaints may occur, including fatigue, irritability, anxiety, and even depression. As in other atopic diseases, the pathophysiology of allergic rhinitis involves specific IgE production after exposure to airborne allergens. The clinical manifestations and underlying immunological mechanisms of the disorder will be discussed later.

CLINICAL DISEASE STATES

Allergic rhinitis is the most common allergic disease, affecting 25 percent of the population. It consists of two forms, seasonal and perennial. Seasonal allergic rhinitis is commonly referred to as "hay fever" or "rose fever" and is triggered by pollens with a typically well-defined season of germination. Perennial allergic rhinitis has similar symptoms, yet involved substances are present year-round, including animal dander, dust mites, and mold. In both forms, allergens interact with mast cells or basal cells in the nasal mucosa. They are then presented by antigen-presenting cells such as dendritic cells and macrophages. $CD4^+$ lymphocytes are stimulated by this presentation to release interleukins including IL-3, IL-4, IL-5, IL-13, and other cytokines that promote local and systemic IgE production by plasma cells. In addition, these cytokines lead to enhanced chemotaxis, inflammatory cell recruitment, proliferation, activation, and prolonged immune cell survival in the airway mucosa.

Within minutes of allergen inhalation in sensitized individuals, IgE antibodies fixed to mast cells and basophils trigger release of acute preformed mediators such as histamine and tryptase in the early-phase response. Shortly afterward, de novo generation of mediators, including cysteinyl-leukotrienes (LTC_4, LTD_5, and LTE_4) as well as prostaglandin D_2 (PGD_2) occurs. These substances cause a pronounced inflammatory response leading to the typical symptoms of paroxysmal sneezing, nasal pruritis and congestion, clear rhinorrhea, and palatal itching.

Over the next four to eight hours, the mediators released during the initial response set off a sequence of events, with enhanced inflammatory responses known as the late-phase response. In this phase, cytokines and various mediators released earlier promote the influx of other immune cells by enhancing expression of vascular cell adhesion molecules (VCAMs) that help traffic circulating eosinophils, neutrophils, and lymphocytes to the nasal endothelium. Although each of these cell types plays a role in the late response, eosinophils appear to be the main effector cell in allergic rhinitis. Nasal obstruction and secretions can lead to secondary effects, including ear and sinus infections, sleep apnea, and asthma exacerbations. Furthermore, the inflammatory cytokines may circulate to the central nervous system, eliciting malaise, irritability, and impaired concentration.

Treatment of allergic rhinitis involves environmental control for indoor allergens, reduction of swelling and congestion by nasal corticosteroids or oral leukotriene receptor antagonists, and relief of rhinorrhea and nasal pruritis by oral or nasal antihistamines. Recalcitrant cases may require desensitization by immunotherapy (allergy shots).

EXPERIMENTAL MODELS

Recent research into the underlying immunological mechanisms of rhinitis has borne new insights into the patho-physiology of allergic rhinitis. Prior understanding favored initial IgE production in regional lymph nodes or bone marrow. Failure of prior experiments to co-localize IgE protein within B cells to the local tissue environment weighed heavily against localized tissue IgE production. In the past ten years, however, a growing body of research has challenged the former dogma that IgE production occurred remotely from the allergen–tissue interface. Studies of local messenger RNA (mRNA) support the hypothesis of local protein synthesis. Durham and colleagues, using a combination of in situ hybridization and immunohistochemistry, showed that cells expressing epsilon–heavy chain mRNA (Cε) were present in the nasal mucosa of allergic individuals, and marked increases of these cells occurred on exposure to allergen. Furthermore, the increases seen in IgE and Cε mRNA after allergen challenge were inhibited by topical corticosteroids, favoring a localized process. In addition, Kleinjan and colleagues used similar techniques to demonstrate finally IgE-producing B cells in the nasal mucosa. Biopsies were obtained from normal subjects and from seasonal and perennial subjects during pollen season and during house dust exposure. The study found no differences in B-cell numbers, either CD19[+] (B cells) or CD138[+] (immunoglobulin-secreting plasma cells) in allergic and normal patients. Allergic patients, however, exhibited significantly greater numbers of IgE-positive B cells than normal patients, and allergen-positive cells were only found in allergics with almost all such cells staining positive for IgE or CD138. The combination of these factors suggests local IgE production may take place in the mucosa during natural allergen exposure.

Other models focus on the eosinophilic inflammation that characterizes allergic rhinitis as well as modulation of the allergic response. Hussain and colleagues sensitized BALB/c mice using Ova intraperitoneally. Subsequent challenge with aerosolized Ova took place. Various outcomes, including nasal symptoms, nasal submucosal eosinophilia, and bone marrow eosinophilia, were measured. Afterward, a subset of mice received CpG oligodeoxynucleotides (ODNs), potent inducers of a T_H1 nonallergenic response. Using enzyme-linked immunosorbent assay, cytokine levels were measured. Findings included elevated IL-4 and IL-5 and suppressed IFN-γ in Ova-sensitized mice compared with ODN-treated mice. In addition, the administration of ODNs abrogated nasal symptoms and upper airway eosinophilia compared with controls. Collectively, these models elucidate the complex immunological basis of allergic rhinitis and demonstrate how manipulation of the immune response can be used clinically as a potential treatment.

Allergic Asthma

OVERVIEW

The human lung provides the fundamental function of gas exchange. As the terminal level of the respiratory tract after the nasal cavity and pharynx, it is constantly exposed to airborne particulate matter. Allergic asthma is the manifestation of a pulmonary immune response to various inhaled substances. Clinically, the cardinal symptoms include (1) generalized but reversible airway obstruction, (2) wheeze, (3) dyspnea, and (4) cough. Symptoms can range from mild to life threatening. Typical allergens include house dust mite, pollen, cockroach epithelium, animal dander, and fungi.

As in allergic rhinitis, recent advances in understanding the immunology of asthma have important therapeutic value, and immune manipulation will likely become an important modality in the treatment of asthma.

Immunology of Asthma

From a histopathological standpoint, the inflammation in allergic asthma involves the entire thickness of the airway. Findings include generalized edema, denudation of the epithelium, subbasement membrane thickening, and smooth muscle and mucous gland hypertrophy. This process begins when dendritic cells, a subset of antigen-presenting cells found in the lung tissue, process inhaled antigens and present them to T lymphocytes through the interaction of the receptor molecule CD28 on T cells and its ligand CD80 (B7.1) on dendritic cells. This interaction results in T lymphocyte development down the T_H2 pathway. T_H2 lymphocytes are characterized by release of a family of proinflammatory cytokines, including IL-3, IL-4, IL-5, IL-13, tumor necrosis factor-α (TNF-α), and granulocyte-macrophage colony-stimulating factor. These cytokines promote development, activation, and survival of eosinophils. In addition, IL-4, IL-5, IL-13, and TNF-α activate endothelial cell adhesion proteins, ICAM-1 and VCAM-1, which assist inflammatory cell movement from blood vessels into the airway. IL-4 and IL-13 are key stimuli of B cells for antigen-specific IgE production, which initiates the allergic cascade. As a whole, these complex immunological processes lead to the pathologic processes that characterize asthma.

Treatment is multifactorial. Environmental measures to eliminate allergen exposure should always be attempted. Inhaled corticosteroids (ICS) remain the mainstay of medical treatment as they down-regulate multiple inflammatory reactions in the lungs. Other adjuncts such as leukotriene receptor antagonists modify significant mediators of allergic inflammation present in asthmatic airways. Newer treatments include monoclonal antibodies directed against IgE (anti-IgE therapy), which have shown some success in decreasing asthma symptoms and the need for oral or inhaled corticosteroids.

Experimental Models

Although our understanding of the pathogenesis of allergic asthma is incomplete, animal models have been of great utility in elucidating the mechanisms of this disease.

A major topic of current research has revolved around airway changes in the chronic asthmatic. This process, known as remodeling, is believed to result in irreversible changes in the lung. McMillan and Lloyd induced acute pulmonary eosinophilia and bronchial hyperreactivity in mice using multiple allergen challenges. They subsequently induced a chronic phase in a subset of mice using Ova challenge. Evaluation at one month after Ova challenge showed significant changes in the Ova-challenged mice. Compared with the acutely challenged mice, the Ova group showed deposition of collagen as well as airway smooth muscle and goblet cell hyperplasia. Cytokine profiles in the chronic phase revealed increases of IL-4, transforming growth factor beta 1 (TGF-$\beta1$), and IFN-γ. These findings strongly support the concept of airway remodeling and reveal a dual T_H1 and T_H2 cytokine profile in the chronic phase of asthma.

Another important focus of asthma research centers on so-called inner-city asthma, an increasing epidemic in developed countries. Many epidemiological studies have shown disproportional rates of asthma in urban, lower socioeconomically stratified patients. Although many socioeconomic factors are thought to play a role, distinct allergic triggers specific to these environments appear to be important. Using recombinant proteins, Sarpong, Zhang, and Kleeberger (2004) evaluated two such allergens, cockroach (Bla g 2) and dust mite (Der f 1), in inbred mouse strain (A/J). Mice were immunized with Bla g 2 and Der f 1 or a combination on days 0 and 7 and were inhalant challenged on day 14. Airway hyperreactivity and airway cellular content were subsequently studied. Findings included dose-related statistically significant increases in airway reactivity and inflammatory and epithelial cell measurements. Compared with individual antigens, however, enhanced inflammatory cell levels and epithelial cell numbers, but not airway reactivity, were noted in the combined group. This model, which has been subsequently validated, has practical implications for preventing asthma.

FOOD ALLERGY AND INTOLERANCE

Perhaps of all allergic reactions, the public, clinicians, and medical personnel misunderstand food allergy most. As little as 1 percent of the U.S. population has true food allergies compared with 20 percent who are perceived to have them. True food allergy is a typical, and sometimes catastrophic, type I, IgE-mediated reaction, which preferably must be proven by in vitro or in vivo testing.

Diagnosis of Food Allergy and Intolerance

The gold standard of food allergy testing is the double-blinded, placebo-controlled food challenge, which will establish whether the patient is truly allergic to a specific food. Because this method of testing for food allergies is time consuming, expensive, and potentially dangerous, in vivo testing is usually performed in food allergy centers. Occasionally, straight food challenges may be tried when the chances of reactions are minimal and the serum IgE (radioallergosorbent test, or RAST) specific for the allergen is low or negative.

Approximately 20 percent of the U.S. population may perceive food as causative reaction in food allergies, whereas the true prevalence of food allergies is approximately 1 percent. Food allergies are usually found in individuals with a strong personal and family history of allergies. Atopic responses are associated with many foods. In children under the age 2, 90 percent of the incriminating foods are eggs, milk, legumes (such as peanuts, which are not nuts), and soy. In adults, fish, shellfish, fruits, and tree nuts might be added to the list.

> Case 9.1 Peanut Allergy
> N.G. is a two-year-old female who was well until the age of seventeen months when she developed a watery, runny nose that persisted throughout the spring but was gone by the summer. She responded well to conventional antihistamines and did well during the summer. In the middle of August, she broke out in hives and wheezing soon after eating a peanut butter sandwich, but the symptoms were reversed with the antihistamine. She had never had peanut butter before that event, but her

mother was a self-described "peanut butter addict" and consumed large amounts during her pregnancy with and breast-feeding of N.G. N.G.'s subsequent skin prick test with peanut revealed a 20 mm by 30 mm wheal and flair response with a markedly elevated RAST to the peanut protein. She has remained peanut free since that time. She is able to eat tree nuts (e.g., almonds and cashews) without a problem because peanuts are not nuts.

Food Intolerance

True allergic reactions (IgE mediated) to food must be differentiated from *food intolerance*, which is rarely multisystemic, not necessarily found among atopic patients, and with no positive skin prick tests or in vitro responses (RAST). A nonallergic reaction that typifies food intolerance would be an acute gastrointestinal response in a lactose-intolerant individual. This patient does not have the enzyme lactase and, therefore, cannot break down sugar lactose in milk and other foods into glucose and galactose. Profound diarrhea or vomiting usually results without any other system involved (respiratory or skin, for example). Food avoidance is the treatment of choice, as it is with food allergy, and over time, food intolerance may resolve. Lactaid is a brand of milk in which the enzyme lactase is added so that the milk may be consumed.

SKIN DISEASES AND ALLERGY

Case 9.2 Skin Reactions

A.A. is a fifty-six-year-old female who was well until she began to develop acute, episodic, or transient swelling of her skin (urticaria), with intense pruritis (itching) and erythema (redness)

that she described as "maddening." She assumed she had food allergies, so she tried to eliminate various substances from her diet, including dairy products, fish, and nuts without any positive response. Eventually, she took antihistamines, with marginal improvement and sought medical attention after a three-month ordeal. An extensive history was taken and allergy tests (all negative) and a variety of serum studies were performed. She was diagnosed with a thyroid abnormality. She was referred to an endocrinologist and did well on therapy, which had nothing to do with an allergic diathesis.

Urticaria and Angioedema

Angioedema and urticaria are two of the more perplexing problems evaluated by physicians, and cases of chronic urticaria (hives of more than six weeks duration) may yield diagnoses in about 20 percent of those evaluated. Perhaps most important in the evaluation is the medical history, followed by understanding whether physical issues such as pressure, cold, and scratching affect the skin. These issues must be carefully explored in the initial questioning of the patient.

Certain types of urticaria may be brought on by physical disruption of mast cells by either cold, scratching, or pressure. There is no IgE mediation of these reactions, unlike those from foods, but histamine release from the cells is common to all. Swelling of the skin due to damage to small blood vessels causes burning and pain of the areas involved and may last for several days. The burning and pain are unrelated to allergies or physical mast cell disruption. These might typically be related to a systemic disorder, and precipitating

Classification	Diagnosis
Plain urticaria	Acute and chronic

Physical urticaria	Aquagenic urticaria
	Cholinergic urticaria
	Cold-induced
	  urticaria
	Delayed-pressure
	  urticaria
	Dermatographism

Angioedema	C_1 esterase inhibitor deficiency

IgG autoantibodies against C_{1q} may be found along with other organ involvement. Fevers, bone pain, and arthralgia may also occur along with the skin involvement.

Swelling of the skin without wheals, or angioedema, may be due to C_1 esterase inhibitor deficiency, and this may be a hereditary or an acquired disease. The reactions may be painful subcutaneous or submucosal reactions initiated by trauma and may involve the gut, causing colic, or the larynx, causing difficulty breathing. This type of angioedema is rare but potentially life threatening.

Case 9.3 Atopic Dermatitis

J.E. is a nineteen-year-old male with a family history of allergies who developed severe pruritis, which is usually worse at night. As a toddler, he had allergic reactions to milk and eggs, which resolved by age 4. In addition, he was a mild asthmatic until puberty. In his mid-teens, he developed a pruritic, crusty rash, which was relieved by corticosteroid creams and antihistamines and resolved somewhat during the summer months, where he lived near the ocean.

After switching to cotton sheets and eliminating his wool blanket, he improved slightly and was finally evaluated by an allergist. Prick skin tests revealed a significant reaction to *dermatophagoides farinae* or dust mite, and subsequently, he covered the sheets, mattress, box spring, and pillows with sealable covers of less than 2 μ of mesh. He also used a mild corticosteroid cream; the scratching stopped, and his skin cleared up.

Case 9.4 Atopic Eczema

Atopic eczema is an inflammatory skin disease characterized by severe pruritis with a chronic, relapsing course. Acute eczema is associated with marked erythema, superficial papulae, and vesiculae, which easily excoriate leading to crusting. It is the most common dermatologic problem for which a dermatologist is consulted. The IgE level in most people with atopic eczema is elevated and is specific to foods and environmental allergens.

Provocative factors of atopic eczema are varied and may include stress, skin irritants, food allergens, environmental allergens, climate, season, and hormones. Avoiding the suspected foods has a mixed response. Often food restriction during a child's early life leaves the child open to detrimental psychological and growth issues during those important developmental years. Fortunately, many food allergies tend to resolve over time; however, in the beginning of avoidance techniques, careful evaluation is mandatory. In addition, excessive amounts of certain foods such as citrus in children and alcohol in adults make eczema worse, and these reactions may be unrelated to an IgE-mediated problem. It seems that food allergy and the intolerance (non-IgE mediated) are important factors in atopic dermatitis.

Box 9.2 Classification of Common Eczematous Skin Diseases

Disease	Feature
Allergic contact dermatitis	Provoked by local contact with allergen
Atopic dermatitis	Extrinsic type (i.e., atopic dermatitis)
Irritant contact dermatitis	Provoked by local contact

Although those with atopic eczema often test positive to various foods and house dust mites, strict avoidance of these allergens does not improve the problem. Although allergies are an important component in atopic eczema, an estimated 90 percent of patients with moderate to severe eczema have staphylococcal infection of the skin. This condition and large insensible water loss make atopic eczema a difficult medical problem.

The effects of the weather, including temperature and humidity, on eczema add to these immunological and nonimmunological factors. A day at the beach may have a positive effect on atopic dermatitis, while a dry, cold winter has the opposite effect. Wet wraps are beneficial because they replace the skin's moisture loss. Corticosteroid creams, hydrotic creams and ointments, and occasional oral antibiotics are the mainstays of treatment. Avoiding allergens, local skin care, and treatment of the pruritis are the best approaches for treating atopic eczema.

Atopic Keratoconjunctivitis

Conjunctivitis is an inflammation of the conjunctiva, the inner eyelid surfaces and the mucous membrane lining the sclera. When the cause is seasonal or perennial (very common), the etiology may be pollen, animals, or dust mites. Prevalence is common, and the treatment usually involves mast cell inhibitors and topical and systemic antihistamines. Topical ophthalmic steroids are usually avoided.

Atopic keratoconjunctivitis is a rare, lifelong problem, seen more commonly in adults with atopic disease such as atopic dermatitis. This facial eczema usually involves the eyelids, and the lid margins usually show chronic inflammation of the lash follicles (blepharitis) and staphylococcal organisms. In addition, the lid margins may thicken and keratonize, and the lids may turn out or turn in. Corneal plaques, cataracts, and defects of the corneal epithelial may lead to loss of sight.

Topical mast cell stabilizers may be used for atopic keratoconjunctivitis, but often topical corticosteroids are required. Facial eczema must be controlled, and the lid margins must be treated. Conventional treatment for seasonal or perennial allergic conjunctivitis is not sufficient. Atopic keratoconjunctivitis may be difficult to manage.

Case 9.4 History Contact Dermatitis

A.A. is a fifty-six-year-old woman who decided, after many years of procrastination, to have her ears pierced. Within four to six weeks of the procedure, she developed protracted pruritis (itchiness) at the site of the piercing, with a crusty rash. She then found she could no longer wear her wedding band or bracelets because of similar reactions.

Patch testing to various allergens, including nickel, was performed. She had a severe forty-eight-hour reaction to nickel, a metal used in jewelry to harden the gold or silver. A.A. could no longer wear her earrings, rings, or bracelets. She could only wear 24-karat gold or .999 fine silver.

Box 9.3 Where Contact Agents are Found

Contact Agents	Where Contactant is Found
Chloroisothiazolinone	Preservatives in creams
Chromate	Leathers and bleaches
Formaldehyde	Cosmetics, newsprint, fabric softeners, wrinkle-resistant clothing
Mercaptobenzothiazole	Rubber products like boots and gloves
Thiuram	Rubber products, clothing dye
Vegetation	*Rhus* (poison ivy), tulips

Contact Dermatitis

Classical contact dermatitis is a Gell and Coombs type IV reaction, mediated by previously sensitized lymphocytes, which is exhibited by raised, very pruritic rash at the sight of the contact. Unlike allergic reactions of a type I, IgE-mediated contact dermatitis, as a type IV reaction, involving low-molecular-weight allergens (less than 1 kDa). These contact allergens are haptens and need to link with proteins in the skin to become allergenic. These haptens may be readily absorbed into the skin, a reaction that renders them antigenic. If the skin is exposed to humidity or warmth, the penetration of the hapten is greater, and the chance of developing contact dermatitis is greater. As these haptens make their way into extravascular spaces, they combine with serum proteins or cell membranes of antigen-presenting cells. The processed antigens is presented by Langerhans cells to T cells leading to a cascade of events that result in an influx of mononuclear cells into the dermis and epidermis, hence dermatitis.

Although most people exposed to these presenting allergens do not develop contact dermatitis, certain substances such as dinitrochlorobezene may sensitize as many as 90 percent of normal individuals, which is why the patient's history with suspected contact dermatitis is important. Among those situations patients need to elucidate are occupation, cosmetics, topical or systemic drugs, recreational activities, effects of holidays, and time course.

Testing for contact dermatitis involves placing a patch of the suspected substance or substances on the back. The area must be kept clean and dry for forty-eight hours, after which the various patches are removed, and the individual areas are evaluated for inflammatory responses. A positive response then characterizes a type IV reaction, and avoidance of the offending allergen is the treatment of choice. Thirty milligrams per day of systemic steroids may be required when large areas of the skin are involved (>25 percent of body surface). Otherwise, corticosteroid creams may be employed; however, avoidance of the contactant is most crucial.

BIBLIOGRAPHY

GENERAL

Adkinson NF Jr, Yunginger JW, Busse WW, et al., eds. Middleton's *Allergy:*

Principles and Practice. 6th ed. Philadelphia, PA: Mosby; 2003.

Janeway CA Jr, Travers P, Walport M, Sholmchik M. *Immunobiology: The Immune System in Health and Disease.* 6th ed. New York: Garland Science; 2004.

Patterson R, et al. eds. *Allergic Diseases: Diagnosis and Management.* 6th ed. Philadelphia, PA: Lippincott-Raven Publishers; 2002.

ANIMAL MODELS

Gronenberg DA, Bielory L, Fischer A, Bonini S, Wahn U. Animal models of allergic and inflammatory conjunctivitis. *Allergy.* 2003;58(11):1101–1113.

Hussain I, Jain VV, Kitagaki K, Businga TR, O'Shaughnessy P. Modulation of murine allergic rhinosinusitis by CpG oligodeoxynucleoides. *Laryngoscope.* 2002;112(10):1819–1826.

Magone MT, Whitcup SM, Fukushima A, Chan CC, Silver PB, Rizzo LV. The role of IL-12 in the induction of late-phase cellular infiltration in a murine model of allergic conjunctivitis. *J Clin Immunol.* 2000;105:299–308.

McMillan SJ, Lloyd CM. Prolonged allergen challenge in mice leads to persistent airway remodeling. *Clin Exp Allergy.* 2004;34(3):497–507.

Sarpong SB, Zhang LY, Kleeberger SR. A novel mouse model of experimental asthma. *Int Arch Allergy Immunol.* 2004;132(4):346–354.

Strait RT, Morris SC, Yang M, Qu X-W, Finkelman FD. Pathways of anaphylaxis in the mouse. *J Clin Immunol.* 2002;109(4):658–668.

10. Immunological Aspects of Skin Diseases

James G. Krueger, M.D., Ph.D., and Lisa Zaba, M.D., Ph.D.

INTRODUCTION

The skin is the largest human organ, and its surface (measuring about 2 square meters) protects the body from invading organisms, toxins, and viruses. Loss of the protective epidermal barrier (secondary to burns or disease states) results in an increased risk of infection from a variety of organisms.

Normal skin may be divided into three major parts: epidermis, dermis, and hypodermis. The epidermis is a stratified, squamous epithelia composed mainly of keratinocytes that differentiate to a physical barrier (the stratum corneum). The dermis is composed largely of collagen and elastin fibers synthesized by dermal fibroblasts. The dermis also contains a rich vascular supply, nerves, and various appendages such as hair follicles, eccrine glands, and apocrine glands. The hypodermis contains subcutaneous adipose tissue with associated vascular and neural elements and contributes the largest bulk of the cutaneous organ.

The skin is also an important immunological organ and is capable of mediating or initiating both innate and acquired immune responses. Keratinocytes synthesize a range of proteins such as defensins that directly kill bacteria. Activated keratinocytes can also rapidly recruit neutrophils and other innate immune cells through release of a large number of mediators such as S100 proteins, chemokines, cytokines, and lipid-derived molecules. Keratinocytes can also activate acquired immunity through synthesis of heat shock proteins that activate dendritic cells (DCs) in the skin.

Normal skin contains at least two resident populations of antigen-presenting DCs Langerhans cells and dermal DCs Langerhans cells are randomly distributed throughout the living cell layers of the epidermis and constitute about 1 percent of all epidermal cells. Although this cell type originates from precursors in the bone marrow, continued proliferation of Langerhans cells in the epidermis appears to sustain steady state levels. However, if large numbers of Langerhans cells are lost from the epidermis (e.g., induced migration after antigen exposure or epidermal damage), bone marrow precursors can replete epidermal stores. Langerhans cells may be identified visually by their characteristic tennis racket–shaped organelles known as Birbeck granules that are a subdomain of the endosomal recycling compartment. CD1a and langerin (CD207) are antigens used to identify Langerhans cells on a molecular level. CD1a is an MHC-like protein that mediates the presentation of nonpeptide antigens to T cells, and langerin (CD207) is an endocytic receptor that recognizes bacterial mannose residues and transports them to the Birbeck granules. Langerhans cells are "immature" DCs that survey the epidermal environment for foreign antigens. If these cells capture an antigen, or are triggered by cytokines or other danger signals, maturation ensues such that the cells up-regulate MHC and co-stimulatory molecules and migrate through dermal lymphatics to skin-draining lymph nodes. Activated, or "mature," Langerhans cells, in turn, activate naïve T cells, inducing T-cell proliferation and differentiation into effector T cells. These Langerhans cell-induced effector T cells home specifically to the skin because they express cutaneous lymphocyte-associated antigen (CLA) that binds to E-selectin on endothelial cells.

Presumably, dermal DCs (HLA-DR$^+$ cells that possess co-stimulatory markers and the integrin CD11c, but lack Birbeck granules, CD1a, and CD207) have a similar potential to activate, mature, and migrate to lymph nodes; however, there is less experimental evidence for this outcome. Potentially, activation of CLA$^+$ T cells is not limited to lymph nodes via Langerhans cell migration but may also occur directly in the skin with activated dermal DCs.

This chapter will explore in detail some skin diseases that have a major immunological component in disease pathogenesis. Two other immune-mediated skin diseases – atopic eczema and contact dermatitis – are dealt with in other chapters.

PSORIASIS

Psoriasis vulgaris is an inflammatory disease of the skin that affects 2–3 percent of people across North America and Europe. Until recently, this disease was thought to be an abnormality in skin cell differentiation, resulting in keratinocyte hyperproliferation. However, work begun in the late 1970s showed evidence that immune

cells accumulating in the skin may play an active role in disease pathogenesis. Selective targeting of activated T cells and immune-related cytokines was then shown to reverse psoriasis in a large number of cases. It is now believed that the epidermal hyperplasia is a consequence of the immune activation of the focal skin lesions. We consider that psoriasis and atopic dermatitis are the most prevalent T-cell-mediated inflammatory diseases in humans.

To understand the cellular features of the psoriasis plaque, a clinical and pathological description of the lesion is warranted. Clinically, the plaque is a red, raised, and scaling (flaking) region of the skin ≥1 cm in size. Usually, many individual lesions cover the skin separated by normal skin. In extreme cases, virtually all of the skin surface can be affected. Histological features include (1) marked thickening of the epidermis with rete elongation, keratinocyte hyperplasia, and incomplete terminal differentiation of keratinocytes (parakeratosis); (2) infiltration of skin lesions by many types of leukocytes; and (3) increased vascular growth (angiogenesis) and dilation of blood vessels (Figure 10.1). Leukocyte alterations in psoriatic skin are extensive and include marked numbers of type I T cells (T$_H$1) and DCs, both activated and nonactivated subsets of each cell type, and neutrophils are present in the stratum corneum in most cases. T cells are mainly skin-homing CLA$^+$ memory cells, either CD4$^+$ T$_H$1 or CD8$^+$ TC1 cells. A subset of CD8$^+$CD103$^+$ T cells is further specialized for epithelial homing through surface expression of the E-cadherin binding integrin αeβ7. Few "allergic" type II T cells (T$_H$2) cells exist in psoriasis skin lesions. Instead, strong T$_H$1 differentiation is suggested from genetic profiling

Normal Skin   **Psoriatic Plaque**

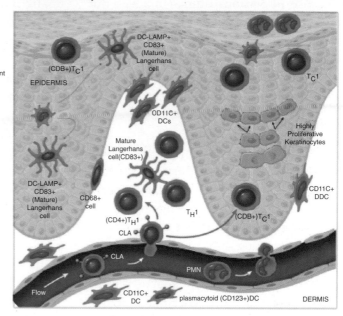

Corneocytes
differentiate
with nucleus
(parakeratosis)

Corneocytes differentiate
without nucleus (orthokeratosis)

granular layer absent

granular layer present

EPIDERMIS

immature
Langerhans Cell

DC-LAMP+
CD83+
(Mature)
Langerhans
cell

(CDB+)T$_C$1

EPIDERMIS

OD11C+
DCs

Mature
Langerhans
cell(CD83+)

T$_C$1

Highly
Proliferative
Keratinocytes

DC-LAMP+
CD83+
(Mature)
Langerhans
cell

CD68+
cell

CD11C+
DDC

(CD4+)T$_H$1

CLA

T$_H$1

(CDB+)T$_C$1

CLA+
T-cell

CLA

PMN

DERMIS

CD11C+
DC

Flow

CD11C+
DC

plasmacytoid (CD123+)DC

DERMIS

Figure 10.1 Schematic drawings of normal skin and psoriatic plaque with infiltrating lymphocytes, Langerhans cells, and proliferating keratinocytes.

of psoriatic lesional skin T cells compared with normal, including increased expression of GATA-3 and STAT-1 transcription factors and T$_H$1-deviating inflammatory cytokines. Furthermore, systemic immune deviation in psoriasis patients is evidenced by the threefold increase in circulating blood T$_H$1 cells compared with normal controls.

On the basis of finding clonal populations of T cells in psoriatic skin lesions, it has been hypothesized that pathogenic T cells are reactive to as yet an unidentified cutaneous antigen(s) and that the process of generating skin-homing effector T cells is initially the same as a normal cellular response. The formation of psoriatic lesions differs from lymphocytic infiltration in acute hypersensitivity reactions in that activation does not resolve spontaneously (as, for example, after the elimination of an infectious agent). Furthermore, chronic lesions contain a significant infiltration of

neutrophils, which is unusual for a "pure" T-cell-mediated response in the skin.

An alternative hypothesis is that, in the genetically programmed psoriatic patient, initial T-cell activation is not necessarily a reaction to a cutaneous antigen but rather to bacterial antigens known to be immunologically cross-reactive with keratinocytes such as the group A streptococcus. Evidence for this pathway is suggested by an elevated immune response to streptococcal antigens in guttate psoriasis and the presence of antigens similar to streptococcal M proteins in the psoriatic lesions.

The model in Figure 10.1 considers mainly the pathogenic activity of T cells in disease pathogenesis, but one must consider the influence of the innate immune response on chronic cellular activation in psoriasis plaques. Yet, the T-cell model has been a working hypothesis on which the therapeutic development of immune-targeted biological drugs has been based.

The use of various animal models, but most especially transplanted human skin on immunodeficient mice, has also been helpful in our understanding of the pathogenic mechanisms involved in the disease.

Animal Models

At the onset, there is no spontaneous model of psoriasis in animals. However, the use of genetically engineered mice or the implantation of psoriasis plaque xenografts in immunodeficient mice has aided greatly in understanding some of the basic mechanisms of skin inflammation as they apply to psoriasis and other inflammatory diseases.

Several types of transcription factors, including STAT-1 and interferon (IFN) regulatory factors (IRFs), convert IFN-induced genes. IRF-1 is a transcriptional activator, whereas IRF-2 suppresses IRF-1 activity. The IRF-2 null mouse chronically overexpresses IRF-1. These mice spontaneously develop inflammatory skin lesions similar to psoriasis, including CD8$^+$ T-cell infiltration in the epidermis, CD4$^+$ T cells in the dermis, and marked epidermal hyperplasia.

IL-12 and IL-23 (related cytokines that share a p40 subunit) stimulate T cells to differentiate and produce IFN-γ. Mice were genetically engineered to express constitutively p40 in the skin by joining the keratin-14 promoter with the p40 gene. These animals developed inflammatory skin lesions with marked epidermal hyperplasia and increased levels of DCs and T-cell-derived cytokines similar to those found in psoriasis lesions. Thus, IL-23 appears to be an important "upstream" inflammatory product leading to possible IFN-γ production and synthesis of "downstream" genes controlled by IFN-γ, STAT-1, and IRFs.

Another approach that has yielded useful information has been to transplant unaffected (nonlesional) skin or lesional skin from a psoriasis patient on severe combined immunodeficiency (SCID) mice. Injection of cytokines into the uninvolved tissue grafts induces some mild hyperplasia, whereas injection of superantigen-activated mononuclear leucocytes obtained from peripheral blood of the same patient induces a full psoriasis phenotype (but without neutrophil infiltration), suggesting that the psoriasis phenotype can be induced in genetically predisposed skin by bacterial antigen-primed leucocytes. When psoriasis lesional skin is grafted, long-term grafts continue to show viable T cells and other infiltrating mononuclear leucocytes. Thus, it appears that viable T cells can continue to expand in situ in skin lesions at a rate that matches the rate of programmed cell death, and one does not need new T cells from the peripheral circulation to perpetuate the lesion.

Perhaps of greater importance has been the observation that when nonlesional "normal" skin from psoriasis patients is grafted onto highly immunodeficient AGR129 mice, the bystander T cells in the graft expand in situ and cause a full-blown psoriatic lesion. Unlike SCID mice, AGR129 mice lack both natural killer (NK) cells and IFN receptors, which may leave them unable to reject graft T cells or create a cytokine environment more conducive to T-cell activation. Either a tumor necrosis factor (TNF) antagonist or anti-CD3 antibodies can block the onset of lesions.

Global View of Psoriasis Through Genomics

Another informative approach to understanding the underlying mechanisms of pathogenesis of the psoriatic plaque has been the study of differences in gene expression detected through transcriptional profiling on 63,000-element gene arrays. Using this technique, it appears that 1,338 genes have altered expression in psoriasis. Having a global view of these differences in gene expression between psoriatic plaques and normal skin background is important because it provides an unbiased means to assess activation pathways in psoriasis. Through genomic analysis, new inflammatory or regulatory cytokine and chemokine products have been identified as overexpressed in psoriatic lesions. Unexpectedly, there is strong expression of numerous lymphoid-organizing chemokines, for example, CCL19, CCL21, and SDF-1 in psoriasis, as expression is normally confined to lymph nodes or formal lymphoid tissues. Most likely, these chemokines orchestrate a striking accumulation of immature dendritic cells (iDCs) and mature dendritic cells (mDCs) in skin lesions; T-cell activation in situ may be regulated through interaction with these DCs in the skin or through release of activating cytokines (such as IL-23) produced by these infiltrating DCs. If one considers that the vascular changes in psoriasis bear a striking resemblance to those in lymph nodes, then the picture of dense perivascular DC/T-cell aggregates and increased expression of lymphoid chemokines suggests that the dermal infiltrates are actually a type of secondary lymphoid tissue.

Genomic profiling permits us to identify which of the many cytokines detected in psoriasis plaques are transcriptional activators. Thus, expression of more than sixty-five genes with increased expression in psoriasis lesions can be linked to IFN-γ and subsequent activation of STAT-1 signaling by this cytokine. For example, the chemokines CXCL9/MIG, CXCL10/IP-10, and CXCL11/I-Tac are STAT-1-regulated products and are synthesized in large part by keratinocytes in plaques. These chemokines direct CXCR3$^+$ T cells to migrate to the epidermis, where they may trigger epidermal hyperplasia as a result of physical damage (disruption of basement membrane and desmosomes) done to epidermal structure through T-cell trafficking or through secreted products.

Interleukin-8 (also induced by IFN-γ) is a key regulatory chemokine for neutrophil trafficking into lesions. Inducible nitric oxide synthase (iNOS) transcription is also regulated by IFN-γ and is highly overexpressed in psoriasis lesions, so that its product (NO, or nitric oxide) may be responsible for either cell damage or vascular dilation in lesions. Hence, IFN-γ plays a key role in leukocyte migration, as well as in epidermal and vascular alterations. The T cells in skin lesions do not become activated to release TNF, IFN-γ, and other cytokines unless triggered by antigen recognition, specific cytokines, or both. Hence, both the clonal nature of these T-cell infiltrates in psoriasis and the ability of CTLA4-Ig to reverse disease activity argue for an ongoing activation of T cells via classical TCR engagement and co-stimulation. Two cytokines produced by activated DCs, IL-12 and IL-23, have been detected in elevated levels in psoriasis lesions. Both of these factors augment IFN-γ production from T cells and may stimulate excessive expansion of T_H1-biased clones. Therefore, in this model, the presence of activated DCs in skin lesions may be as important in sustaining disease activity as are T-cell infiltrates. Long-term disease persistence in the skin (individual plaques can last for years without suppression by therapy) has been hypothesized to be a consequence of organized lymphoid tissue that forms in these inflammatory skin lesions.

Insights into Psoriasis Pathogenesis from Treatments

In 2003, on the basis of many observations that T cells play an important role in the pathogenesis of psoriasis, two T-cell-targeting biologics, alefacept and efalizumab, were initially tested for activity in psoriasis and are now approved by the U.S. Food and Drug Administration (FDA). Alefacept is a fusion protein that contains the extracellular domain of LFA-3 fused with immunoglobulin constant region domains. This agent binds to CD2, which is expressed at high levels on memory T cells. Although this binding interaction with CD2 could inhibit normal LFA-3/CD2 signaling, successful therapeutic outcomes with this agent are most closely associated with depletion of T cells from psoriasis skin lesions and, to a lesser extent, depletion of memory T cells (CD8 > CD4) from the circulation.

Efalizumab is a humanized monoclonal antibody that binds to the alpha subunit (CD11a) of the integrin lymphocyte functional antigen (LFA-1). LFA-1 is expressed at high levels on T lymphocytes, while other integrins are specific for monocytes, macrophages, neutrophils, and DCs. Thus, LFA-1 blockade with efalizumab, specifically targets T cells, and alters T-cell function in several ways: (1) prevents firm adhesion of T cells to inflamed (ICAM$^+$) endothelium and thus blocks entry of cells from the circulation; (2) prevents binding of T cells to ICAM$^+$ keratinocytes, thus reducing trafficking of cells into the epidermis; and (3) reduces T-cell activation, with attendant cytokine release, either directly or by blocking DC/T-cell immune synapse formation.

Although alefacept and efalizumab are potent immune therapies, only 25–30 percent of treated patients experience maximal disease improvement after a twelve-week treatment course. For unknown reasons, responses to these targeted agents are more variable than to more general immunosuppressive treatments. Possible explanations include variable expression of redundant T-cell activation pathways, restrictions in the access of large molecules to relevant T-cell pools, or more complex interactions between T cells and other types of leukocytes that contribute to disease pathogenesis in different patients. Genetic/genomic heterogeneity of humans seems likely to underlie the variable response to molecule-specific antagonists, but more consistent improvements in disease are seen with less selective T-cell antagonists, for example, cyclosporine, suggesting that psoriasis is fundamentally caused by cellular immune system disregulation. In general, suppression of T-cell-mediated inflammation – functionally defined as genomic suppression of IFN-γ, STAT-1, and downstream genes regulated by STAT-1 in psoriasis skin lesions – leads to objective improvement or clearing of disease, whereas failure to suppress these inflammatory genes leads to continuing disease activity. A review of therapeutic trials with many different agents indicates that there are no documented cases in which T cells and associated inflammatory genes were reduced without corresponding improvements in disease-defining epidermal hyperplasia. Hence, no data argues against the fundamental hypothesis that activation of the cellular immune system triggers psoriasis.

Another therapeutic approach in psoriasis has been to antagonize inflammatory cytokines. Although an antibody to IL-8 was administered to psoriasis patients with moderate improvement in disease activity, the first major success of the anticytokine approach was antagonizing TNF with the chimeric antibody infliximab. Subsequently, etanercept, a TNF/lymphotoxin antagonist fusion protein, consisting of the extracellular domain of TNF-R2 and immunoglobulin constant region domains, was shown to improve psoriasis. This agent is now an FDA-approved drug for treating psoriasis and psoriatic arthritis. The success of these trials suggests the need to consider psoriatic inflammation in a broader context than just IFN-γ release from activated T cells. Although TNF is often considered a key cytokine of innate immune responses, activated type I T-cells co-synthesize IFN-γ and TNF. Many different inflammatory genes, including IL-8 and iNOS, which are central mediators in psoriasis, have composite promoters for both STAT-1 and NFκB transcription factors that are activated by IFN-γ and TNF, respectively. Thus, the extent to which many type I genes are transcribed may be determined by combined levels of TNF and IFN-γ in the lesions. A recent study shows that etanercept induces strong suppression of type I inflammatory genes in psoriasis lesions, consistent with the view that T-cell-mediated pathways are being modulated by TNF inhibition. One should also add that TNF stimulates differentiation and activation of DCs, cells that present antigen to T cells. Thus, interference with DCs may break DC/T-cell immune synapses necessary for psoriasis pathogenesis.

Pathogenic Insights Provided by Genetics

Several genetic susceptibility loci have been associated with an increased risk of developing psoriasis, but the identity of susceptibility genes has been elusive. Finally, a susceptibility region (PSORS2) has been mapped to a discrete DNA sequence. PSORS2 is shown to encode a mutated binding site for the transcription factor RUNX1. Two adjacent genes, SCL9A3R1/EBP50 and RAPTOR, each associated with activation-related signal transduction, may be affected in a way that leads to T-cell activation or keratinocyte hyperplasia, but more work is needed to understand fully the functional consequences of this mutation.

In summary, psoriasis vulgaris can be viewed as a cell-mediated autoimmune disease characterized by interaction between DCs, T cells, and inflammatory cytokines. In this reaction, there is transcriptional activation of a broad set of inflammation-producing gene products that change trafficking of leukocytes and growth patterns of resident skin cells. Although evidence suggests that type I T cells are probably reacting with an autoantigen in diseased skin, this is not yet proven. Alternatively, the psoriasis could be a disease of an overactive innate immune system or underactive T regulatory pathways. The use of animal models, the study of cell types in the lesions, the use of genomics to detect transcriptional profiling, and clinical trials have all been useful in understanding the disease process; however, a good deal of work still needs to be done to treat this serious disease of the skin.

ALOPECIA AREATA

Alopecia areata (AA) is most likely a T-cell-mediated disease of a skin appendage, the hair follicle, and thus can be classified as an inflammatory skin disease. The condition is quite common because about 1.7 percent of the population experience an episode of AA during their lifetime. AA may be focal, affecting only one small region of the skin

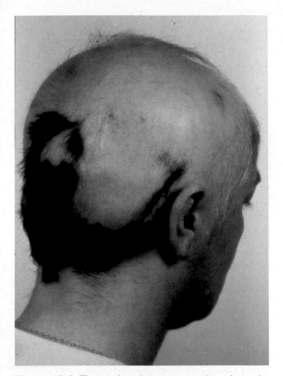

Figure 10.2 The patient has nonscarring alopecia areata covering >90 percent of his scalp. White tufts of hair near the temples are evidence of hair regrowth during active inflammation in the hair bulb, which inhibits pigment transfer from melanocytes to keratinocytes and hair.

of focal hair loss. These pathognomonic exclamation point hairs are broader at their distal ends, hence the name.

Although the exact mechanism of pathological events is still unknown, there is a growing body of evidence indicating that it is a T-cell-mediated autoimmune disease as follows:

1. The mononuclear infiltrate surrounding the hair follicle is primarily composed of CD4 and CD8+ T cells as well as macrophages.
2. Type I T cells produce IFN-γ, which is associated with increased expression of HLA-DR, HLA-ABC, and ICAM-1 in the follicular epithelium, resulting in increased leukocyte trafficking from blood into the hair follicle.
3. Hair regrowth is reproducibly induced by immunosuppressive drug treatment, including local corticosteroid injections and the use of systemic cyclosporine.
4. Lesional scalp from AA patients grafted onto SCID mice regrows, coinciding with the loss of the infiltrating lymphocytes in the graft. Furthermore, hair loss can be transferred to human scalp explants in SCID mice by injection of lesional T cells.

(Figure 10.2), or more generalized total hair loss from the scalp (alopecia totalis) or scalp and body (alopecia universalis).

Normal hair growth cycle can be broken down into three phases (1) anagen growth phase lasting three or more years, (2) catagen transitional period lasting two to four weeks, and (3) telogen phase when the hair follicle advances from the inferior segment of the follicular sheath into the isthmus and is eventually shed, either by traction or from being pushed out by a new hair in anagen phase. Hairs affected by AA end the anagen phase prematurely and enter into telogen, resulting in precipitous hair shedding. Because AA does not result in destruction/scarring of the hair follicle, "lost" hairs may eventually grow back, first appearing as "exclamation point" hairs along the border

Circulating autoantibodies to follicular structures have been reported in biopsies of AA patients but have also been reported in normal controls. These autoantibodies have also been seen in C3H/HeJ mice and DEBR rats but do not appear pathogenic in either mice or humans. Also one cannot transfer AA by injection of patient IgG into human skin explants.

In contrast, C3H/HeJ mice develop spontaneous hair loss with aging and demonstrate many features of AA, including inflammatory infiltrates and response to intralesional steroids. More important, grafts from C3H/HeJ mice when implanted into C3H/SmNCPrkd (SCID/J) mice do not result in hair loss, which emphasizes the role of the host immune system. In common with human AA, there is elevated expression of MHC class I and II antigens and ICAM-1 in the skin of these animals, and they respond to topical immunotherapy like humans.

As in many other autoimmune diseases, there is a genetic susceptibility to the disease. AA has HLA associations with DQB/*03 and possibly HLA-A. These associations suggest a role for CD4$^+$ T cells in AA but association with HLA, ABC was not examined in these studies, thus excluding the possible role of CD8$^+$ T cells. Autoimmune diseases result from many factors, and it is probable that AA is polygenic with multiple potential routes of genetic susceptibility. In addition to HLA genes, there is known genetic polymorphism in cytokine receptors and antigen-processing molecules. Thus, genetics alone is unlikely to supply a complete explanation of disease development.

If there is a T-cell-mediated component to this disease coupled with a genetic susceptibility, what antigens stimulate this T-cell activation? Among the recent hypothesis has been the suggestion that the autoantigen in AA is the melanocyte. Evidence that supports this conclusion includes the clinical observation that with disease activity pigmented hairs are lost more quickly then nonpigmented/white hairs. Second, melanocytes are a significant component of the hair bulb, which is the site of the immunological attack. Finally, there is an association of AA with vitiligo – a disease of focal melanocyte ablation. Supportive evidence can also be found in the animal models. Using SCID mice with skin grafts obtained from AA patients, melanocyte-associated peptides are capable of activating lesional T cells to induce hair loss. However, melanocyte antigens may not be the only autoantigens capable of stimulating these cells.

Treatment at present is related to the observation that AA appears to be mediated by a T_H1 response with production of IFN-γ. Psoriasis also has a T_H1 response. IL-10, which inhibits T_H1 responses, was found to be effective in psoriasis in a phase II clinical trial. On the basis of these results and a small trial in AA, the use of IL-10 in intralesional AA might be warranted. The same might be said of alefacept and monoclonal antibodies that are directed against CD11a (LFA-1) or CD4 cells. All of these immunomodalities are presently available and could be considered as potential new therapeutics if an appropriate risk-to-benefit equation is established in clinical trials.

ANTIBODY-INDUCED BULLOUS SKIN LESIONS

This group of skin diseases includes pemphigus vulgaris, bullous pemphigoid, dermatitis herpetiformis, and several other relatively rare blistering disorders. Although uncommon, these are serious, sometimes fatal, skin diseases. The group is unified by production of autoantibodies to different adhesion proteins/structures within the epidermis or basement membrane zone at the epidermal–dermal junction.

Pemphigus Vulgaris

This is the most serious of these disorders, and before the introduction of steroids, it was often fatal. The usual age of onset is between forty and sixty years old, but it may occur in any age group. Clinically, it often begins with ulceration of the oral mucosa followed by formation of widespread flaccid weepy bullae. Most patients with *Pemphigus vulgaris* have circulating antibodies to desmosomal adhesion molecules such as desmoglein 3, which disrupts intercellular connections within the epidermis. This results in the loss of normal epithelium and detachment of cells. The titer of this antibody often but not always correlates with disease activity.

Direct immunofluorescence of the perilesional skin is diagnostic and the IgG class of antibodies and C3 complement are seen at the site of the lesions (Figure 10.3). Further support for the direct role of autoantibodies in this disease is the fact that sera from pemphigus patients will produce pemphigus-like lesions in monkeys and mice. Furthermore, IgG fractions from these sera will induce epithelial cell detachment in human skin cultures.

The main treatment has been the use of systemic corticosteroids. The initial dose

Figure 10.3 Immunofluorescent photograph of a frozen section of psoriasis plaque using serum from a patient with pemphigus vulgaris. Note the clear binding of anti-desmoglein-3 antibodies in the patient's serum binding to desmoglein-3 protein that is present in desmosomes cementing epidermal cells together.

must be high to suppress new lesions and may reach 100 mg/day. Once new blister formation is under control, the dose can be attenuated. Other forms of antibody suppressive treatments have been used, such as azathioprine and low doses of methotrexate, and even plasmapheresis has been successful in removing circulating antibodies, especially if the disease becomes steroid resistant. More recently, depletion of B cells with the monoclonal CD20 antibody rituximab has shown efficacy in difficult cases.

Bullous Pemphigoid

The condition is clinically similar to pemphigus, but the blisters are subepidermal not intraepidermal. This disease occurs more often in an older age group (usually sixty years or older) and is characterized by large tense bullae on thighs, arms, and abdomen. IgG immune complexes and C3 are visualized by indirect immunofluorescence as a continuous linear band along the basement membrane, detectable in 75–90 percent of patients with active disease.

Although it is believed that autoantibodies to a basement membrane protein cause these blisters, experimental demonstration of this association is more difficult than with pemphigus. Sera from these patients do not produce pemphigoid lesions in monkeys and mice. Second, the antibodies remain detectable during remission, and the titers do not correlate with disease activity. Treatment is similar to that described for pemphigus, but the doses needed to suppress lesions are usually lower.

Dermatitis Herpetiformis

The lesions in this condition are usually smaller than those seen in pemphigus, are extremely itchy, and are seen on exterior surfaces of elbows, knees, buttocks, necks, and shoulders. Visually, the lesions resemble herpetic papules; however, the herpes virus is not involved in this condition. The age group is quite different from that of pemphigus (twenty-five to forty years old) but it may occur at any age. IgA is the major class of antibody detected, deposited in a granular fashion in the tips of the dermal papillae, forming subepithelial bullae. However, unlike pemphigus, no circulating autoantibodies to skin are seen in the sera of these patients. An interesting and as yet unexplained observation is that many of the DH patients have a concomitant enteropathy similar to celiac disease. Clinically, they do not have the symptoms of celiac disease and the associated condition is usually only demonstrable by jejunal biopsy. About 30 percent of these patients have antibodies to gliadin and endomysium in their sera. They also have an increased risk of lymphoma (like celiac disease patients) and a genetic component exhibited by a markedly increased inheritance of HLA-B8, DR3-DQ2 haplotypes.

Dermatitis herpetiformis responds to a strict gluten-free diet, which may need to be in force for several years before the lesions heal. Reintroduction of gluten results in the reappearance of the lesions, indicating the important role of gluten in the condition. Yet the presence of IgA deposits in the skin and their immunological basis remain unknown.

FUTURE DIRECTIONS FOR RESEARCH

Inflammatory diseases of the skin are an exciting and evolving field of research in which basic research frequently translates into clinical applications. Accessibility of human skin biopsies and intersection with biopharma production of immune-modulating therapies increases research velocity and immediacy. Current "hot" topics for researchers studying psoriasis, for example, include the newly defined TH17 T cell, and immunomodulating effects of innate antimicrobial peptides contributing to disease initiation and maintenance. Since the advent of effective immune-modulating therapies targeting T cells, and the discovery of a large IFN-γ signature in psoriatic lesions, psoriasis has been known as a T_H1-mediated disease. T_H17 cells producing IL-17 and IL-22, first discovered in animal models of autoimmunity, have now been found to promote psoriasis disease pathogenesis, both through IL-17-dependent leukocyte migration, and through IL-22-dependent keratinocyte hyperproliferation. Current questions in the field include defining the relationship between T_H1 and T_H17 cells in humans: Are they synergistic or antagonistic? Are they both involved in initiation and maintenance and is blocking one or both subsets most effective for patient therapy? Another current topic of research is the role of innate antimicrobials, including β-defensins and cathelicidins, as upstream versus downstream inflammatory mediators. LL-37 cathelicidin was recently found to bind ribonucleic acids and initiate plasmacytoid DC activation through TLR9. Activated plasmacytoid DCs produce large quantities of IFN-α, which leads to downstream myeloid DC activation and subsequent T-cell activation. However, both IL-17 and IL-22 are potent inducers of keratinocyte-elaborated antimicrobial peptides, forming a potential for positive feedback and continued inflammation. Unanswered questions include the temporal relationship between innate antimicrobial peptides and T-cell adaptive immunity, as well as the genetic basis for this breakdown in tolerance and immune regulation.

In summary, inflammatory diseases of the skin are an important and exciting area of research. Working with other researchers in both academia and industry rapidly moves the field from the bench to the bedside. Researching inflammatory skin diseases also allows for collaboration with other related fields where the immune system is deviated – as is the case for skin cancer.

BIBLIOGRAPHY

SUGGESTED READING

Chamian F, Krueger JG. Psoriasis vulgaris: an interplay of T lymphocytes, dendritic cells, and inflammatory cytokines in pathogenesis. *Curr Opin Rheumatol.* 2004;16:331–337.

Kalish RS, Gilhar A. Alopecia areata: autoimmunity – the evidence is compelling. *J Investig Dermatol Symp Proc.* 2003;8:164–167.

Krueger JG. Treating psoriasis with biological agents. *Sci Med.* 2002;8:149–161.

Lew W, Bowcock AM, Krueger JG. Psoriasis vulgaris: cutaneous lymphoid tissue supports T-cell activation and "type 1"

inflammatory gene expression. *Trends Immunol.* 2004;25:295–305.

LANDMARK PAPERS

Asadullah K, Sterry W, Stephanek K, et al. IL-10 is a key cytokine in psoriasis. Proof of principle by IL-10 therapy: A new therapeutic approach. *J Clin Invest.* 1998;101(4):783–794.

Cicardi M, Agostoni A. Hereditary angioedema. *N Engl J Med.* 1996;334(25): 1666–1667.

Gilhar A, Ullmann Y, Berkutzki T, Assy B, Kalish RS. Autoimmune hair loss (alopecia areata) transferred by T lymphocytes to human scalp explants on SCID mice. *J Clin Invest.* 1998;101:62–67.

Gottlieb SL, Gilleaudeau P, Johnson R, et al. Response of psoriasis to a lymphocyte-selective toxin ($DAB_{389}IL$-2) suggests a primary immune, but not keratinocyte, pathogenic basis. *Nat Med.* 1995;1: 442–447.

Kalish RS, Johnson KL, Hordinsky MK. Alopecia areata: autoreactive T cells are variably enriched in scalp lesions relative to peripheral blood. *Arch Dermatol.* 1992;128:1072–1077.

McElvee KJ, Boggess D, King LE Jr, Sundberg JP. Experimental induction of alopecia areata-like hair loss in C3H/HeJ mice using full-thickness skin grafts. *J Investig Dermatol.* 1998;11:797–803.

11. Experimental Approaches to the Study of Autoimmune Rheumatic Diseases

Dalit Ashany, M.D., and Mary K. Crow, M.D.

INTRODUCTION

The ultimate objective of biomedical research is to gain new understanding of the mechanisms of disease such that advances in treatment, and ultimately prevention and cure, are applied to that disease. However, progress is complicated by the inherent heterogeneity of human populations, even among those diagnosed with a particular disease. Even when appropriate study populations can be defined, access to the most relevant tissues and respect for patient privacy and autonomy present challenges to unfettered human-subject research. Although recent large-scale genomewide association studies in patients with systemic autoimmune diseases have identified candidate disease susceptibility genes, in vitro systems and experimental models are required to characterize the immunopathogenic significance of those genes and their products. Once targets for potential new therapies are identified, initial testing for toxicities of those therapeutics in humans is rarely appropriate. These limitations are among those that have led investigators to identify and to develop useful animal models that closely mimic human disease. Such models have been a particular focus of research relevant to the autoimmune rheumatic diseases. Although the use of animal models will always be limited by the likelihood of genetic and molecular distinctions between humans

and lower mammals, current data from the analysis of the genomes of mice and man, including study of disease susceptibility loci, indicate that important hints regarding disease mechanisms can be gleaned from study of animal models. This chapter will review the major animal models investigators are using to explore the mechanisms of autoimmune rheumatic diseases, emphasizing the degree of fidelity of those models to the relevant human disease. The most frequently studied mammal, the mouse, will be the focus of discussion.

TYPES OF ANIMAL MODELS

Spontaneous

Mouse strains that exhibit spontaneous development of syndromes that closely resemble human autoimmune rheumatic diseases have been identified by experienced investigators carefully observing mouse colonies. In addition, some efforts to induce mutation using chemical mutagens have generated mice that express immune system defects or pathology that provide clues to human diseases with similar problems. Advantages of spontaneous models of disease are that the phenotype is generally quite reproducible from animal to animal (although, in some cases, the disease is only partially penetrant) and development of the disease does not require intervention by the investigator.

A disadvantage of spontaneous models is that the disease often takes months to develop, slowing the pace of investigation.

Inducible

Some of the most useful animal models are those that are induced by the investigator by administration of a drug, an antigen, an adjuvant, an antibody, or through surgical manipulation of the immune system. For example, demethylating drugs alter the structure of chromatin, resulting in increased accessibility of positive or negative regulatory elements in gene promoters or enhancers and subsequent alteration of the gene expression profile of the animal, sometimes resulting in disease. Removal of the thymus at day 3 after birth has been demonstrated to promote development of several organ-targeted autoimmune diseases, most likely based on removal of an important regulatory T-cell population. Induction of immune system activation, as in the pristane model of lupus, can lead to altered patterns of cytokine production and autoimmunity. In some cases, autoimmune disease can be simply transferred from one animal to another by administration of an autoantibody or autoreactive T-cell population. Under these circumstances, the cells and molecules of the immune system that are required for disease expression can be identified and the investigation narrowed to one or at least a more narrow range of immune system components. The contribution of background genetic factors to development of a disease phenotype can also be studied in inducible animal models.

Transgenic and Knockout

Many investigators have used the technology that generates animals that either overexpress or are deficient in a single gene to investigate the relevance of that gene product to development of a disease phenotype. This approach has been particularly fruitful in the study of lupus, with transgenic and knockout mice demonstrating that any number of genetic modifications that alter self-antigen accessibility or threshold for immune system activation can lead to production of the classic lupus autoantibody, anti-DNA antibody, and deposition of those autoantibodies in the kidney, another characteristic of human lupus. Deficiencies in the complement system, members of which help to clear apoptotic debris and solubilize immune complexes; increased or decreased expression of cell surface molecules, kinases, phosphatases, or adaptor molecules relevant to intracellular signaling and that modulate the threshold for lymphocyte activation; and altered expression of death pathway molecules, such as *Fas*, can result in increased targeting of the immune response toward self components and manifestations of autoimmunity. An advantage of these sophisticated animal systems is that the modification is often restricted to one gene, or at least a small genomic region adjacent to the gene of interest, allowing the study of the impact of that particular molecular product and its relevant pathway on disease expression. However, there are inherent dangers in relying solely on transgenic and knockout models. That the gene of interest is absent during embryonic and fetal development means that other gene products can take over some of the functions of the modified gene, obfuscating the predicted phenotype. The role of a gene in development of a disease can also be overestimated if background genomic factors in the neighborhood of the modified gene also contribute to disease. Finally, the fact that overexpression or deletion of a given gene results in a disease phenotype does not necessarily indicate that the same human gene is altered in the corresponding human disease. In fact, few of the genes that result in disease when modified in murine systems have been confirmed as disease genes in humans. Nonetheless, the transgenic and knockout approaches help to identify important pathways for further study and that may be eventually targeted therapeutically.

Congenic

Like the transgenic and knockout approaches, congenic mice have proved very useful in studying the specific contributions of narrow genomic regions to aspects of disease pathology. The utility of congenic mouse strains, in which a segment of a chromosome is bred into a desired genetic background, is nicely illustrated by the NZM 2410 strain. That mouse model has allowed identification of at least three chromosomal loci that confer distinct immune system alterations, which when present together result in severe lupus-like disease. As in the case of the transgenic and knockout models, gene sequences in the chromosomal segment of interest can interact with background genes to complicate interpretation of the role of gene products in the congenic region.

RHEUMATOID ARTHRITIS

Introduction and Epidemiology

Rheumatoid arthritis (RA) is the most common inflammatory arthritis. Its incidence worldwide is estimated to be between 0.5 and 1 percent of the general population.

Certain populations, such as the Pima Indians in North America, have a much higher incidence of RA (about 5 percent) than the general population. RA is one of many chronic inflammatory diseases that predominate in women. The ratio of female to male patients is estimated to be from 2:1 to 4:1.

Etiology and Pathogenesis

The etiology of RA has not been elucidated although a variety of studies suggest that a combination of environmental and genetic factors is responsible; a contribution of either one is necessary but not sufficient for full expression of the disease. A genetic component is demonstrated by studies of monozygotic twins, in whom the concordance rate is perhaps 30 to 50 percent when one twin is affected, compared with 1 percent for the general population. The immunogenetics is under intense study although there is a clear risk factor in the class II MHC haplotype of an individual. Additional genes associated with RA include *PTPN22* and *STAT4*.

The major pathology of RA is localized to the joints. The synovial membrane surrounding the joints becomes highly vascular and infiltrated with virtually all cellular components of the immune system. T and B lymphocytes are highly represented and form lymphoid aggregates where B cells differentiate to antibody-forming cells. Poorly controlled production of pro-inflammatory cytokines, such as tumor necrosis factor (TNF) and interleukin-1 (IL-1), promote recruitment of additional inflammatory cells, and production of metalloproteinases contributes to tissue damage. The presence of immune complexes in joint fluid and direct deposition of those complexes on the surface of cartilage support a direct role for autoantibodies in some aspects of RA inflammation. Among the autoantibody specificities that have been implicated in RA pathogenesis are rheumatoid factor, an antibody with specificity for the Fc portion of IgG, and anticyclic citrullinated peptide antibodies, which have been shown in some cases to precede development of clinical disease by years.

Clinical Features

RA usually has a slow onset over the course of weeks to months. The initial symptoms may be systemic with individuals presenting with fatigue, malaise, puffy hands, or diffuse musculoskeletal pain with joints becoming involved later. Articular involvement is usually symmetric although an asymmetric presentation with more symmetry developing later in the course of disease is not unusual (Figure 11.1). Morning stiffness that persists for at least one hour is characteristic of the disease and is related to the accumulation of edema fluid within inflamed tissues during sleep. The joints most commonly involved first in RA are the small joints of the hands and feet, including the metacarpophalangeal joints, proximal interphalangeal joints, metatarsophalangeal joints, and the wrists. Larger joints generally become symptomatic after small joints although patients can also present initially with large-joint involvement.

Although RA is primarily a disease of the joints, it is also clearly a systemic disease that can cause a variety of extraarticular manifestations involving major organ systems. A full discussion of these is beyond the scope of this chapter; however, they include the development of rheumatoid nodules, subcutaneous nodules occurring on the extensor surfaces; pulmonary involvement, including pleuritis, bronchiolitis obliterans, or interstitial fibrosis; and ocular involvement, including scleritis, episcleritis, and vasculitis. Extra-articular manifestations of RA occur most often in

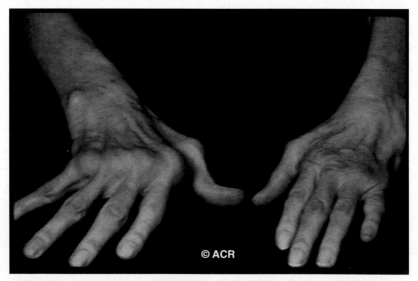

© ACR

Figure 11.1 Metacarpalphalangeal joint swelling and ulnar deviation in a patient with rheumatoid arthritis. © 1972–2004 American College of Rheumatology Clinical Slide Collection. Used with permission.

seropositive patients with more severe joint disease.

Treatment of RA

Patients with RA have variable courses, ranging from those who progress rapidly to complete destruction of joints if left untreated, to those who, with few pharmacologic interventions, smolder along with minimal disease that leaves cartilage functional and activities of daily living unchanged from the premorbid state. The challenge for physicians is to determine into which category a patient falls. Treatment choices include nonsteroidal anti-inflammatory drugs (NSAIDs), which are useful to help control some of the inflammatory signs of RA but do not prevent progression of the disease. A large class of drugs known as DMARDs (disease-modifying antirheumatic drugs) includes hydroxycholoroquine, an agent that has been shown to have anti-inflammatory properties in the disease but does not prevent erosive arthritis. Other DMARDs include those that have been shown to prevent joint destruction, which include sulfasalazine, methotrexate, leflunomide, and azathioprine. In recent years, the development of biologics targeting specific cytokines, immune cells, and immune receptors have provided additional potent therapeutics with which to treat RA. In this category are three different drugs that target the TNF cytokine (etancercept, adalimumb, and infliximab), an IL-1 receptor antagonist (anakinra), an anti-CD20 antibody that selectively depletes B cells (rituximab), and a selective co-stimulation modulator that inhibits T-cell activation by binding to CD80 and CD86, thereby blocking CD28 interaction (abatacept).

ANIMAL MODELS OF RHEUMATOID ARTHRITIS

No animal model is regarded as a high-fidelity replicate of human RA. However, several models that variably use T cells or antibodies that target the joint, or that induce monocyte activation and inflammation, have been used to study distinct aspects of the disease phenotype.

Animal models of arthritis can be used to understand elements of the arthritic process in patients. Recent therapeutic approaches in patients with RA, including the use of biological agents, are based on initial findings in murine models of experimental arthritis, although final proof of concept must come from clinical studies. Animal models are powerful tools for studying pathological changes in articular cartilage and bone in great detail and can be used to evaluate mechanisms of erosive processes. Although, in general, more inflammation drives more destruction, the uncoupling of inflammation and erosion can be seen as well, and different mediators are involved in these processes.

COLLAGEN-INDUCED ARTHRITIS

Collagen-induced arthritis (CIA) is an example of an inducible animal model for human RA. In this model, the disease is induced in susceptible strains of animals by immunization with cartilage type II collagen. The resulting disease is a T-cell-dependent, antibody-mediated autoimmune disease directed against the type II collagen immunogen. Similar to RA, CIA is characterized by massive infiltration of synovial joints by inflammatory cells and hyperplasia of the synovial membrane (pannus). In addition, the disease is characterized by both cartilage and bone destruction as seen in RA.

Both collagen-specific T and B lymphocytes are involved in the induction of CIA. The effector mechanisms that lead to joint tissue destruction are less well understood, and a number of inflammatory cell types have been implicated. These include fibroblast-like synoviocytes, bone marrow–derived macrophages, granulocytes, and dendritic cells as well as lymphocytes. Pro-inflammatory cytokines (IL-1β, TNF) and various chemokines are involved in the pathogenesis of the immune-mediated joint damage observed in both CIA and RA. Another similarity between RA and CIA is that the development of synovial inflammation is associated with pronounced angiogenesis with growth of high endothelial venules.

In contrast to RA, where large numbers of T lymphocytes accumulate in the inflamed synovium, few T cells are found in the synovium of CIA. Another difference between collagen arthritis and RA is that the former is more highly destructive than RA and in contrast to RA has a marked sensitivity to suppression of inflammation and joint destruction by NSAIDs such as indomethacin. In contrast to the female preponderance in RA, males are more susceptible than females in murine CIA.

ADJUVANT ARTHRITIS

Adjuvant arthritis is the oldest studied model of polyarthritis. It is induced by intradermal injection of complete Freund's adjuvant, containing heat-killed mycobacteria, in susceptible rat strains, mostly Lewis rats. Arthritis develops within two weeks. The active component in bacteria is the cell wall peptidoglycan.

Histopathological features are primarily a periarthritis, with marked periostitis

rather than synovitis, and massive inflammation in the bone marrow. Immune-complex deposition in the cartilage is not a characteristic feature, and cartilage destruction is limited in early disease.

Adjuvant arthritis has a pure T-cell-driven pathogenesis, and passive transfer of T cells from diseased animals can induce arthritis. The joint inflammation is thought to reflect the generation of a T-cell reaction to bacterial epitopes cross-reacting with endogenous bacterial fragments continuously present in synovial tissues or with cartilaginous antigens. Similar to RA, TNF and IL-1 have been shown to play a role in pathogenesis. Treatment with anti-TNF or anti-IL-1 therapy blocks inflammation and tissue destruction in the model, with the most optimal blockade occurring with combination therapy. As seen in CIA, NSAIDs are effective inhibitors of cartilage and bone destruction in this model and this represents a significant difference from human RA.

Adjuvant-induced arthritis is severe but self-limited, and the rat recovers within a few months. This is a general shortcoming of most animal models when compared with the chronic process of human RA. An additional feature of adjuvant-induced arthritis is that once the rats undergo spontaneous remission the animal can no longer be reinduced to develop disease. This resistance has made the model suitable for studies in regulation of T-cell tolerance.

ANTIGEN-INDUCED ARTHRITIS

Antigen-induced arthritis is a model of RA that is induced by immunizing animals with a foreign antigen, usually bovine serum albumin, and subsequently injecting the same antigen into a joint. As a result, a pronounced T-cell-dependent immune complex-mediated arthritis develops that is severe but self-limited. The advantage of this model is that a defined part of the pathogenesis leading to arthritis is addressed and the arthritis remains confined to the injected joint, enabling comparison with a contralateral control joint of the same animal.

The histopathology of antigen-induced arthritis has many characteristics of human RA. These include granulocyte-rich exudates in the joint space, thickening of the synovial lining layer, and at later stages a predominantly mononuclear infiltrate in the synovium, which later includes numerous T cells and clusters of plasma cells. Intense immune complex formation is seen in superficial layers of the articular cartilage, which may contribute to localized cartilage destruction. Early loss of proteoglycan, followed by pannus formation and cartilage and bone erosion, is a common finding, and these characteristics are close to those found in human RA.

The arthritis produced is chronic and is thought to be due to prolonged antigen retention in the joint tissue in combination with antigen-specific T-cell-mediated delayed hypersensitivity. Prolonged antigen retention in the joint occurs by antibody-mediated trapping and charge-mediated binding. This principle is also of importance in the recently developed KRN model of arthritis in which anti-glucose-6-phosphate isomerase (GPI) antibodies stick to GPI antigen trapped at cartilage surfaces and contribute to chronicity and destruction.

Unlike the other mouse models described so far, elimination of TNF and IL-1 is poorly effective in suppressing joint inflammation, pointing to a substantial role for other mediators of inflammation in this form of arthritis. Elimination of IL-1, however, did yield impressive protection against cartilage destruction.

The model of antigen-induced arthritis is most suited to studies into the mechanism of cartilage destruction, as induced by a mix of immune complexes and T-cell reactivity. The model is useful for the study of the regulation of local T-cell hyperreactivity against a retained foreign antigen in comparison with similar events against self antigens as seen in CIA.

K/BxN (KRN) MODEL

This spontaneous mouse model of arthritis was generated by crossing the T-cell receptor (TCR) transgenic mouse line (known as KRNxC56Bl/6) with the nonobese diabetic mouse strain. Autoantibodies that arise in the K/BxN mouse recognize the ubiquitously expressed intracellular enzyme GPI. The novel feature of this model is the development of a small-joint arthritis where the driving antigen has been elucidated and where the autoantibodies generated are pathogenic and transfer disease to other strains of mice.

The antibodies recognize endogenous GPI, which seems to associate preferentially with the cartilage surface. This may explain the dominance of joint pathology in these mice, although GPI is also abundant at other sites of the body. Activation of complement through the alternative pathway is crucial in these mice, and variable susceptibility in different mouse strains may largely be attributed to varying activity of complement and level of expression of Fcγ receptors on phagocytes among the different strains.

Although anti-GPI antibodies are found in some RA patients in moderate levels, the role of these antibodies in disease pathogenesis remains to be defined. The role of IL-1 and TNF in the pathogenesis of KRN arthritis is similar to other murine models. IL-1-deficient mice do not develop arthritis and TNF-deficient mice have a more variable course.

SYSTEMIC LUPUS ERYTHEMATOSUS

Introduction and Epidemiology

Systemic lupus erythematosus (SLE) is an autoimmune disease in which the immune system targets intracellular particles that contain both nucleic acids and nucleic acid-binding proteins. Virtually all components of the immune system have been implicated in SLE, with B-cell hyperactivity, antigen-presenting cell activation, T-cell dysfunction, and altered cytokine profiles documented. The consequence of this broad scope of autoimmune manifestations is a multisystem disease with the potential for affecting many organs, including kidney, brain, heart, skin, and joint. Studies exploring the prevalence of SLE in the continental United States have reported rates of disease ranging between 14.6 and 50.8 per 100,000. The disease occurs predominantly in women of childbearing age, with a female to male ratio of approximately 10:1, suggesting a role for hormonal factors in the pathogenesis of the disease. The incidence of disease also appears to vary among different races. In the United States, for example, African American women have an increased relative risk of disease compared with Caucasian women.

Etiology and Pathogenesis

Multiple factors are associated with the development of SLE, including genetic, racial, hormonal, and environmental factors. Recent genomewide association studies of single-nucleotide polymorphisms have identified gene variants that show a significant association with SLE in patients of European descent. These include *HLA-DRB1*, *ITGAM*, *IRF5*, *PXK*, *PTPN22*, *FCGR2A*, *STAT4*, *BLK*, and *BANK1*. While the functional correlates of these gene variants have yet to be characterized, most components of the innate and adaptive immune responses contribute to lupus pathogenesis. Current understanding of the disease implicates self-reactive B cells and helper T cells in the production of autoantibodies, with cytokines, particularly IFN-α, promoting augmented antigen-presenting cell function and immune system activation.

One proposed mechanism for the development of autoantibodies involves a defect in apoptosis or clearance of apoptotic cells, leading to a disturbance in immune tolerance. The redistribution of cellular antigens during apoptosis leads to a display of cytoplasmic and nuclear antigens on the cell surface, enhancing immune reactivity to antigens, which are normally protected intracellularly. Activation of antigen-presenting cells by IFN-α might promote presentation of autoantigens to self-reactive T cells. Immune complexes form in the microvasculature, leading to complement activation and inflammation. Antibody–antigen complexes deposit on the basement membranes of skin and kidneys. In active SLE, this process has been confirmed based on the presence of complexes of nuclear antigens such as DNA, immunoglobulins, and complement proteins at these sites. Immune complexes containing nucleic acids also play an important role in lupus pathogenesis based on their capacity to stimulate toll-like receptors and amplify production of IFN-α. Gene targets of IFN-α include pro-inflammatory mediators, chemokines, and cytokines, and activation of those mediators can result in recruitment of inflammatory cells to target tissue, resulting in target organ damage.

Clinical Features

Systemic lupus erythematosus is a chronic autoimmune disease that can affect almost any organ system. Its presentation and course are highly variable, ranging from indolent to fulminant. Constitutional symptoms, including fatigue, fever, and arthralgia are often present during presentation or recurrent SLE flares. Arthritis of the small joints of the hands, wrists, and knees may occur. Multiple cutaneous manifestations of SLE include malar rash, an erythematous rash over the cheeks and nasal bridge; photosensitivity; and discoid lesions, which are plaquelike eruptions with follicular plugging and scarring, among others (Figure 11.2).

The kidney is the most commonly involved visceral organ in SLE. Glomerular disease usually develops within the first few years after onset and is usually asymptomatic. Acute nephritic disease may manifest as hypertension and hematuria. Nephrotic syndrome may cause edema, weight gain, or hyperlipidemia. Acute or chronic renal failure may cause symptoms related to uremia and fluid overload.

Neuropsychiatric manifestations of SLE are widely variable. Headache is the most common neurological symptom, often with migraine or complex migraine features. Cognitive disorders may be variably apparent in patients with SLE. Formal neuropsychiatric testing reveals deficits in 21–67 percent of patients with SLE. Psychosis related to SLE may manifest as paranoia or hallucinations. Other neuropsychiatric

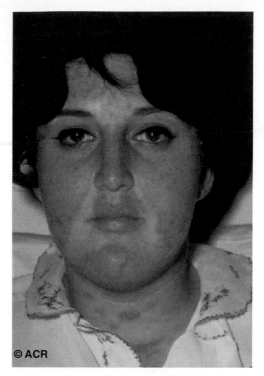

© ACR

Figure 11.2 Malar rash in a patient with systemic lupus erythematosus. © 1972–2004 American College of Rheumatology Clinical Slide Collection. Used with permission.

manifestations of SLE include delirium, seizures, strokes, and transient ischemic attacks and movement disorders. The etiology of these is not always clear but may be related to vasculitis or presence of antiphospholipid antibodies.

Other organ systems that may be involved in SLE include the cardiopulmonary system, with episodes of pleuritis and pericarditis being the most common manifestations, as well as the hematopoietic system in which various cytopenias due to antibody-mediated peripheral cell destruction occur.

Treatment of SLE

Managing SLE is challenging because no interventions can result in cure, exacerbations of disease can occur after months of stable maintenance treatment, and undesirable side effects of the therapies can be significant. Careful and frequent monitoring of patients is important in selecting management plans, monitoring efficacy, and changing treatments. The physician must first decide whether a patient needs treatment and, if so, whether conservative management is sufficient or aggressive immunosuppression is necessary. For manifestations that are not life or organ threatening such as rash, musculoskeletal disease, or mild serositis, conservative management with NSAIDs, topical or low-dose glucocorticoids, or hydroxychloroquine are mainstays of treatment. For severe manifestations of disease such as renal or central nervous system disease, immunosuppression with high-dose steroids and cytotoxic agents such as cyclophosphamide, mycophenolate mofetil, or azathioprine is a therapeutic alternative. Most recently, studies investigating the role of the anti-CD20 monoclonal antibody rituximab, co-stimulatory blockade with abatacept and blockade of the cytokines IFN-α, IL-6, and B-lymphocyte stimulator in controlling various manifestations SLE are being actively pursued in clinical trials.

Animal Models of SLE

Several murine strains have served as classic models of lupus-like disease, with each having many features that mimic immunological and pathological aspects of human lupus. Although several spontaneous mouse models of lupus have striking similarities to human SLE, none of the animal models reproduces human SLE perfectly. What makes these animal models particularly interesting to study is that the differences may reflect different forms of the human disease.

NZB x NZW F1 (B/W F1) LUPUS MODEL

The F1 hybrid is the earliest recognized spontaneous model of lupus. The mouse was developed from a cross between NZB mice, which develop a spontaneous autoimmune disease resembling hemolytic anemia, and NZW mice, which are phenotypically normal. The B/W F1 strain is one of the best-studied models of human SLE and is considered by many to be the murine model most closely resembling human SLE. The disease is characterized by autoantibodies, including antinuclear antibodies (ANAs), IgG autoantibodies to double-stranded DNA (dsDNA), as well as lupus erythematosus (LE) cells, representing phagocytic cells that have engulfed antibody-opsonized cell debris. Death results from a severe glomerulonephritis (GN) due to the deposition of immune complexes, including those containing anti-DNA antibodies. The disease is more severe and occurs earlier in female mice than in their male counterparts.

The B/W F1 is a good representative of human SLE because female B/W F1 mice manifest similar autoantibody profiles, and the disease develops in the absence of any known disease-accelerating gene, unlike other mouse models. Production of anti-dsDNA antibodies in this mouse, as in human SLE, is thought to be T-cell dependent as suggested by the IgG isotype, by somatic mutations in the antibody genes, and by experiments in which depletion of T cells suppresses antibody production and ameliorates disease. As is true for humans with lupus, the correlation between nephritis and anti-DNA antibody levels is not universal. In addition to anti-dsDNA antibodies, the mice develop other autoantibodies found in human disease, including those that bind single-stranded (ssDNA), transfer RNA (tRNA), polynucleotides, histones, and nucleic acid–protein complexes. Anti-erythrocyte antibodies occur in 35–57 percent of B/W F1 females, but the mice rarely develop hemolytic anemia. Consistent with the important pathogenic role for IFN-α in human lupus, disease and death are accelerated in B/W F1 mice who receive IFN-α.

MRL/*LPR* LUPUS MODEL

MRL/MpJ-Fas*lpr* (MRL/*lpr*) is another spontaneous model of SLE. The MRL/*lpr* mouse has a genetic mutation, termed lpr (lymphoproliferation), which leads to massive lymphoid organ enlargement and severe early-life lupus-like disease. The congenic MRL/+/+ strain lacks the mutation and develops a mild lupus-like disease. MRL/*lpr* mice exhibit many clinical manifestations found in human SLE. Autoantibodies produced by these mice are similar in spectrum to those seen in human lupus, including anti-dsDNA and anti-Sm antibodies. The mice also make rheumatoid factors. MRL/*lpr* mice develop proliferative GN at an early age (4–5 months), and renal failure is the presumed primary cause of death in these mice.

Although the exact mechanisms involved in the pathogenesis of lupus nephritis are as yet unclear, there is general agreement that disease is mediated by glomerular deposition of autoantibodies as immune complexes formed in situ or by direct binding of the antibodies to an intrinsic renal antigen or a self-antigen deposited in the kidney. This deposited immunoglobulin then induces renal injury primarily through complement activation, leading to recruitment and activation of inflammatory mediators. These mechanisms appear to exist in both human and murine lupus. However, a recent study in MRL/*lpr* mice suggested that the production of autoanti-

bodies was not required for renal disease. Mice that expressed a mutant transgene that did not permit secretion of circulating immunoglobulin still developed renal disease, suggesting that immunoglobulin-expressing B cells might also participate in the disease process either as antigen-presenting cells or as part of the local inflammatory process.

In contrast to B/W F1 mice, both male and female MRL/*lpr* mice develop high serum levels of immunoglobulins, ANAs, and immune complexes, as well as disease. Other antibodies in their repertoire include IgG2a anti-chromatin, anti-RBCs, anti-thyroglobulin, antilymphocyte, anti-ribosomal P, and anti-RNA polymerase I.

Polyarthritis occurs in MRL/*lpr* mice in some but not all colonies. The prevalence varies between 15 and 20 percent. The arthritis is a destructive arthropathy, characterized by synovial cell proliferation with early subchondral bone destruction and marginal erosions. This is unlike the nonerosive arthritis that occurs in some patients with SLE.

Unlike human SLE, MRL/*lpr* mice are characterized by massive lymphadenopathy and splenomegaly, which is due to a defect in the *fas* gene, a key mediator of apoptosis. The *fas* defect alone is sufficient to induce autoantibody production but is not sufficient to induce renal disease. This is demonstrated in experiments in which the *lpr* gene is bred onto a normal background, resulting in congenic *lpr* mice that produce autoantibodies but do not develop renal disease. Thus, genes in the MRL background, independent of *fas*, are necessary for disease development, including renal disease, in MRL/*lpr* mice. *Fas* defects in humans are generally not seen in patients with SLE, although a population of patients with genetic defects in the *fas* gene develop a disease known as autoimmune lympho-proliferation syndrome, characterized by massive lymphadenopathy along with some autoimmune features.

BXSB LUPUS MODEL

The BXSB mouse is a recombinant inbred strain that spontaneously develops an autoimmune syndrome similar to human SLE. This mouse model is characterized by the production of autoantibodies, hypergammaglobulinemia with class switching to IgG3 and IgG2b, hypocomplementemia, splenomegaly, and GN. BXSB mice develop a wide range of autoantibodies to nuclear components, typical of SLE, including ANAs, anti-dsDNA, anti-ssDNA, and antichromatin antibodies, with accompanying splenomegaly and lymphadenopathy. In addition, a small proportion make anti-erythrocyte antibodies.

The unique features of BXSB mice are that their disease is much worse in the male than the female, and the disease-accelerating gene responsible for that difference (called *Yaa* for Y chromosome autoimmunity accelerator) is located on the Y chromosome and manifests in a male mortality of 50 percent by the age of six months. These mice have recently been documented to have a duplicated segment of the X chromosome that has been translocated to the Y chromosome. That segment includes *TLR7*, encoding a toll-like receptor that responds to ssRNA. The female BXSB mouse gets late-life lupus with death occurring at fourteen months. This suggests that additional genes contribute to disease in female mice.

By three months of age the mice have elevated levels of circulating immune complexes and hypocomplementemia. They are the only lupus mouse strain that has serum levels of C4 that diminish as clinical disease appears. Death is caused by immune complex GN. Histologically, the disease is more exudative than in other mouse models, with neutrophils invading glomeruli along with IgG and C3 deposition, proliferative changes in mesangia and endothelial cells, and basement membrane thickening. The progression from nephritis to death is rapid. Of the most widely studied SLE mouse models, the BXSB has the most fulminant disease.

NZM2410 MODEL

The NZM2410 mouse is another spontaneous model of SLE and is a congenic recombinant inbred strain (termed NZM for New Zealand Mixed) produced by inbreeding (NZB × NZW)F1 × NZW backcross progeny. This mouse strain displays systemic autoimmunity with a highly penetrant, early-onset acute GN. The mice develop GN with a penetrance of about 85 percent and a 50 percent mortality at about six months of age. This represents an earlier onset of disease than that of B/W F1 mice.

The NZM2410 mouse strain differs significantly from the classical B/W F1 model and human SLE, where there is a strong female preponderance, in that both males and females develop the disease equally. It is possible either that the genomic regions responsible for the strong gender dimorphism in B/W F1 were not included in NZM2410 or that NZM2410 contains a collection of homozygous susceptibility alleles that are so severe that they can override the effects of sex hormones on the immune system.

Linkage analysis of susceptibility to GN and ANA production in the NZM2410 strain by Morel and Wakeland (2000) have identified three prominent loci termed *Sle1*, *2*, and *3* that are strongly associated with lupus susceptibility. Subsequent congenic strains made by moving each locus onto the lupus-resistant C57Bl/6J (B6) background have determined (1) that *Sle1* mediates a spontaneous loss of immunological tolerance to nuclear antigens; (2) that *Sle2* lowers the activation threshold of the B-cell compartment and mediates polyclonal/polyreactive antibody production; and (3) that *Sle3* mediates a dysregulation of the T-cell compartment that potentiates polyclonal IgG antibody production and decreases activation-induced cell death in CD4 T cells. *Sle1* and *Sle3* in combination revealed that these two susceptibility genes are sufficient to mediate the development of severe humoral autoimmunity and fatal lupus nephritis on the B6 background. B6 bicongenic mice with these two alleles spontaneously develop high titers of autoantibody directed against a broad spectrum of nuclear chromatin autoantigens and die of kidney failure (penetrance >55 percent) due to autoimmune GN within twelve months of age.

The lethal phenotype produced by the combination of *Sle1* and *Sle3* on the B6 background was somewhat surprising, in that both of these genes are derived from the relatively unaffected NZW strain. This suggested that their severe autoimmune phenotypes must be suppressed in some manner by the NZW genome. Genetic analysis of this epistatic suppression in NZW identified the presence and locations of four SLE suppressor loci (designated *Sles1* through *Sles4*) that account for the absence of fatal disease in NZW.

Murine chromosome 1 contains the *Sle1* locus as well as other loci of lupus susceptibility. This region in humans, specifically 1q41-q42, also shows evidence of linkage with SLE, including the production of antichromatin antibodies. Thus, important susceptibility genes for autoimmunity appear to be conserved between mice and humans, supporting approaches to look for candidate human SLE-associated genes based on mouse studies.

SJÖGREN'S SYNDROME

Introduction and Epidemiology

Primary Sjögren's syndrome (SS) is a systemic autoimmune disease that targets the exocrine glands (Figure 11.3). It is characterized by xerostomia (dry mouth), xerophthalmia (dry eyes), and is usually accompanied by production of autoantibodies specific for the Ro RNA-binding protein. SS is a common autoimmune disorder. Prevalence estimates range from approximately 0.5 to 5 percent. Approximately, one-half of all cases of SS are primary and the remainder occur as secondary SS. Secondary SS is defined as the former definition of primary Sjögren's in the presence of another autoimmune connective tissue disorder such as RA or SLE. Similar to most autoimmune disorders, most cases (approximately 90 percent) occur in women. The majority of cases occur in midlife; however, the disorder is also seen in children and the elderly.

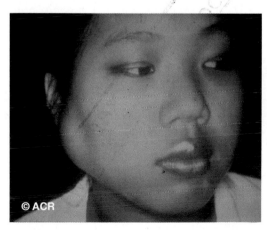

Figure 11.3 Parotid gland swelling in a patient with Sjögren's syndrome. © 1972–2004 American College of Rheumatology Clinical Slide Collection. Used with permission.

Etiology and Pathogenesis

Sjögren's syndrome has a strong immunogenetic component. Like many other autoimmune disorders, HLA studies have identified associations with MHC haplotypes. Studies have demonstrated that -DR2 and -DR3 associations in Sjögren's are secondary to linkage disequilibrium with HLA-DQ alleles. Genetically defined allelic markers have subsequently identified a large number of polymorphisms involving the HLA DRB1/DQA1/DQB1 haplotype, which adds to the complexity of the genetic background of SS. These polymorphisms have been shown to vary with ethnicity, clinical manifestations, and, importantly, with the autoantibody response. Similar to the situation in SLE, IFN-α has been implicated in SS pathogenesis based on expression of interferon-induced genes in salivary gland tissue and increased type I interferon activity in serum.

Salivary gland pathology shows infiltration with perivascular collections of T and B lymphocytes. The cells form distinct aggregates, termed foci, in periductal and periacinar locations that can result in replacement of epithelial structure. In rare cases, patients with SS develop non-Hodgkin's B-cell lymphoma.

Clinical Features

The most common clinical manifestations of SS are ocular and oral. Patients most often perceive xerophthalmia as a foreign body-type sensation manifested by scratchiness, grittiness, or irritation. Patients with xerostomia will complain of a parched sensation in the mouth, which often extends to the throat. Eating can be difficult without supplemental fluids. The reduction in salivary volume and loss of the antibacterial properties of saliva in the dry mouth accelerate tooth decay. Unexplained rampant dental caries may, in fact, be the first sign of a dry mouth. Other xeroses such as dry skin and dry vaginal mucosa leading to irritation and dyspareunia may also occur.

Extraglandular manifestations of SS include musculoskeletal symptoms, with arthralgias and transient synovitis occurring in 54 to 84 percent of patients. Pulmonary involvement, which most commonly is cough due to xerotrachea, occurs in approximately 50 percent of patients. Mild autoimmune hepatitis has been reported to occur in approximately one-quarter of primary SS patients, with smooth muscle antibodies seen in 7 to 33 percent. Antimitochondrial antibodies have been reported in 7 to 13 percent of patients, suggesting an association of primary SS with primary biliary cirrhosis (PBC).

Neurologic disease is perhaps the most common significant extraglandular manifestation of SS and can involve the cranial nerves, peripheral nerves, and rarely the central nervous system. Clinical reports suggest that half of SS patients have some form of neurological involvement, with estimates ranging from 22 to 76 percent.

Treatment of Sjögren's Syndrome

For the majority of patients, the mainstay of treatment for Sjögren's disease is external replacement of moisture. Patients should be encouraged to use tear substitutes often, and a variety of over-the-counter preparations are available. For xerostomia, artificial salivas are available, but these are generally not very successful and most patients find them unpalatable. Patients whose symptoms of dryness are not optimally controlled by moisture replacement should be considered for treatment with secretory stimulants. There are two approved agents available for use as secretagogues in SS: pilocarpine (Salagen) and cevemiline (Evoxac). Both agents have been shown, in controlled clinical trials, to increase salivary flow rate significantly in SS. There are no disease-modifying drugs that have been demonstrated to have specific efficacy for SS. Minor musculoskeletal symptoms usually respond to NSAID therapy. Because erosive joint disease is rare, therapy with DMARDs is usually unnecessary; however, hydroxychloroquine has been used to treat fatigue, arthralgia, and myalgia in primary SS. Cranial and peripheral neuropathy may be treated with low-dose tricyclic antidepressants or gabapentin. Symptomatic cases resistant to the previously mentioned therapies may be treated with intravenous gammaglobulin. Central nervous system manifestations, which are felt to be due to Sjögren's, should be treated aggressively with high-dose oral or pulse intravenous corticosteroid and daily or monthly intravenous pulse cyclophosphamide.

Animal Models of Sjögren's Syndrome

Nonobese diabetic mice have been used predominantly as a model of autoimmune diabetes mellitus, but they also develop an autoimmune exocrinopathy characterized by hyposecretion of saliva and acinar cell atrophy.

MRL+/+ and MRL/*lpr* mice spontaneously develop lacrimal and salivary gland inflammation and have been used as models for SS.

IQI/Jic (IQI) mice are a model of primary SS, unlike the animal models above that are autoimmune-prone mice that develop SS-like pathology associated with other autoimmune conditions, such as lupus, inflammatory arthritis, or insulitis. IQI mice spontaneously develop autoimmune infiltration of lymphocytes into the lacrimal and salivary glands, leading to dacryoadenitis and sialoadenitis. The incidence of the disease is higher in females than in males. Sialoadenitis in female mice can be detected from two months of age onward and significant progression of the lesions is observed after nine months of age. Inflammatory lesions occurring at young ages mainly consist of CD4$^+$ T cells with lesser abundance of CD8$^+$ T cells, B cells, and macrophages, and the proportions of B cells and plasma cells are elevated in accordance with increasing magnification of the lesions. Production of ANAs, one of the prominent pathophysiological features in patients with SS, is also observed in old IQI mice. Moreover, IQI mice develop inflammatory lesions in the lung, pancreas, and kidney in addition to the lacrimal and salivary glands that are similar to those in patients with primary SS. Thus, this murine model may be the most suitable for the investigation of the pathogenesis of SS, with progression from oral and ocular disease to a systemic disorder.

PROGRESSIVE SYSTEMIC SCLEROSIS

Introduction and Epidemiology

Progressive systemic sclerosis (PSS) is a disorder of connective tissue clinically characterized by thickening and fibrosis of the skin (scleroderma) and by distinctive forms of involvement of internal organs, including the heart, lungs, kidneys, and gastrointestinal tract. The hallmarks of the disease are autoimmunity and inflammation, widespread vasculopathy (blood vessel damage), affecting multiple vascular beds, and progressive interstitial and perivascular fibrosis. The etiology is unknown. The incidence of systemic sclerosis is estimated to be between eighteen and twenty individuals per one million persons per year. All age groups may be affected, but the onset of disease is highest between the ages of thirty and fifty years old. Systemic sclerosis is three to four times more common in women than in men, with women of childbearing age at peak risk.

Etiology and Pathogenesis

The pathogenesis of systemic sclerosis involves an interplay between obliterative vasculopathy in multiple vascular beds, inflammation, and autoimmunity, and progressive fibrosis. Vascular injury and activation are the earliest and possibly primary events in the pathogenesis of PSS. This is suggested by histopathological evidence of vascular damage that is present before fibrosis, and clinical manifestations, such as Raynaud's phenomenon, an episodic and reversible cold-induced vasospasm of the fingers and toes, that precede other disease manifestations. Additional manifestations of PSS-associated vasculopathy include cutaneous telangiectasia, nail-fold capillary alterations, pulmonary arterial hypertension, gastric antral vascular ectasia, and scleroderma renal crisis with malignant hypertension. In late-stage PSS, there is a striking paucity of small blood vessels in lesional skin and other organs. Endothelial cell injury might be triggered by granzymes, endothelial cell-specific autoantibodies, vasculotropic viruses, inflammatory cytokines, or reactive oxygen radicals generated during ischemia/reperfusion.

Clinical Features

Patients with systemic sclerosis have a wide array of symptoms and difficulties, ranging from complaints related to specific internal organ involvement as well as the symptoms of a chronic catabolic illness. Raynaud's phenomenon is the initial complaint in approximately 70 percent of patients with systemic sclerosis. Peripheral vasoconstriction in response to cold is physiologic, and individuals with Raynaud's, no matter the cause, have undue intolerance to environmental cold. The digital arteries of patients with systemic sclerosis exhibit marked intimal hyperplasia as well as adventitial fibrosis. Severe narrowing (more than 75 percent) of the arterial lumen results, which may be sufficiently severe to account for Raynaud's phenomenon. The skin thickening of systemic sclerosis begins on the fingers and hands in nearly all cases. The skin initially appears shiny and taut and may be erythematous at early stages (Figure 11.4). The skin of the face and neck is usually involved next and is associated with an immobile and pinched facies. The skin change may stay restricted to fingers, hands, and face and may remain relatively mild. Extension to the forearms is often followed by rapid centripetal spread to the upper arms, shoulders, anterior chest, back, abdomen, and legs (diffuse scleroderma).

Involvement of the gastrointestinal tract is the third most common manifestation of systemic sclerosis. Impaired function of the lower esophageal sphincter is associated with symptoms of intermittent heartburn,

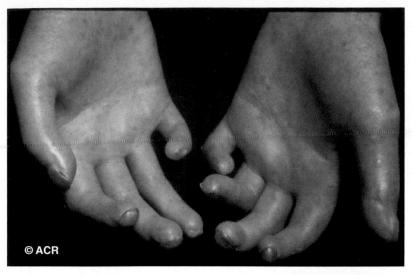

Figure 11.4. Skin tightening and distal necrosis in a patient with systemic sclerosis. © 1972–2004 American College of Rheumatology Clinical Slide Collection. Used with permission.

typically described as a retrosternal burning pain. Complications of chronic esophageal reflux include erosive esophagitis with bleeding, Barrett's esophagus, and lower esophageal stricture. Small-bowel involvement is encountered in patients with longstanding disease. Symptoms include intermittent bloating with abdominal cramps, intermittent or chronic diarrhea, and presentations suggestive of intestinal obstruction.

Pulmonary involvement is the leading cause of mortality and a principal source of morbidity in systemic sclerosis. Pathological processes operative in scleroderma lung include combinations of vascular obliteration, fibrosis, and inflammation. Patients with diffuse scleroderma are at risk for progressive interstitial fibrotic lung disease and pulmonary arterial hypertension. The clinical onset of pulmonary involvement is frequently insidious and characterized by progressive dyspnea on exertion, limited effort tolerance, and a nonproductive cough. Other organs involved in systemic

sclerosis include the musculoskeletal system, with arthralgias, arthritis, and myositis as potential manifestations, as well as the heart and kidney.

Treatment of Progressive Systemic Sclerosis

No drug therapies are available for the management of systemic sclerosis that have been proven to enhance survival, prevent internal organ involvement, or slow, halt, or improve deterioration of function of involved organs, including the skin. In the absence of such agents, management is directed at treating manifestations of the disease. NSAIDs are generally useful in managing arthralgias and myalgias, although occasional patients require low-dosage oral glucocorticoids. Symptoms of reflux esophagitis are typical of systemic sclerosis but generally amenable to therapy with H2 blockers and protein pump inhibitors. Pulmonary involvement has generally not been considered amenable to therapy. A patient in whom there is evidence of pulmonary interstitial inflammation might be treated with glucocorticoids and immunosuppressive agents. A recent double-blind, randomized, placebo-controlled trial to determine the effects of oral cyclophosphamide on lung function and health-related symptoms in patients with evidence of active alveolitis and scleroderma-related interstitial lung disease reported a significant but modest beneficial effect on lung function, dyspnea, thickening of the skin, and health-related quality of life. Pulmonary hypertension has emerged as a principal cause of morbidity and mortality in late systemic sclerosis. Centrally infused prostacyclin (epoprostenol) improves both short- and long-term hemodynamics, as well as the quality of life and survival. Studies have demonstrated that treatment with the oral endothelin receptor anatagonist bosentan is well tolerated in PSS patients with interstitial lung disease and is effective for treatment of severe pulmonary hypertension in study patients. Scleroderma renal crisis demands prompt recognition of the diagnosis and aggressive treatment of the accompanying accelerated hypertension. Angiotensin-converting enzyme inhibitors such as captopril and enalapril are mechanistically ideal to treat the hyperreninemic hypertension of scleroderma renal crisis and are the treatment of choice.

Animal Models of Progressive Systemic Sclerosis

The pathogenesis of PSS involves a triad of small-vessel vasculopathy; inflammation, and autoimmunity; and interstitial and vascular fibrosis in the skin, lungs, and multiple other organs. Various animal models have been investigated as spontaneous or inducible models for SSC. Although none of them reproduce all three pathogenetic components of the disease, some models do recapitulate selected phenotypic features. Two useful animal models of PSS include bleomycin-induced skin fibrosis and the chronic graft-versus-host disease system, which results in skin fibrosis. In addition, the tight skin (Tsk-1) mouse has been proposed as a model for PSS based on skin pathology that is similar to that of the human disease, with increased accumulation of collagen and glycosaminoglycans in the skin and production of serum autoantibodies. The gene mutated in the Tsk-1 mouse is *fibrillin-1*, whose product can form a part of elastic fibers.

POLYMYOSITIS

Introduction and Epidemiology

Polymyositis (PM) is an inflammatory muscle disease characterized by injury and death of muscle cells and resulting in severe weakness. Polymyositis is considered to be an autoimmune disease based on the presence of autoantibodies with characteristic specificities, including those reactive with tRNA synthetases. In addition, infiltration of T cells, predominantly CD8+ cytotoxic T cells, may contribute directly to muscle damage. PM is a rare disease and only a few epidemiological studies have been published. The reported incidence ranges between two and eight new cases per million people per year.

Etiology and Pathogenesis

The idiopathic inflammatory myopathies, including PM, are believed to be immune-mediated processes possibly triggered by environmental factors in genetically susceptible individuals. This hypothesis is based on the recognized association with other autoimmune and collagen vascular diseases, the prevalence and type of circulating autoantibodies, animal models, immunogenetic observations, specifics of the inflammatory changes in muscle, and the treatment response to immunosuppressive agents. Autoantibodies associated with PM include the anti-tRNA synthetase antibodies (anti-Jo-1 and others) as well as antibodies directed against the signal recognition particle. In PM, $CD8^+$ cytotoxic T cells invade muscle fibers that express MHC class I antigens, leading to fiber necrosis via the perforin pathway.

Clinical Features

The main symptoms of PM are weakness affecting primarily the proximal muscles. The onset is typically subacute, occurring over several weeks, with patients complaining of increasing fatigue in rising from a chair, lifting their arms, climbing steps, or combing their hair. The neck extensor muscles may be involved causing difficulty in holding up the head. In severe advanced cases, the respiratory and oropharyngeal muscles are involved causing dysphagia and respiratory difficulties. Myalgias are less frequent than muscular weakness, and when present, accompany the weakness. The most common clinical signs are decreased strength in the proximal muscles, contractures, and late in the course of the disease, muscular atrophy, which occurs in up to 40 percent of cases. Dysphagia occurs in one-third of cases and is due to involvement of the oropharyngeal muscles or involvement of the striated muscle fibers of the upper esophagus. Pulmonary symptoms are due to weakness of the thoracic muscles or interstitial lung disease. Fibrosis is radiologically demonstrated in 5–10 percent of cases and is often associated with anti-tRNA synthetase antibodies such as anti-Jo-1.

Treatment of Polymyositis

Glucocorticoids are the standard first-line medication for patients with idiopathic inflammatory myopathy. Initially, prednisone is given in a single dose of 1 to 2 mg/kg per day. Regular evaluations of muscle strength and serum enzymes should be performed during treatment. Ideally, the initial steroid dosage is maintained until strength and creatine kinase values have returned to normal and have remained normal for four to eight weeks and then tapered. If a patient fails to respond to glucocorticoid therapy or if a patient has had some improvement but the level of strength has reached a plateau, additional therapy with either the immunosuppressive agent azathioprine or methotrexate is added. Another therapeutic option is intravenous immune globulin, which is being used increasingly to treat inflammatory myopathies. This therapy is associated with little toxicity but is extremely expensive. Controlled trials involving larger numbers of patients are needed to prove a benefit for this and other therapies in PM.

Animal Models of Polymyositis

Several animal models have been developed that may prove useful for understanding the pathogenesis of PM. Experimental autoimmune myositis (EAM) can be induced by immunization of rodents with skeletal muscle homogenate and adjuvant. Similarly, Lewis rats immunized with purified skeletal muscle myosin develop EAM with the same pattern and severity as EAM induced by whole-rabbit skeletal-muscle homogenate. Multiple inflammatory lesions are detected histopathologically in various muscle groups in animals immunized with either preparation. Dendritic cells presenting pyruvate kinase M1/M2 peptide 464-472 to T cells have also been effective in inducing EAM in BALB/c mice, with >40 percent of the mice developing pathological changes in skeletal muscle similar to those seen in human PM.

PM can also be induced in mice by viral infection. Intraperitoneal inoculation of Coxsackie B1 virus, Tucson strain, into young mice can result in proximal hindquarter weakness that persists for more than ten weeks. The myositis persists long after the virus is cleared and in the presence of neutralizing antibody, suggesting that the immunological response is contributing to pathology.

A possible murine model of inflammatory myositis has resulted from a genetic deficiency in a member of the synaptotagmin family, comprising Ca2$^+$ sensors involved in cell membrane fusion. Syt VII is a ubiquitously expressed synaptotagmin previously implicated in plasma membrane repair and *Trypanosoma cruzi* invasion, events mediated by the Ca2$^+$-regulated exocytosis of lysosomes. Mice that are Syt VII deficient have an inflammatory myopathy, with muscle-fiber invasion by leukocytes and endomysial collagen deposition. This pathological picture is associated with elevated creatine kinase release and progressive muscle weakness as well as a strong ANA response.

SERONEGATIVE SPONDYLOARTHROPATHY

Introduction and Epidemiology

Ankylosing spondylitis (AS) and related spondyloarthropathies are characterized by sacroiliitis and inflammation of the intervertebral discs in the lumbar spine, as well as an enthesitis at sites of ligamentous insertions into bone. Patients with AS develop calcification of the ligamentous insertions, back stiffness, and pain. The immunologic basis of the specific locations of inflammation in this disorder is not understood, but a strong association of the disease with particular HLA alleles, particularly HLA-B27, suggests a possible role for antigen presentation to T cells in the immunopathogenesis. The prevalence of AS closely parallels the frequency of HLA-B27. Among whites, the estimated prevalence rate of AS is 197 per 100,000 in the United States. AS, in general, is diagnosed more frequently in males. Females, however, may have milder or subclinical disease. AS is more common in males with a male to female ratio of 3:1. The age of onset of AS is usually from the late teens to age 40.

Etiology and Pathogenesis

The exact etiology of AS is unclear. The strong association with most subtypes of HLA-B27 supports the hypothesis that the disease is due to a genetically determined immune response to environmental factors in susceptible individuals. HLA-B27 is present in 80 to 98 percent of white patients with AS, in contrast to only about 8 percent of the general population. The arthritogenic peptide hypothesis postulates that AS results when external antigenic challenge activates autoreactive T cells that recognize endogenous peptides presented by HLA-B27. In normal situations, the HLA-B27 molecule on the surface of the antigen-presenting cells presents endogenously derived peptides to CD8$^+$ T cells. These peptides, which are usually nine amino acids long and have arginine in position 2, are mostly self-derived, but they may also be of viral or bacterial origin. Recent studies also suggest that the intracellular handling of molecular complexes that include HLA-B27 molecules may activate an inflammatory stress response and contribute to disease.

Clinical Features

Back pain is the most common symptom and the first manifestation in approximately 75 percent of patients with AS. The inflammatory back pain of AS has particular features that differentiate it from mechanical back pain. These include insidious onset of the pain occurring over months or years, generally with at least three months of symptoms before presentation. Symptoms include morning stiffness lasting at least thirty minutes, improvement of symptoms with moderate physical activity, and diffuse nonspecific radiation of pain into both buttocks. Patients often experience stiffness and pain that awakens them in the early morning hours, a distinctive symptom not generally found in patients with mechanical back pain. Tenderness at tendon insertion points due to enthesitis, an inflammatory reaction, is a common complaint. Typical tender sites include the costosternal junctions, spinous processes, iliac crests, greater trochanters, ischial tuberosities, tibial tubercles, or heels (Achilles tendinitis or plantar fasciitis). AS is also characterized by a number of extra-articular manifestations including uveitis, occurring in 25–35 percent of patients during the course of the disease. Manifestations of cardiac involvement include ascending aortitis, aortic valve incompetence, conduction abnormalities, cardiomegaly, and pericarditis. In rare situations, aortitis may precede other features of AS. Aortic incompetence was noted in 3.5 percent of patients who had the disease for fifteen years and in 10 percent after thirty years. Cardiac conduction disturbances are seen with increasing frequency with the passage of time, occurring in 2.7 percent of those with disease of fifteen years' duration and in 8.5 percent after thirty years.

Treatment of Ankylosing Spondylitis

AS is a relatively mild disease for most patients with a good functional prognosis. The majority of patients do not experience significant extraskeletal manifestations, except for acute anterior uveitis. Usually, the eye disease can be well managed with eye drops containing corticosteroids to reduce inflammation and with pupil-dilating, atropine-like agents to prevent or diminish synechiae. The objectives for treatment of AS are to relieve pain, stiffness, and fatigue and to maintain good posture and good physical and psychosocial functioning. Physiotherapy provided as exercises is effective in improving thoracolumbar mobility and fitness, at least in the short term (up to one year). Until recently, no drug had been shown to significantly influence the course of spinal disease and retard the process of ossification in AS. Similarly, there was no evidence to suggest that any of the conventional DMARDs, including sulfasalazine and methotrexate, altered or inhibited the inflammation seen in the spine and entheses in AS. Recently, the introduction of anti-TNF agents in the treatment of AS can be regarded as a definite advantage in the therapy of this disease. Both infliximab and etancercept have been shown to improve signs and symptoms of disease. Continuous treatment is necessary in most patients. More than two-thirds of the patients stay on therapy after one year. Guidelines for the use of anti-TNF therapies have recently been developed. The new therapeutic modalities identify important clinical questions to be answered by further research. Clearly, infliximab and etanercept have disease-modifying properties, but their long-term safety and disease-controlling effects in terms of improvement or maintenance of function, as well as the prevention of structural damage, still have to be demonstrated.

Animal Models of Seronegative Spondyloarthropathy

HLA-B27 transgenic rats and strains of HLA-B27 transgenic β2-microglobulin-deficient mice develop a multisystem inflammatory disease affecting the joints, skin, and bowel with strong similarity to human spondyloarthritis. This model supports a direct mechanistic role for that MHC product in the disease, although the details of that mechanism have not been elucidated.

As is the case for other autoimmune rheumatic diseases, antigen-induced murine models are proving useful in study of AS. Aggrecan and versican are large proteoglycan molecules that are present in the intervertebral disc and hyaline cartilages of the sacroiliac joint, as well as in entheses. Versican is generally absent from cartilage tissue except in the sacroiliac joint but is concentrated in ligaments and the annulus of the intervertebral disc. Immunization of BALB/c mice with versican results in an AS-like pathology, including sacroiliitis, enthesitis, and discitis. Those mice develop an ankylosis of the spine similar to that seen in AS. It has also been noted that immunity to versican can induce uveitis, a clinical feature of the human disease.

Future Directions of Research

Significant progress in characterizing the underlying immunopathogenic mechanisms of rheumatic diseases is being stimulated by accelerated success in defining disease susceptibility genes using high-throughput single-nucleotide polymorphism analysis. In addition, increased focus on the activation of the innate immune response, resulting in activation of molecular pathways involved in either production of type I interferon or TNF, is leading to new understanding of the effect of those cytokines on altered immunoregulation and inflammation and has substantially advanced development of new targeted therapies.

Future advances in rheumatic disease research are likely to derive from functional studies related to disease-associated genes identified in the large-scale studies. The regulation of innate immune system activation, alterations in function of cell surface molecules, and signaling pathways that control the threshold for lymphocyte activation and regulation of the complement system are areas for further study that may identify functional correlates of the genes characterized in recent collaborative projects. The regulation of cytokine production, with a particular emphasis on the type I interferon pathway, will be an important topic that can link genetics and translational research that is based on careful clinical characterization in association with laboratory investigations. The use of the experimental murine models described in this chapter will represent an important approach to elucidating the mechanisms through which gene variants and altered immune function result in tissue damage and disease consistent with the pathology that occurs in humans. Future studies should be aimed at identifying molecular targets that can be practically modulated using new therapeutics, with animal studies serving to speed translation to humans.

BIBLIOGRAPHY

SUGGESTED READING

Briani C, Doria A, Sarzi-Puttini P, Dalakas MC. Update on idiopathic inflammatory myopathies. *Autoimmunity*. 2006;39(3):161–170.

Christner PJ, Jimenez SA. Animal models of systemic sclerosis: insights into systemic sclerosis pathogenesis and potential therapeutic approaches. *Curr Opin Rheumatol*. 2004;16:746–752.

Crow MK. Collaboration, genetic associations, and lupus erythematosus. *N Engl J Med*. 2008;358(9):956–961.

Hahn BH. Animal models of systemic lupus erythematosus. In: Wallace DJ, Hahn BH, eds. *Dubois' Lupus Erythematosus*. 6th ed. Philadelphia, PA: Lippincott Williams & Wilkins; 2002:339.

Holmdahl R, Andersson M, Goldschmidt TJ, Gustafsson K, Jansson L, Mo JA. Type II collagen autoimmunity in animals and provocations leading to arthritis. *Immunol Rev*. 1990;118:193–232.

Holmdahl R. Experimental models for rheumatoid arthritis. In: Firestein GS, Panayi GS, Wollheim FA, eds. *Rheumatoid Arthritis New Frontiers in Pathogenesis and Treatment*. New York, NY: Oxford University Press; 2000:39.

Jorgensen TN, Gubbels MR, Kotzin BL. New insights into disease pathogenesis from mouse lupus genetics. *Curr Opin Immunol*. 2004;16:787–793.

Kono DH, Theofilopoulos AN. Genetics of systemic autoimmunity in mouse models of lupus. *Int Rev Immunol*. 2000;19:367–387.

Lauwerys BR, Wakeland EK. Genetics of lupus nephritis. *Lupus*. 2005;14:2–12.

Morel L, Wakeland EK. Lessons from the NZM2410 model and related strains. *Int Rev Immunol*. 2000;19:423–446.

Nagaraju K, Plotz PH. Animal models of myositis. *Rheum Dis Clin North Am*. 2002;28:917–933.

Theofilopoulos AN, Dixon FJ. Murine models of systemic lupus erythematosus. *Adv Immunol*. 1985;37:269–390.

Van den Berg WB. 2004. Animal models. In: St. Clair EW, Pisetsky DS, Haynes BF, eds. *Rheumatoid Arthritis*. Philadelphia, PA: Lippincott Williams & Wilkins; 2004.

Varga J, Abraham D. Systemic sclerosis: a prototypic multisystem fibrotic disorder. *J Clin Invest*. 2007;117(3):557–567.

Wakeland EK, Liu K, Graham RR, Behrens TW. Delineating the genetic basis of systemic lupus erythematosus. *Immunity*. 2001;15:397–408.

Zhang Y. Animal models of inflammatory spinal and sacroiliac joint diseases. *Rheum Dis Clin North Am*. 2003;29:631–645.

12. Immunological Aspects of Cardiac Disease

John B. Zabriskie, M.D., Allan Gibofsky, M.D., J.D., Wesley C. Van Voorhis, M.D., Ph.D., Frederick S. Buckner, M.D., and Noel R. Rose, M.D., Ph.D.

INTRODUCTION

Although the vast majority of cardiac diseases relate to the presence of atherosclerosis in the vessels supplying blood and oxygen to the heart, there are certain conditions in which immunological events play an important role. This chapter will concentrate on the immunological aspects of these diseases. We will also discuss the animal models associated with each of these disorders with particular emphasis on whether these models help us to understand further the immunological aspects of these conditions.

RHEUMATIC FEVER

Acute rheumatic fever (ARF) is a delayed, nonsuppurative sequela of a pharyngeal infection with the group A streptococcus. A latent period of two to three weeks follows the initial streptococcal pharyngitis. The latent period remains the same for each individual patient in the event of a recurrence. This suggests that the patient has already been exposed to more than one streptococcal infection in the past. The onset of disease is usually characterized by an acute febrile illness, which may manifest itself in one of three classical ways: (1) The patient may present with migratory arthritis predominantly involving the large joints of the body. (2) There may also be concomitant clinical and laboratory signs of carditis and valvulitis, or carditis and valvulitis may be the only signs of an acute episode. (3) There may be involvement of the central nervous system, manifesting itself as Sydenham's chorea. The clinical episodes are self-limiting but damage to the valves may be chronic and progressive, resulting in cardiac decompensation and death.

Although both the severity and mortality of the disease have dramatically declined since the turn of the century, recent reports indicate a resurgence in this country (Veasy et al. 1987) and in many military installations in the world, reminding us that ARF remains a public health problem even in developed countries. In addition, the disease continues essentially unabated in many of the developing countries. Estimates suggest 10–20 million new cases per year in those countries where two-thirds of the world's population lives.

Epidemiology

The incidence of ARF actually began to decline long before the introduction of antibiotics into clinical practice, decreasing from 250 to 100 patients per 100,000 population from 1862 to 1962 in Denmark (see Figure 12.1). Why the decline occurred is not entirely clear, but better hygiene, improved economic conditions, and less crowding were certainly important factors.

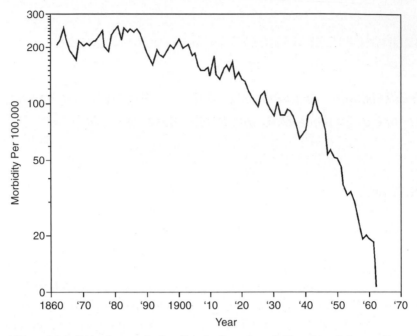

Figure 12.1 Data demonstrating the decline of mortality rates of rheumatic fever long before the advent of penicillin and then the precipitous drop after its introduction.

The introduction of antibiotics in 1950 rapidly accelerated this decline, until by 1980, the incidence ranged from 0.23 to 1.88 patients per 100,000, primarily in children and teenagers in the United States. A notable exception has been in the Australian aborigines (125/100,000) and the native Hawaiian and Maori populations (both of Polynesian ancestry), where the incidence continues to be 13.4/100,000 hospitalized children per year.

Whether certain M-type strains are more "rheumatogenic" than others remains controversial. Certain investigators have stated that M protein types 5, 14, 18, and 24 are mainly associated with outbreaks, but in the large series collected in the Great Lakes Naval Station of ARF during World War II, the main strains were types 17, 19, and 30. In the Caribbean and in Latin America, the main ARF strains are 11 and 41. Thus, whether certain strains are more "rheumatogenic" than others remains

unresolved. What is true, however, is that a streptococcal strain capable of causing a well-documented pharyngitis is generally capable of causing ARF.

Pathogenesis

Although there is little evidence for the direct involvement of group A streptococci in the affected tissues of ARF patients, a large body of epidemiological and immunological evidence indirectly implicates the group A streptococcus in the initiation of the disease process: (1) It is well known that outbreaks of ARF closely follow epidemics of either streptococcal sore throats or scarlet fever. (2) Adequate treatment of a documented streptococcal pharyngitis markedly reduces the incidence of subsequent ARF. (3) Appropriate antimicrobial prophylaxis prevents the recurrences of disease in known patients with acute ARF.

A note of caution is necessary concerning documentation (either clinically or microbiologically) of an antecedent streptococcal infection. The frequency of isolation of group A streptococci from the oropharynx is extremely low during the acute stage of rheumatic fever even in populations with limited access to antibiotics. Further, there appears to be an age-related discrepancy in the clinical documentation of an antecedent sore throat. In older children and young adults, the recollection of a streptococcal sore throat approaches 70 percent; in younger children, this rate approaches only 20 percent. Thus, it is important to have a high index of suspicion of ARF in children or young adults presenting with signs of arthritis or carditis even in the absence of a clinically and microbiologically documented sore throat.

Another intriguing, yet unexplained observation has been the invariable association of ARF only with streptococcal pharyngitis. Although there have been many outbreaks of streptococcal skin infections (impetigo), ARF almost never occurs following infection with these strains. Furthermore, in Trinidad, where both impetigo and ARF are concomitant infections, the strains colonizing the skin are different from those associated with ARF and did not influence the incidence of ARF.

Group A Streptococcus

Figure 12.2 is a schematic cross section of the group A streptococci. Many of the antigens present in the group A streptococcus cross-react with antigens present in mammalian tissues: a concept we call molecular mimicry. Thus, antibodies present in the sera of ARF patients bind to cardiac tissue or cells in the caudate nucleus or to human kidney tissues. The controversial question is whether any or some of these antibodies play a role in initiating the disease process. This will be discussed in more detail in the etiology section. For a more detailed discussion of these cross-reactions, the reader is referred to several excellent reviews of this subject matter.

Although, numerous attempts to produce antibodies to this capsule have been unsuccessful, more recently reports have emerged demonstrating high antibody titers to hyaluronic acid using techniques designed to detect nonprecipitating antibodies in the sera of immunized animals. Similar antibodies have been noted in humans. The data establishing the importance of this capsule in human infections have been almost nonexistent, although Stollerman has commented on the presence of a large mucoid capsule as being one of the more important characteristics of certain "rheumatogenic" strains.

Genetics

That ARF might be the result of a host genetic predisposition has intrigued investigators for over a century. It has been variously suggested that the disease gene is transmitted in an autosomal dominant fashion, in an autosomal recessive fashion with limited penetrance, or that it is possibly related to the genes conferring blood-group secretor status.

Renewed interest in the genetics of ARF occurred with the recognition that gene products of the human MHC (major histocompatibility complex) were associated with certain clinical disease states. Using an alloserum from a multiparous donor, an increased frequency of a B-cell alloantigen was reported in several genetically distinct and ethnically diverse populations of ARF individuals and was not MHC related.

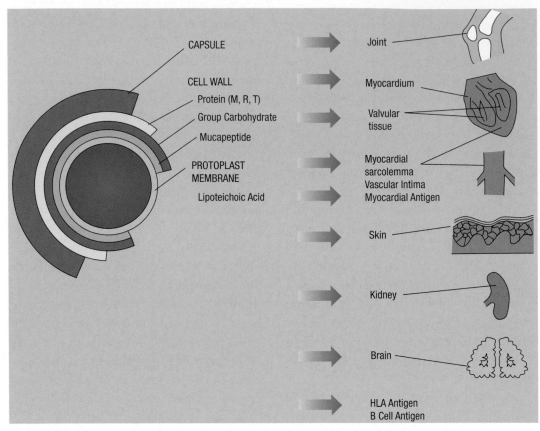

CAPSULE

CELL WALL
  Protein (M, R, T)
  Group Carbohydrate
  Mucapeptide

PROTOPLAST
MEMBRANE

Lipoteichoic Acid

Joint

Myocardium

Valvular
tissue

Myocardial
sarcolemma
Vascular Intima
Myocardial Antigen

Skin

Kidney

Brain

HLA Antigen
B Cell Antigen

Figure 12.2 Schematic representation of the various structures of the group A streptococcus. Note the wide variety of cross-reactions between its antigens and mammalian tissues.

Most recently, a monoclonal antibody (D8/17) was prepared by immunizing mice with B cells from an ARF patient. A B-cell antigen identified by this antibody was found to be expressed on increased numbers of B cells in 100 percent of rheumatic fever patients of diverse ethnic origins and only in 10 percent of normal individuals. The antigen defined by this monoclonal antibody showed no association with or linkage to any of the known MHC haplotypes, nor did it appear to be related to B-cell activation antigens.

These studies are in contrast to other reports in which an increased frequency of certain human leucocyte antigens (HLAs) was seen in ARF patients. There are marked differences in the increased frequency of the HLAs, depending on the racial features of the patient group. These seemingly conflicting results concerning HLA and RF susceptibility prompt speculation that these reported associations might be of class II genes close to (or in linkage disequilibrium with) but not identical to the putatative RF susceptibility gene. Alternatively, and more likely, susceptibility to ARF is polygenic, and the D8/17 antigen might be associated with only one of the genes (i.e., those of the MHC encoding for the D-related [DR] antigens) conferring susceptibility. Although the full explanation remains to be determined, the presence of the D8/17 antigen does appear to identify a population at special risk of contracting ARF.

Etiologic Considerations

A large body of both immunological and epidemiological evidence has implicated the group A streptococcus in the induction of the disease process. Yet, the precise pathological mechanisms involved in the process remain obscure. At least three main theories have been proposed.

The first theory is concerned with the question of whether persistence of the organism is important. Despite several controversial reports, no investigators have been able to consistently and reproducibly demonstrate live organisms in rheumatic fever joints, cardiac tissues, or valves.

The second theory focuses on whether deposition of toxic products is required. Although an attractive hypothesis, little or no experimental evidence has been obtained to support this concept. Renewed interest in extracellular toxins has recently emerged with the observation that certain streptococcal pyrogenic exotoxins (A and C) may act as superantigens. These antigens may stimulate large numbers of T cells through their unique bridging interaction with T-cell receptors of specific Vβ types and class II MHC molecules. This interaction is clearly distinct from conventional antigen presentation in the context of MHC. Once activated, these cells elaborate tumor necrosis factor, gamma interferon, and a number of interleukin moieties, thereby contributing to the initiation of pathological damage. Furthermore, it has been suggested that in certain disease states such as rheumatoid arthritis, autoreactive cells of specific Vβ lineage may "home" to the target organ. Although this is an attractive hypothesis, no data concerning the role of these superantigens in ARF have been forthcoming.

Perhaps the best evidence to date favors the theory of an abnormal host immune response (both humoral and cellular) in the genetically susceptible individual to those streptococcal antigens cross-reactive with mammalian tissues. The evidence supporting this theory can be divided into three broad categories:

1. Employing a wide variety of methods, numerous investigators have documented the presence of heart-reactive antibodies (see Figure 12.3) in ARF sera. The prevalence of these antibodies has varied from a low of 33 percent to a high of 85 percent in various series. Although these antibodies are seen in other individuals (notably those with uncomplicated streptococcal infections that do not go on to rheumatic fever and patients with poststreptococcal glomerulonephritis), the titers are always lower than that seen in rheumatic fever and decrease with time during the convalescent period (Figure 12.4).

   In terms of diagnosis and prognosis, it is important to observe that these heart-reactive antibody titers decline over time. By the end of three years, these titers are essentially undetectable in patients who had only a single attack (see Figure 12.4) This pattern is consistent with the well-known clinical observation that recurrences of rheumatic fever most often occur within the first two to three years after the initial attack and become rarer five years after an initial episode.

   As illustrated in Figure 12.5, this pattern of titers also has prognostic value. During the two- to five-year period after the initial attack, patient M.P.'s heart-reactive titers dropped to undetectable levels. However, with a known break in prophylaxis starting in year 6, at least two streptococcal infections occurred,

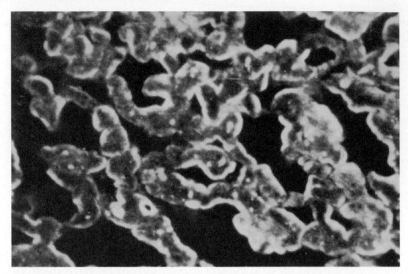

Figure 12.3 Photomicrograph of immunofluorescent staining of heart sections with a serum from an acute rheumatic fever patient followed by a fluorescein-tagged antihuman IgG goat serum. Note the intense sarcolemmal staining pattern of the serum. Identical results were obtained with rabbit sera immunized with Group A streptococcal cell walls but not Group D walls.

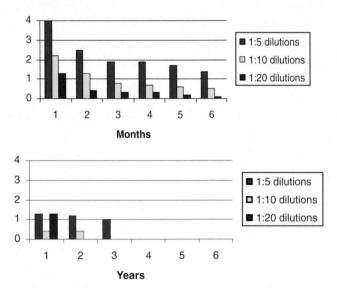

Figure 12.4 Serial heart-reactive antibody titers in forty patients with documented acute rheumatic fever. Note the slow decline of these titers over the first two years after the initial episode and the absence of these antibodies five years after the initial attack.

as evidenced by rise in antistreptolysin O (ASO) titers during that period. Of note was the concomitant rise in heart-reactive antibody titers. The final infection was followed by a clinical recurrence of classical rheumatic carditis complete with isolation of the organism, elevated heart-reactive antibodies,

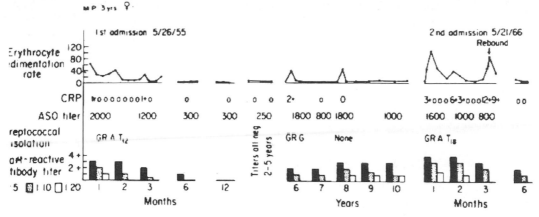

Figure 12.5 Heart-reactive antibody titers and laboratory data obtained from a patient with rheumatic fever who had two well-documented acute attacks eleven years apart. Note absence of the heart-reactive antibody during years 2 to 5 and its reappearance during years 6 to 10 after evidence of two intercurrent streptococcal infections secondary to breaks in penicillin prophylaxis (see ASO titers). High titers of heart-reactive antibody appeared with the second attack. CRP, C reactive protein. Reprinted from Kelley's Textbook of Rheumatology, chapter 103, copyright Elsevier 2006.

and acute-phase reactants eleven years after the initial attack.

2. Sera from patients with ARF also contain increased levels of antibodies to both myosin and tropomyosin, as compared with sera from patients with pharyngeal streptococcal infections that do not develop ARF. These myosin-affinity purified antibodies also cross-react with M protein moieties (known to share amino acid homology with myosin), suggesting this molecule could be the antigenic stimulus for the production of myosin antibodies in these sera.

3. Finally, as indicated earlier, autoimmune antibodies are a prominent finding in another major clinical manifestation of ARF, namely, Sydenham's chorea, and these antibodies are directed against the cells of the caudate nucleus. The titers of this antibody correspond with clinical disease activity.

4. In all cases in which autoreactive antibodies are seen (heart, brain, cardiac valves, kidney), they can be absorbed with streptococcal antigens, notably those streptococcal antigens of the M protein that share homology with human myosin, tropomyosin, keratin, and so on.

At a cellular level, there is now ample evidence for the presence of both lymphocytes and macrophages at the site of pathological damage in the heart valves in patients with ARF (see Figure 12.6). The cells are predominantly CD4[+] helper lymphocytes during acute stages of the disease (4:1). The ratio of CD4[+]/CD8[+] lymphocytes (2:1) more closely approximates the normal ratio in chronic valvular specimens. A majority of these cells express DR antigens. A potentially important finding has been the observation that macrophage-like fibroblasts present in the diseased valves express DR antigens and might be the antigen-presenting cells for the CD4[+] lymphocytes. Increased cellular reactivity to streptococcal antigens has also been noted in the peripheral blood mononuclear cell preparations of ARF patients when compared with these cells isolated from

Composition of the Mononuclear Celllular Infiltrates in Acute and Chronic Active Rheumatic Valvulitis

Patient	Type of valve	Type of valvulitis"	Percentage of mononuclear cells				Percentage of Leu 4 + T cell		Leu 3a/ Leu 2a ratio
			HLA-DR+	63D3+	Leu 16+	Leu 4+	Leu 3a+	Leu 2a+	
Acute valvulitis									
1	Mitral	Acute	58.9	42.6	5.1	49.5	75.6	23.9	3.1
2	Mitral	Acute	49.8	43.1	6.9	43.1	58.7	34.3	1.9
	Aortic	Acute	52.7	51.0	3.9	38.1	65.9	26.5	2.3
3	Mitral	Acute	63.9	42.0	5.5	52.4	75.4	18.9	4.0
4	Aortic	Acute	68.1	56.0	7.4	33.7	71.6	22.0	3.3
Chronic valvulitis									
4	Mitral	Chronic active	49.4	47.4	7.4	44.3	53.7	38.8	1.4
5	Mitral	Chronic active	48.8	39.1	1.4	53.9	45.2	51.5	0.9
	Aortic	Chronic active	67.8	35.0	4.0	36.8	47.5	49.1	1.0
6	Mitral	Chronic active	41.8	23.4	8.0	65.9	57.3	33.3	1.7
	Aortic	Chronic active	69.6	48.7	6.2	30.1	58.2	32.6	1.8
7	Mitral	Chronic active	55.4	24.2	8.1	59.8	64.9	24.7	2.6
8	Mitral	Chronic active	80.4	34.1	13.4	44.4	44.8	50.9	0.9
9	Mitral	Chronic active	46.1	29.6	0.8	65.6	61.6	33.3	1.8

"Determined in the frozen valve samples studies

Figure 12.6 Composition of the mononuclear cellular infiltrates in acute and chronic rheumatic valvulitis. Note the increased CD4/CD8 ratios in acute cases of ARF compared with the more normal CD4/CD8 ratios in chronic more inactive disease patients. Reprinted from Kemeny, et al. (1989) with permission from Elsevier. Kemeny E, Grieve T, Marcus R, Sareli P, Zabriskie JB. Identification of mononuclear cells and T cell subsets in rheumatic valvulitis. *Clin Immunol Immunopathol.* 1989;52:225–237, table 3, p. 231.

nephritis patients. This abnormal reactivity peaks at six months after the attack but may persist for as long as two years after the initial episode. Once again, the reactivity was specific only for those strains associated with ARF, suggesting an abnormal humoral and cellular response to streptococcal antigens unique to rheumatic fever–associated streptococci.

The observation that lymphocytes obtained from experimental animals sensitized to cell membranes but not cell walls are specifically cytotoxic for syngeneic embryonic cardiac myofibers in vitro further strengthens support for the potential pathologic importance of these T cells. In humans, normal mononuclear cells primed in vitro by M protein molecules from a rheumatic fever–associated strain are also cytotoxic for myofibers, but specificity solely for cardiac cells was lacking in the human studies. Similar studies have not yet been performed using lymphocytes from active ARF patients.

A new and potentially interesting chapter is unfolding concerning this manifestation of rheumatic fever. It has been known for years that often the early symptoms of chorea may present as emotional or behavioral changes in the patient and only later do the choreiform motor symptoms appear. Years after the choreiform symptoms subsided a number of chorea patients presented with behavioral disorders such as tics or obsessive-compulsive disorders (OCD).

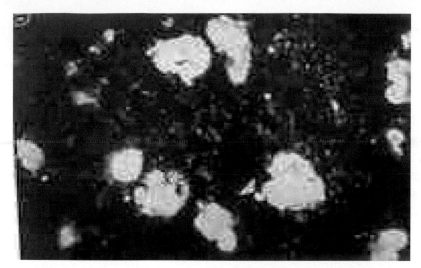

Figure 12.7 Immunofluorescent micrograph of frozen sections of normal human caudate nucleus showing positive staining of large neurons. The serum used was obtained from a child with prolonged active chorea.

These earlier observations coupled with the known presence of antibrain antibodies in the sera of Sydenham's chorea patients (see Figure 12.7) raised the question of whether a prior streptococcal infection (or infection with other microbes) might induce antibodies cross-reactive with brain antigen(s) involved in neural pathways associated with behavior. Two recent papers indicate a strong association of the D8/17 B-cell marker with children with OCD. While Swedo and colleagues selected patients on the basis of a strong history of prior streptococcal infections, Murphy and colleagues noted a strong association of the marker with OCD patients without a history of streptococcal infections. These preliminary studies suggest that streptococci and probably other microbes may induce antibodies, which functionally disrupt the basal ganglia pathways leading not only to classical chorea but also to other behavioral disorders in these children without evidence of classical chorea.

Second, the use of the D8/17 monoclonal antibody has also proved helpful in the differential diagnosis of ARF from other disorders. In our hands, all rheumatic fever patients express abnormal levels of D8/17-positive B cells, especially during the acute attack. In those cases where the diagnosis of ARF has been doubtful, presence of elevated levels of D8/17-positive B cells has proven to be helpful in establishing the correct diagnosis.

Animal Models of Rheumatic Fever

Although investigators over the past sixty to seventy years have tried to understand the pathogenetic mechanisms involved in the initiation and progression of ARF, to date we still do not have a clear picture of the factors involved in the microbe-host relationship.

The most significant drawback to our understanding is that the relationship of the group A streptococcus to this disease is primarily human, and animal models have not been helpful to date. As elegantly pointed out by Krishna and Iyer in a recent chapter devoted to these models, the design of the animal models has closely paralleled the prevailing hypothesis at any given time. These have involved (1) whether persistent and subclinical infection by the organism was a factor, (2) whether direct injury to the myocardium or valves by streptococcal toxins was involved, or (3) whether streptococcal antibodies cross-reactive with human tissues can initiate immune-mediated injury. Unfortunately, none of these approaches have yielded any unequivocal evidence of the classic lesions of ARF. Furthermore, none have clearly demonstrated the known clinical features of the human disease such as a prior streptococcal pharyngitis followed by a latent period followed by clinical and pathological signs of an ARF episode.

However, since the 1970s, observation in ARF patients both in circulatory blood samples and serum as well as studies in tissues removed from ARF and RHD patients have strengthened the concept that an abnormal response to streptococcal antigens at a cellular and humoral level in the genetically susceptible host results in the clinical and laboratory signs of ARF. Further studies have revealed the following: (1) heart-reactive antibodies cross-reactive with streptococcal antigens are present in the sera of these patients; (2) the number of $CD4^+$ cells are increased both in the plasma and tissues of ARF patients compared with CD8; (3) the total number of B cells is increased compared with age-matched controls; (4) the inflammatory cytokines such as TNF-α, IL-2, and IL-1 are elevated in the acute phase and return to normal levels after the episode; and (5) group A streptococci secrete several exotoxins called SPEA, SPEB, and SPEC, which are called superantigens because they bind to the lateral side of TCR and the MHC stimulating a large release of cytokines that could initiate the ARF process. Furthermore they are even capable of deleting certain TCR alleles, possibly inducing loss of self-tolerance and the induction of self-reactive autoantibodies.

All of these observations coupled with the unique association of group A streptococcal infections in humans versus animals suggest that introduction of human genes in mice or rats to create transgenic animals may be more helpful in understanding the human rheumatic fever process. These animals are now available for study mainly based on the long-term commitment to transgenic mice by Dr. Chella David. These mice contain the gene for human $CD4^+$ cells and genes for several different MHC molecules. These mice are more susceptible to the lethal efforts of the superantigen toxins (similar to humans) when compared with nontransgenic littermates, but to date, no studies have been carried out to determine how these mice might react to oral infection with several different group A streptococcal M types, particularly with respect to myocardial and valvular damage. The gene for human B-cell production may also be needed to complete the pathological findings seen in human disease.

Whether these human gene introductions are sufficient to mimic the human disease is not known. But the creation of these and other transgenic models may well be more fruitful since all natural models tested so far have had little success.

Streptococcal Vaccine Candidates

As early as the 1930s, researchers were pursuing the study of streptococcal vaccinations, with the injection of whole-killed group A streptococci and cell walls, thereof culminating in injections of partially purified M protein extracts in the 1970s. However, all interest, especially by the pharmaceutical companies, ceased at that point because the U.S. Food and Drug Administration (FDA) proclaimed that one could work on streptococcal vaccines as long as no streptococcal component was used! The FDA was afraid that induction of antibodies cross-reactive with human tissues, especially cardiac tissues, could be detrimental to the vaccinee. However, it was soon apparent that many individuals had antibodies cross-reactive with a variety of human tissues and were perfectly normal. In the past decade, the restriction was removed on the condition that toxicity studies in animals did not reveal any deletion effects in the animals when injected with a streptococcal vaccine candidate.

This ushered in the search for an effective, safe, and inexpensive group A streptococcal vaccine, and there are now at least four prominent candidates with more in the "pipeline." This area has recently been reviewed in *New Generation Vaccines* (chapter 57) and will only briefly be summarized here.

1. Perhaps the most advanced candidate is by Dale and colleagues (1996), which is synthetic peptide sequences of a variety of M protein types taken from the variable region of the M protein and hooked together by linkers. This has induced protective immunity in animals to a number of different M protein types and is safe for use in humans. Clinical trial of its efficacy to prevent streptococcal infections is currently under way.

2. The use of the C-repeat constant region of the M protein advanced by Fischetti (1989) produces protection against *oral* colonization of the throat by group A streptococci.

3. A surface protein called C5 peptidase, which is present on the surface of all group A and group B streptococci, produces antibodies that block both the colonization of group A and group B streptococci in oral colonization studies.

4. The streptococcal group A carbohydrate (CHO) as proposed by Zabriskie and colleagues has been purified and used as an immunogen to protect against streptococcal infections. This vaccine candidate promotes phagocytosis of group A streptococci of several different M types, will protect against infection using passive and active immunization studies, and also protects against oral colonization. Table 12.1 summarizes all the studies on these four candidates and it can be seen that the variable region of the M protein and the CHO molecule offer the most convincing evidence for a protective vaccine against group A streptococcal infections.

Directions for Future Research

Obviously, the most active area for streptococcal research in the future will be the development of a good group A streptococcal vaccine. Several good candidates are present and more will be studied and evaluated in the future. There are also candidates such as the hyaluronic acid capsule (see Figure 12.2) and many other surface antigens, including the T antigen (similar in many cases but not identical to the M antigen) and others still unknown. It is an exciting area and the production of a safe and inexpensive efficacious vaccine will be the desired goal, especially in

Table 12.1 Summary of Functional Properties of 4 Group A Streptococcal Vaccine Candidates

Candidates	I	II	III	IV
Variable Region M Protein	+	+	+	+
Constant Region	–	–	–	–
C_5 Peptidase	–	+	ND	ND
Group A CHO	+	+	+	+

I. Phagocytosis

II. Prevention of colonization

III. Passive Protection

IV. Active Protection

countries that do not have a well-developed health care system.

Yet our understanding of the basic mechanisms involved in the transition from a relatively mild pharyngeal infection with group A streptococci followed by a latent quiescent period and then followed by ARF with or without carditis or the appearance of Sydenham's chorea is still an important goal because the appearance of the arthritis or acute damage to the valvular tissue is clearly associated with infection of the group A streptococcus. It is the only infectious disease of its type in which we at least know the causative organism. Do superantigens play a role in this transformation? Are particular cytokines and lymphokines present during the quiescent period? Are cellular mechanisms at work, and if so, what cells are involved? These questions are important because the answers to those questions in ARF may hold keys to unlocking other rheumatic diseases (see Chapter 11) as well as our basic understanding of host-microbial relationships in other "presumed" autoimmune diseases.

Those are the difficulties in these studies. The disease is now seen most frequently in developing countries (Africa, South America, India, China, etc.), but careful and well-funded collaborations with clinicians and researchers in these countries could be rewarding. Another fascinating challenge has been the obvious change both in the organism's ability to cause these complications but also in the severity of the disease. One might argue that this is secondary to better health care and medical care and better nutrition in these countries. However, in many poor countries, there really is no health care system in place nor has nutrition improved significantly in the past sixty years; yet, the disease is milder. In some ways, it is similar to diseases such as measles, which is not a particular problem in most populations but can be devastating in those populations that have never been exposed to the agent. Over time, even in these populations, the disease has decreased in severity as herd immunity to the agent increases.

Finally, one of the most intriguing, unresolved questions has been the possible association of the group A streptococcus with behavioral disorders such as OCD, tics, Tourette's syndrome, and anorexia nervosa. Even as early as the 1890s, Osler observed in his textbook of medicine that many of his former Sydenham's chorea patients (a well-known neurological manifestation of a streptococcal infection) often were later seen as patients in the behavioral disorder clinics. One can also expand these concepts to other organisms in which there may be shared antigenicity between microbial and mammalian antigens.

Summary

ARF remains one of the few autoimmune disorders known to occur as a result of infection with a specific organism. The confirmed observation of an increased frequency of a B-cell alloantigen in several populations of rheumatics suggests that it might be possible to identify individuals susceptible to ARF at birth. If so, then from a public health standpoint, these individuals would be prime candidates for immunization with any streptococcal vaccine that might be developed in the future. In addition, careful monitoring of streptococcal disease in the susceptible population could lead to early and effective antibiotic strategies, resulting in disease prevention. Finally, in individuals previously infected, who later present with subtle or nonspecific manifestations of the disease, the presence or absence of the marker could be useful in arriving at a diagnosis.

The continued study of ARF as a paradigm for microbial-host interactions also has important implications for the study of autoimmune diseases in general and rheumatic diseases in particular. Further insights into this intriguing host–parasite relationship may shed additional light into those diseases in which the infection is presumed but has not yet been identified.

CHAGAS' DISEASE

Chagas' disease is named after the Brazilian physician Carlos Chagas who first discovered the parasite responsible for the signs and symptoms of the disease. The causative agent is the hemoflagellate protozoan *Trypanosoma cruzi*. This protozoan parasite is transmitted to the blood-sucking reduviid bug vector when the reduviids take a blood meal from animals or humans who are infected with circulating *T. cruzi*. When the infected bug takes a subsequent blood meal, it usually defecates on the skin of the next victim and deposits *T. cruzi* as well. The individual then becomes infected either by the feces deposited at the site of the puncture or inadvertent contamination of a mucous membrane of the human secondary to hand contamination with organisms. The distribution of the arthropod vectors is limited to the Western Hemisphere and is widely distributed in the southern United States, Mexico, and Central America. The reduviid vectors are common in most South American countries, especially Brazil, Argentina, Bolivia, and Chile. Chagas' is a disease primarily of the poor largely because the reduviid bugs favor living in adobe mud or enter poor housing through cracks or holes in the walls and thatched roofs.

Mode of Transmission and Epidemiology

An estimated 20 million people are currently infected with *T. cruzi*, and approximately 100 million people are at risk of infection. The endemic area of Chagas' disease is huge, stretching from Mexico to southern Argentina, but is limited to the Western Hemisphere. The incidence, prevalence, and severity of Chagas' disease and *T. cruzi* infection seem to be higher in South America than Central America; this may be due to differences in vector behavior or strain variation of *T. cruzi* or differences in disease recognition and reporting.

T. cruzi is transmitted by blood-feeding reduviid insect vectors, vertically from mother to child, or by blood transfusions. Vector transmission is responsible for most of *T. cruzi* infections, and most of this transmission is secondary to the deposit of infected feces and urine by the reduviid bug at the time of the blood meal. As an alternative, humans have been reported to be infected by accidental oral ingestion of reduviid bugs, which presumably release metacyclic trypomastigotes to invade the oral mucosal cells. Parasites persist in the blood of seropositive asymptomatic individuals, and blood from these individuals can transmit infection in approximately 12 percent to 25 percent of transfusions. Blood transfusion transmission has become less frequent as blood banks in endemic areas screen blood with serologic tests to determine whether the blood is likely to be contaminated with *T. cruzi*. However, some areas do not routinely screen donors for *T. cruzi* infection. Congenital transmission occurs in approximately 1 percent of pregnancies of infected women, but the incidence is higher if the woman is infected during pregnancy. Infection of the fetus probably occurs transplacentally in months 5 to 9 of pregnancy.

The reduviid vectors that transmit *T. cruzi* are members of the order Hemiptera, family Reduviidae, and subfamily Triatominae. Although there are more than 100 species of triatomines, few are epidemiologically significant as vectors of *T. cruzi* to humans. Species that colonize housing (domiciliary app.) are important in transmission to humans in the southern part of South America. *Triatoma infestans* is the principal vector responsible for the most transmissions in these "southern cone" countries of South America.

Many reduviid species live in wild habitats and do not invade housing; thus, they do not come in contact with humans and are not important in transmission to humans, although they are important in the propagation of *T. cruzi* in nature. Some sylvatic species (e.g., *Triatoma dimidiata* and *Rhodnius prozlixus*) can inhabit both wild habitants and housing, and these sylvatic species are important in human transmission in the northern part of South America and in Central America.

Host–Parasite Interaction and Host Susceptibility

INNATE IMMUNE RESPONSE

Upon inoculation into tissues of the mammalian host, *T. cruzi* infects local cells where it multiplies intracellularly as amastigotes. At this early point in infection, the host depends on its innate immune response to microorganisms, which is primarily mediated by macrophages and natural killer (NK) cells. Unactivated (resting) macrophages, however, have little ability to kill *T. cruzi* and serve as important host cells for parasite replication. Within two hours of macrophage invasion, the majority of *T. cruzi* have escaped the phagosome and exist free in the host cytoplasm. It is assumed that by rapidly escaping the phagolysosome, *T. cruzi* is able to avoid degradation by intracellular microbicidal enzymes in the unprimed macrophage. A variety of stimuli are capable of priming macrophages for antitrypanosomal activity, with IFN-γ being particularly potent. The addition of a complex mixture of cytokines, including interleukins (IL-2, IL-3, IL-4, and IL-5) to IFN-γ leads to even greater macrophage trypanocidal activity. Anti-IL-4 antibodies added to the mixture were capable of neutralizing the effect, but the combination of IFN-γ and purified IL-4 was no better than IFN-γ alone.

Lipopolysaccharide significantly increases the trypanocidal effect of IFN-γ on macrophages, apparently through a mechanism not solely mediated by the stimulation of TNF production. Another cytokine that is effective at priming macrophages for trypanocidal activity in vitro is granulocyte-macrophage colony-stimulating factor.

Serum taken from an uninfected human does not lyse trypomastigotes, but serum taken from infected patients does lyse trypomastigotes. Thus, the complement system requires the participation of the acquired immune response to *T. cruzi* to become operational. Parasite lysis by immune serum occurs primarily via the alternative complement pathway. This means that the complement cascade is initiated by direct association of complement components (C3) with the parasite surface, rather than by fixation of complement by antibody Fc receptors. In fact, Fab and F(ab)$_2$' prepared from chagasic patients' sera (which are incapable of fixing complement) were nearly as efficient as intact immunoglobulin G (IgG) in complement lysis assays with trypomastigotes. This implied that the effect of immune antibodies on complement lysis of trypomastigotes was a function of the specificity of the antigen-binding sites, rather than complement fixation by bound antibodies. In other words, there was a surface component on the parasites that, when neutralized by immune sera, rendered the parasites susceptible to complement lysis.

Antibodies directed to a 160-kDa protein correlated with the capacity of the serum for complement-mediated lysis of trypomastigotes. Subsequent work led to the [purification and characterization of the specific parasite product, gp160. This glycoprotein bound the complement component C3b and inhibited C3 convertase formation, thus inhibiting activation of the alternative complement pathway. It is membrane bound and shares genetic and functional similarities to the human complement regulatory protein, decay accelerating factor. Further work indicated that this protein also bound human C4b, a component of the classical pathway C3 convertase, and therefore may restrict classic complement activation. The *T. cruzi* complement regulatory protein is stage specific in that it is only expressed by mammalian forms of the parasite. A recent study reported that stable transfection of *T. cruzi* epimastigotes (which are susceptible to complement lysis by normal serum) with the complementary DNA for the *T. cruzi* complement regulatory protein conferred complement resistance.

TISSUE TROPISM

Why does *T. cruzi* preferentially parasitize muscle and nerve tissue? Arguing teleologically, the host immune response needs to control the parasite infection but not at the cost of destroying vital organs (i.e., heart and peripheral nerves). The down-regulatory immune responses may be more exuberant in these critical tissues where even minor injury can be fatal and regenerative capacity is limited (e.g., the cardiac conduction system). *T. cruzi* may have evolved to preferentially infect these tissues as relatively immune-privileged sites. Several other parasites that preferentially infect muscle tissue or nervous tissue include toxoplasmosis, trichinella, Taenia species (beef and pork tapeworms), and sarcocystis. Each of these species depends on a carnivorous-definitive host ingesting the meat of an intermediate host to complete its life cycle. There is no evidence, however, that consumption of *T. cruzi*–infected tissues plays a role in this parasite's life cycle. Thus, the predilection for growth in muscle and nervous tissue is more likely to be related to a strategy for long-term parasite survival in the host, rather than a strategy related to direct transmission to secondary hosts.

IFN-γ induction of macrophage trypanocidal activity is associated with the production of hydrogen peroxide. However, treatment of activated macrophages with catalase, superoxide dismutase, or sodium benzoate to scavenge respiratory burst metabolites failed to inhibit trypanocidal activity in vitro, suggesting an oxygen-independent mechanism of *T. cruzi* destruction. Subsequent studies have revealed the importance of nitric oxide (NO) production in the killing mechanism in murine systems. Macrophages primed with IFN-γ produce NO, and the addition of an inhibitor to NO synthase blocks the trypanocidal activity. Levels of extracellular L-arginine (the substrate for NO production) modulate the trypanocidal activity of macrophages. NO may be directly toxic to *T. cruzi*; however, it reacts with superoxide (O_2^-) to yield peroxynitrite ($ONDO^-$), which is highly toxic to *T. cruzi*. In vivo, inducible nitric oxide synthase (iNOS) is induced at the protein and messenger RNA levels, and NO is released during acute infection in coincidence with secretion of IFN-γ and TNF. The administration of inhibitors of NO production leads to greater susceptibility of *T. cruzi*–infected mice. Mice carrying disruption of the iNOS genes are highly susceptible to *T. cruzi* infection. The IFN-γ–induced, NO-dependent mechanism of macrophage killing of *T. cruzi* can be inhibited by the addition of interleukin-10 or transforming growth factor-β in vitro.

NK cells participate in the innate immune response to *T. cruzi* infection, and NK cells secrete IFN-γ after incubation with *T. cruzi* in vitro. This was shown by culturing splenocytes from athymic nude mice with *T. cruzi* and detecting the secretion of IFN-γ, then demonstrating that the pretreatment of the splenocytes with anti-NK1.1 monoclonal antibody blocked the IFN-γ production. Since IFN-γ activates macrophages to kill *T. cruzi*, the role of NK cells in *T. cruzi* infection would be expected to be protective. In fact, a relatively *T. cruzi*–resistant strain of mouse was rendered highly susceptible to infection by pretreatment with anti-NK1.1 antibodies. Thus, NK cells appear to be an early source of IFN-γ that helps control parasite replication before the acquired immune response becomes predominant. NK cells may also be involved in the immune response later in infection, since they are present in inflammatory lesions of muscle in experimental mice 270 days after infection.

ANIMAL MODELS

Trypanosoma cruzi multiplies and disseminates throughout the host before a specific antiparasitic immune response is mounted. In mice, parasites first become apparent in blood approximately five to seven days after infection and rise in numbers until three or four weeks into infection when the mice either die or the infection is controlled by the immune response (Figure 12.1). RAG knockout mice, which are deficient in both B- and T-cell function, have similar levels of parasitemia compared with wild-type mice until day 13 of infection, at which point the parasitemia level becomes higher in the RAG knockouts. This indicates that the acquired immune response has little effect until about two weeks into the infection. Although anti–*T. cruzi* antibodies are detectable at about day 7 in murine models, protective antibodies are not present until several weeks later. This was shown in experiments in which antibodies taken from acutely infected mice were not protective against *T. cruzi* infection in immune-naïve mice. However, experimental mice or rats that received sera from animals that survived acute infection experience a significant decrease in parasitemia level and mortality following a challenge with virulent parasites.

The importance of IgG in the humoral immune response was first demonstrated by Castelo Branco. The protective component of serum from chronically infected mice could be removed by staphylococcal protein A (which absorbs IgG). Furthermore, the purified IgG component from whole serum was capable of conferring protection. Both IgG subclasses 1 and 2 are capable of clearing *T. cruzi*. Antibodies mediate protection from *T. cruzi* by opsonization, complement activation, and antibody-dependent cellular cytotoxicity.

T cells have a protective role in the acquired immune response to *T. cruzi*. Experiments in mice showed that T-cell activation correlated with resistance to infection. Passive transfer of T cells from mice immunized against *T. cruzi* conferred resistance in mice challenged with *T. cruzi*. Deficient T-cell function is associated with increased sensitivity to infection. This has been shown in nude mice; thymectomized mice; mice treated with cyclosporine A, anti-CD4, and anti-CD8; and mice genomically deleted of CD4, CD8, β_2-microglobulin, TAP-1, or MHC molecules. The increased susceptibility associated with deficient T-cell function is most apparent during acute infection. Mice that are depleted of T cells (CD4$^+$ or CD8$^+$) after they have survived the acute infection do not have altered parasitemia or longevity. The declining role of T cells and the importance of humoral immunity in controlling infection after the acute stage are schematically illustrated (Figure 12.1).

The presence of parasite-specific T cells has been demonstrated for both CD4$^+$ and CD8$^+$ T cells. Nickell and colleagues isolated CD4$^+$ T cells from spleens of infected mice that proliferate to *T. cruzi* antigen in a HLA-restricted fashion. The CD4$^+$ T-cell line recognized an undefined trypomastigote antigen(s), did not cross-react with *Leishmania* spp. or *Toxoplasma gondii*, and was able to passively protect syngeneic recipients from lethal *T. cruzi* challenge infection. Kahn and Wleklinski isolated and cloned CD4$^+$ T cells from *T. cruzi*–infected mice that proliferate and secrete cytokines in response to the surface protein, SA-85, a member of the sialidase superfamily. The MHC class II epitope in this protein was mapped to a 20-amino acid sequence. Nickell and associates were able to isolate CD8$^+$ T cells from infected mice that lysed parasite-infected target cells in an MHC-restricted manner. The parasite antigens involved in the stimulation of CD8$^+$ T cells were not characterized. However, Wizel and colleagues detected class I–restricted CD8$^+$ T cells from spleens of infected mice that lyse target cells, presenting epitopes from the *trans*-sialidase family of proteins. These cytotoxic lymphocytes passively transferred protection against challenge infection.

The inflammatory infiltrates in *T. cruzi*–infected experimental animals have been analyzed for cellular surface markers. Mirkin and colleagues studied tissues from C3H/HeN mice during acute, early chronic, and late chronic infection. The inflammatory infiltrates consisted mainly of lymphocytes (60–90 percent) and macrophages (10–40 percent). The lymphocytes primarily carried the T-cell marker, Thy1.2. Both CD4$^+$ and CD8$^+$ T cells were present in the infiltrates of skeletal muscle, sciatic nerve, and spinal cord. The general trend was for a slight predominance of CD8$^+$ cells over CD4$^+$, particularly during the early chronic and late chronic stages. Sun and Tarleton also found that Thy1.2$^+$ cells were the major lymphocyte population in tissues (cardiac and skeletal muscle) during acute infection. CD8$^+$ T cells (47–59 percent) dominated over CD4$^+$ T cells (9–19 percent). B cells and macrophages each represented less than 1 percent of the cells in the inflammatory infiltrates. Tissues from humans with chronic chagasic cardiomyopathy were similarly analyzed. As with mice, T cells were the primary cell type in the inflammatory infiltrates, with a greater proportion of CD8$^+$ cells than CD4$^+$. Many of the CD8$^+$ T cells expressed granzyme A. The extent that the tissue lymphocytes are directed toward parasites and parasite antigen as opposed to self-targets (i.e., autoimmunity) has not been fully clarified (see "Pathogenesis and Modulation of Immune Function" section).

T cells in *T. cruzi* infection perform a variety of antiparasitic functions. They provide helper T-cell function by stimulating B cells to produce parasite-specific antibody. Nickell and colleagues showed that a T-cell line derived from the spleens of *T. cruzi*–infected mice was able to induce normal spleen cells to produce parasitic-directed antibodies when stimulated in vitro with *T. cruzi* antigen. The activation of helper T-cell function is supported by the predominance of IgG2a and IgG2b antibodies in *T. cruzi* infection, which are typical of CD4$^+$ T-cell-dependent responses. T cells produce cytokines in *T. cruzi* infection, which mediate important antiparasitic functions. CD8$^+$ T cells lyse *T. cruzi*–infected host cells, which presumably interrupts the parasite life cycle, thus limiting its replication. Interestingly, mice genetically deficient for genes controlling perforin or granzyme B–mediated

cytolytic pathways had parasitemia and mortality rates similar to wild-type mice, suggesting that cytolytic function, in fact, may not be the protective effector mechanism of CD8$^+$ T cells. Wizel and coworkers showed that *T. cruzi*–specific CD8$^+$ T cells produce IFN-γ and TNF-α upon stimulation, thus raising the possibility that these cells mediate their effects by cytokine release.

Pathogenesis and Modulation of Immune Function

PATHOGENESIS

The pathogenesis of acute Chagas' disease is not in dispute. On standard histopathological study, inflammatory lesions are found to co-localize with abundant parasites, demonstrating that inflammatory damage is directed to the parasite. The pathophysiology of chronic Chagas' disease is still in question, but the competing (nonexclusive) views are that disease results from an autoimmune response directed at the affected organ systems or from damage resulting from inflammation related to the persistence of the parasite. Supporting the autoimmune hypothesis are observations that live *T. cruzi* parasites have been difficult to demonstrate in involved organs by conventional histological study and that autoimmune T cells and antibodies develop during infection with *T. cruzi*. Furthermore, autoimmune antibodies and autoimmune T cells have been associated with chronic Chagas' disease or lesions. Some *T. cruzi* antigens molecularly mimic affected host tissues. It is hypothesized that the chronic infection leads to loss of tolerance and, combined with antigenic mimicry, results in specific autoimmune attack of cardiac, gut, and peripheral nervous tissues.

The other hypothesis is that progressive inflammation directed at parasites that reside in target organs cause the pathologic damage of chronic infection. Studies that support this hypothesis have found that parasite antigens and DNA can be detected in many chronic inflammatory infiltrate and that parasitologic treatment of chronically infected animals or humans tends to lead to improvement and resolution of disease. The evidence for the competing theories of chronic Chagas' disease pathogenesis is discussed in detail in the next section. Since the autoimmune and parasite-directed pathogenesis theories are not mutually exclusive and since evidence exists to support each of them, it seems likely that both mechanisms could be pathogeneic in chronic Chagas' disease.

AUTOIMMUNITY AND PATHOGENESIS OF CHAGAS' DISEASE

The theory of autoimmunity leading to damage in chronic Chagas' disease is supported by a number of observations. First, few parasites can be demonstrated in the inflammatory lesions by conventional histological study. This observation suggests the disease may not be driven solely by reaction to the parasite. Second, only 10 percent to 30 percent of chronically infected people develop Chagas' disease, although most can be shown to have chronic parasitemia. This suggests that, in addition to chronic *T. cruzi* infection, some other factor(s) determines which individual develops disease. Susceptibility to autoimmune disease could be the host factor that determines who develops disease. Third, chronic Chagas' disease is very organ specific, generally limited to the heart, nervous tissues, or innervation of the gut. Since the parasite can reside in almost any cell type, the organ specificity of Chagas' disease suggests that additional specificity of Chagas' disease is imposed during infection, perhaps by the particular autoimmune response that is generated by chronic *T. cruzi* infection. Fourth, the long lag time from infection to disease could be necessary to generate disease by autoimmunity. Fifth, the presence of autoimmune T cells and antibodies in infected individuals, especially when they are associated with disease, is evidence that autoimmunity may play a role in pathogenesis. It should also be noted that each of these properties of chronic Chagas' disease could be due to parasite-directed pathogenesis, as discussed below.

Autoimmune antibodies are easily demonstrated in *T. cruzi*-infected individuals. Antibodies to myocardium and nervous tissues are found in high levels in persons and mice infected with *T. cruzi* compared with those that are not. Since the myocardium and nervous tissues are key organs that are damaged in chronic Chagas' disease, finding antibodies to these tissues could mean that these antibodies cause autoimmune damage to these tissues. As an alternative, antigens from myocardium and nervous tissues are probably exposed by the damage of infection of these organs, and antibodies may be generated to these tissues without being pathogenic.

Many of the autoantibodies found in the sera of *T. cruzi*–infected persons and mice are so-called natural autoantibodies, which can be found in low levels in the serum of normal humans and mice. The "natural autoantibodies" are directed against proteins that are highly conserved in evolution and are not necessarily an indication of autoimmune disease. The high levels of natural autoantibodies after *T. cruzi* infection may be the result of the polyclonal lymphocytic proliferative response that occurs during acute infection. Levels of natural autoantibodies do not correlate with diseases in individuals who are chronically infected with *T. cruzi*.

MOLECULAR MIMICRY IN CHAGAS' DISEASE

Molecular mimicry of host antigens by parasite antigens has been found to generate autoantibodies that are found in chronic *T. cruzi* infection (See table 12.2). Autoimmune pathogenesis by molecular mimicry requires breakdown in tolerance of the immune system to self-antigens. A breakdown in tolerance could occur in response to chronic *T. cruzi* infection or because of the polyclonal lymphocyte proliferative response that occurs early after infection. Although many molecular mimicry epitopes have been described, only a few have been shown to correlate with disease in chronic *T. cruzi* infection.

For example, high levels of antibodies to rodent endocardium, blood vessels, and interstitium (EVI) have been found in the sera of *T. cruzi*–infected individuals and the mammalian host and were absorbed by epimastigote antigens, thus demonstrating cross-reactivity. However, these EVI antigens shown to be directed against α-galactose epitopes were specific for murine laminin and not human laminin. Furthermore, anti-EVI antibodies (α-galactose/laminin) or other autoantibodies have not been shown to transfer disease to noninfected animals.

Perhaps more interesting (in terms of the organs infected) has been a protein found on the surface of trypomastigotes in association with the flagellum, Fl-160. This protein molecularly mimics myenteric plexus and peripheral neurons. These antibodies are found in 30 percent of individuals with chronic Chagas' disease; yet, they do not appear to correlate with disease activity in these patients. In addition, T-cell responses to this protein have not been seen in individuals with Chagas' disease, and passive transfer of these immune T-cells was not consistently effective.

Another peptide of interest has been the ribosomal Po protein (R13 peptide), which has been shown to cross-react with a functional protein on human B1-adenergic receptors. Antibodies to this receptor via immunization with the R13 peptide have led to electrocardiographic (ECG) changes in mice that are similar to those seen in chronic Chagas' carditis but no changes in digestive symptoms have been noted.

Antibodies to an interesting *T. cruzi* protein called B13 is seen in the sera of all patients with chronic Chagas' cardiomyopathy and this antibody cross-reacts with human cardiac myosin but in only 17 percent of asymptomatic individuals. Furthermore, T cells directed to both B13 and myosin have been detected in biopsy specimens from persons with chronic Chagas' cardiomyopathy. These results suggest that antibody and T cells directed to cardiac myosin may be pathogenic in chronic Chagas' cardiomyopathy. However, in animal models transfer of antibody and T cells directed to myosin have not been reported to lead to pathogenic changes. Perhaps the mouse model may not be correct and as in rheumatic fever the introduction of myosin in the Lewis rat may be a better animal model.

PARASITE-DIRECTED PATHOGENESIS

Since the studies reporting that autoimmunity may be involved in the inflammatory infiltrates of chronic Chagas' disease are not conclusive, the alternative theory is that parasites residing in chronically infected host tissue may cause chronic

Table 12.2 Molecular Mimicry Antigens of *Trypanosoma Cruzi*

T. Cruzi Antigen	Cross-reactive Mammalian Antigen	Pattern of Mammalian Reactivity	Mammalian Species	Relationship to Disease
(α1-3)-galactose	Murine laminin	Endocardium, blood vessels, and interstitium	Rodent, not human	None
Sulfated glycolipids	Sulfagalactosyl-ceramide	Neurons, astrocytes	Mouse	Not tested
Neutral glycosphingolipids	Cardia-neutral-glycosphingolipids	Heart muscle	Mouse	Not tested
GP50/55 kDa	P28 kDa	Activated T and B lymphocytes	Mouse, human	Not tested
Amastigote cell-surface and epimastigote cytoplasmic (CE5 Mab)	P60, p32 kDa	Central and peripheral neurons	Rodent, human	Not tested
p58, p35 kDa (5H7 & 3H3 Mabs)	P58, p37	Central and peripheral neurons, glia	Rodent	Not tested
150-kDa surface trypomastigote antigen		Striated and smooth muscle including smooth muscle of cardiac arteries	Human, mouse	Not tested
FL-160, 160-kDa flagellar-associated surface protein of trypomastigotes	p48 kDa	Myenteric plexus and peripheral nerve axons	Rodent, human	Antibodies to FL-160 found in 30 percent of those infected with *T. cruzi* but no relationship with disease
Microtubule-associated protein	Microtubule-associated protein	Fibroblasts, brain cells	Mouse, bovine	Not tested
B13, 140, and 116-kDa proteins	Cardiac myosin	Heart ventricle	Human, mouse	Antibodies correlate with cardiac disease, autoreactive T cells from cardiac lesions
Ribosomal P protein	Ribosomal P protein	All mammalian cells	Human	High levels of antibodies to R13 peptide correlate with Chagas cardiomyophy

(continued)

Table 12.2 *(continued)*

T. Cruzi Antigen	Cross-reactive Mammalian Antigen	Pattern of Mammalian Reactivity	Mammalian Species	Relationship to Disease
Ribosomal PO protein (R13 peptides)	β_1-adrenergic receptor	Heart	Human	Not tested, though antibodies found in 47 percent of chagasic heart disease patients and levels of anti-R13 correlate with cardiomyopathy
Ribosomal 23-kDa protein	Ribosomal 23-kDa protein		Human	No correlation of antibody levels with cardiac disease
p25-kDa Epimastigote protein	Heart sarcolemma	Heart	Human, rodent	Antibody levels with cardiac disease
Microsomal and membrane antigens	p71, 65, 59, 45, 44, 34, 30–27 kDa	Myocardium and skeletal muscle	Human, hamster	Not tested

Adapted with permission from Buckner FS, Van Voorhis WC. Immune response to *Trypanosoma cruzi*: control of infection and pathogenesis of Chagas' disease. In: Cunningham MW, Fujinami RS, eds. *Effects of Microbes on the Immune System*. Philadelphia, PA: Lippincott-Raven Press; 2000:5 69–591.

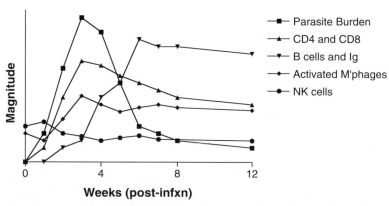

Figure 12.8 Relative magnitude of immune response mediators and parasite burden during acute *Trypanosoma cruzi* infection in the mouse. Adapted with permission from Buckner FS, Van Voorhis WC. Immune response to *Trypanosoma cruzi*: control of infection and pathogenesis of Chagas' disease. In: Cunningham MW, Fujinami RS, eds. *Effects of Microbes on the Immune System*. Philadelphia, PA: Lippincott-Raven Press; 2000:5 69–591.

Immunological Aspects of Cardiac Disease

disease by either damaging tissues directly or focusing the inflammatory response in host tissues. Many of the properties of chronic Chagas' disease cited in support of the autoimmune hypothesis may also be possible with parasite-directed pathogenesis. Parasites may be difficult to demonstrate in the lesions but that may be due to limitations of present techniques. We do know that chronically infected individuals harbor parasites, and the fact that not all chronically infected individuals develop chronic disease may reflect parasite burden, strain differences, or host variation in the immune response. The organ specificity may be due to tropism of the parasite for cardiac and neuronal tissues. Thus, the long lag time to develop disease may be due to the slowly progressive damage that is required to generate clinical disease.

Two other factors support the parasite-directed damage. First, immunosuppression exacerbates, not ameliorates, the disease process and causes worsening of the pathologic lesions of Chagas' disease. However, one could argue that loss of the immune response permits continued growth of the organism and damage. The second factor is that treatment with antiparasitic drugs in early Chagas' disease markedly lessened the progression to chronic disease, although the number of patients assigned to treatment versus placebo groups was small.

Future Directions of Research

Clearly, more evidence is needed to support or refute the autoimmune hypothesis of Chagas' disease. In animal models, transfer of immune cells or sera without parasites and recapitulation of cardiac disease would be one convincing line of evidence. Animal experiments in which chronic *T.*

cruzi infection could be cured with chemotherapy would provide a model to evaluate whether parasites need to persist for the chronic pathology to occur. In humans, nonrandomized study of patients treated with benznidazole indicates that cardiac complications are reduced compared with untreated individuals, suggesting that the pathology may be parasite driven. A prospective randomized trial is needed to cure humans of parasites and then observe whether cardiac disease remits or fails to develop. For this to work, better drugs and better ways to detect chronic infection and to assess the cure of infection are required. In addition, in humans, better correlations between clinical cardiac disease and autoimmune phenomena are needed. Finally, therapeutic trials to interrupt autoimmune cardiac damage are needed, but this will require further research to learn the best way to intervene.

Conclusions

These findings support the importance of the parasite in generating chronic Chagas' disease and the search for more effective and less toxic antiparasitic therapeutics. However, autoimmune mechanisms may potentiate or may even be necessary for the parasite-directed pathogenesis of chronic *T. cruzi* infection. Further understanding of these autoimmune mechanisms could suggest immunomodulatory therapy that could act as an adjunct to antiparasitic therapy to help reduce the damage of chronic Chagas' disease.

OTHER IMMUNE-MEDIATED MYOCARDIAL DISEASES

A suggestive antecedent viral infection leads to immune-mediated heart-muscle disease. These diseases may be conveniently divided into two main categories: myocarditis and dilated cardiomyopathy (DCM). We will not discuss drug- or allergy-mediated myocarditis or myocardial damage related to ischemic heart disease.

Myocarditis

The major features of myocarditis are disturbances in heart rhythms, congestive heart failure, or cardiogenic shock. ECG changes include nonspecific ST-Twave changes, while two-dimensional echocardiograms reveal (1) normal ventricular size but decreased contractility early in the disease and (2) later heart enlargement with thinning of the muscle in chronic cases. In addition, both ventricles may be affected in chronic cases. None of the clinical features described are diagnostic for myocarditis, and until the use of the endomyocardial biotome, the diagnosis could only be established with certainty by postmortem examination.

The incidence of the disease varies from 1 to 10/100,000. The reasons for this wide discrepancy may be related to exposure to the different types and strains of cardiotropic viruses as well as genetic differences in host populations. Many patients recover spontaneously inter supportive treatment but the five-year survival of biopsy-proven giant cell myocarditis is only 56 percent, and in pediatric patients, the mortality rates may be even higher.

Dilated Cardiomyopathy

DCM is a chronic form of heart disease characterized by right ventricular dilation and impaired contraction. The clinical spectrum varies from asymptomatic cardiomopathy to severe congestive heart failure. Patients may also display signs or symptoms of arrhythmias, systemic pulmonary vein congestion, triple gallup rhythms, and mitral or tricuspid regurgitation. Once the diagnosis is established, the outcome is poor, with a five-year mortality of 46 percent. In 1985 in Minnesota, the prevalence was 36.5/100,000, and African Americans and males were associated with increased risk. In Sweden, the incidence was 10/100,000.

It is uncertain how many cases represent progression from myocarditis to DCM since in general the endomyocardial biopsy is not routinely performed in DCM patients. Some reports have indicated that there is a relationship between the two, but biopsies in both diseases are needed to prove or disprove this concept.

Etiologic Considerations

In both myocarditis and DCM, there appears to be an association with prior Coxsackie virus infections. In children and infants with DCM, significantly increased titers of neutralizing antibody to the virus has been found. In addition, Coxsackie virus B–specific nucleic acid sequences have been found in the heart tissues of a small number of these patients. Furthermore, using polymerase chain reaction (PCR) techniques, many children with suspected myocarditis were PCR positive for several viral agents in endomyocardial biopsies (twenty-six of thirty-eight samples from thirty-four patients), and the viral sequences were more often adenoviral than enteroviral.

Autoimmune Considerations

As in other immune-mediated diseases of the heart, many investigators have now explored the role of autoantibodies to the heart as an explanation for the disease. Using cardiac tissue from rats and humans (either frozen tissue or isolated myocytes), immunofluorescence studies showed the antibody localized on the myocyte, giving a sarcolemmal, myolemnal pattern or on the striations, producing a fibrillar pattern. Whether these two patterns represent different forms of the disease is unclear because both patterns were seen in the sera of mice immunized with cardiac myosin. The specificity of these patterns is unclear because many normal sera gave the same pattern in one series (91 percent of patients vs. 35 percent of controls). Another series was more specific where 59 percent of acute myocarditis patients where positive versus 0 percent of healthy controls.

Perhaps more sensitive has been the use of the Western immunoblot technique. Here 97 of 103 samples exhibited positive reactivity but no single pattern was seen to be unique in either group. However, myocarditis sera reacted more to myosin heavy chain, while cardiomyopathy sera reacted more to muscle actin. Again, many normal sera also reacted to these antigens but in lower titers. Further techniques such as enzyme-linked immunosorbent assay (ELISA), using purified cardiac myosin heavy chain material, may be needed for clinical evaluation of these antibodies.

Using a variety of well-defined cardiac cytoskeletal proteins (myosin, laminin, and β_1-adrenergic receptors) as well as mitochondrial components such as adenosine nucleotide translocator (ANT) and branched-chain ketodehydrogenase (BCKD), ELISA studies have revealed that autoantibodies to ANT were elevated in 24/32 patients with DCM. Control sera were within normal limits.

These results show that many patients with myocarditis and with DCM develop autoantibodies to a number of cardiac constituents. Large-scale evaluation is necessary before one can conclude that the detection of any single antibody, or group of antibodies, is sufficiently sensitive and specific to replace the endomyocardial biopsy as a primary diagnostic tool.

None of these antibodies to cardiac antigens is known to play a direct pathogenetic role in the disease. However, the presence of antibodies to β_1-adrenergic receptors in DCM and Chagas' disease is highly suggestive of a direct pathogenetic effect, since the antigen is accessible on the surface of the myocardiocyte. β_1-adrenergic receptor antibodies can induce apoptosis in isolated adult cardiomyocytes and antibodies activating the receptors are associated with reduced cardiac function in chronic heart failure. Antibodies to the mitochondrial antigens, ANT and BCKD, may also have adverse consequences on cardiac function. It is not clear, however, whether these antibodies have access to their target antigens in vivo.

Genetic Features

Because of the possible autoimmune origin of myocarditis and DCM in humans, and the well-documented association of experimental myocarditis with MHC in mice (Rose et al. 1988) a number of studies to determine the relationship with the human MHC (HLA) have been carried out. Several investigators have reported that DCM patients had an increased frequency of HLA-DR4 and a decreased frequency of HLA-DR6. The largest study to date reconfirmed these findings and also found that DR4-Dqw4 haplotype conferred heightened risk of disease.

A predominance of myocarditis in males has been reported in a number of studies. The proportion of male patients is about 60 percent. In this respect, myocarditis differs from most autoimmune diseases, which predominantly affect females.

Environmental Features

Myocarditis has both infectious and non-infectious causes. Acute myocarditis is associated with infections of many types, including bacterial, rickettsial, viral, mycotic, protozoan, and helminthic. As stated previously, several viruses have been implicated in this disease and, in some cases, multiple viruses may be detected in the heart. In Europe and North America, among the most common agents are the enteroviruses and the adenoviruses. It has been reported that Coxsackie virus group B infections were associated with at least half of the acute cases of myocarditits and by immunofluorescence, the Coxsackie virus B antigen was found in the myocardium of 30.9 percent of routine autopsy specimens of myocarditis. Serotype B3 is identified most frequently.

Animal Models

Since enteroviruses have been most often implicated in human myocarditis and DCM, animal models with these agents have been used to investigate the pathogenic mechanisms of these diseases. Although infections with Cox Sackie Virus B3 are relatively common in humans, the development of clinically significant cardiac disease in humans is uncommon, suggesting that differences in host response may be crucial. These differences may be related to genetic factors or may relate to virus-specific receptors on host tissue.

Thus, mice with a wide variety of genetic backgrounds have been used to study the viral host relationships related to human disease.

All strains of mice tested developed acute myocarditis starting two or three days after CB3 infection. The disease reached its peak on day 7 and gradually resolved, so that by twenty-one days after infection the heart was histologically normal. In a few strains of mice, however, the myocarditis persisted. Further studies resolved CB3-induced myocarditis into two distinct phases. The first phase occurred during the first week after infection and was characterized by focal necrosis of myocytes and an accompanying focal acute inflammatory response with a mixed-cell infiltrate, consisting of polymorphonuclear and mononuclear cells. The second phase of CB3-induced myocarditis becomes evident about nine days after infection and is fully manifested by fifteen to twenty-one days after infection. Histologically, the inflammatory process was diffuse rather than focal and consisted mainly of mononuclear interstitial infiltrate. Little or no myocyte necrosis was evident at that time. Infectious virus could be cultured only during the first phase of disease; no virus was isolated after day 9. Heart-reactive autoantibodies were present in all strains that developed the second phase of myocarditis. Only certain inbred strains of mice developed this secondary autoimmune myocarditis. Susceptibility was determined primarily by non-H-2-background genes, although H-2-encoded differences influenced the severity of the autoimmune response initiated by molecular mimicry between the virus and heart antigens. Available evidence suggests that the autoimmune response depends on virus-induced damage to the heart since it was observed that transgenic mice expressing IFN-γ in their pancreatic beta cells failed to develop CB3-induced myocarditis, even though the virus proliferated in other sites. This work challenges the concept of molecular mimicry as the mechanism initiating the autoimmune response and suggests that it is due to a "bystander effect." The virus infections may serve as an adjuvant for the cardiac antigens liberated during the viral infection of the heart.

The presence of autoantibodies in the late phase of CB3-induced myocarditis provided the opportunity to evaluate the pathogenic significance of the immune response. The first step was to characterize the cardiac antigen, and it was found that cardiac myosin heavy chain was the major antigen. Knowing this, Rose and colleagues demonstrated that purified mouse cardiac myosin injected with complete Freund's adjuvant (CFA) produced lesions that resembled the late phase of CB3-induced myocarditis. Furthermore, only strains of mice that were genetically susceptible to the disease produced these lesions, whereas resistant strains did not. One can also induce the disease with peptides derived from the cardiac myosin molecule.

Cellular immunity also played a role in that autoreactive T cells were present in the lesions. Two types of cytotoxic T cells were discovered. One was specific for CB3-infected myocytes, and one was specific for uninfected myocytes. The latter reactivity was probably a result of the appearance of novel determinants expressed on the myocyte following altered myocyte metabolism. With regard to the myosin-specific T cells, mice depleted of $CD4^+$ or $CD8^+$ T cells failed to develop myocarditis after myosin immunization. Both humoral and cellular responses to cardiac myosin participate in the lesion as antibody plus complement is deposited in the hearts of these mice.

Recent investigations have focused on the critical role of the initial, innate immune response in switching from harmless autoimmunity to a pathogenic autoimmune response. Administration of pro-inflammatory cytokines, IL-1 or TNF-α, to genetically resistant B10A mice confers susceptibility to myocarditis after challenge with CB3 or murine myosin in CFA. However, antibody to TNF-α or IL-1 receptor antagonist prevents or delays the onset of myocarditis in genetically susceptible A/J mice, leading to the conclusion that these early inflammatory mediators are required for autoimmune myocarditis.

Myocarditis can be induced in mice by other viruses, including mouse cytomegalovirus (CMV), a herpes virus. Sublethal mouse CMV infections of BALB/c mice induce inflammation of the heart similar to that seen in the CB3-induced disease in mice. Infectious virus was not detected in the heart after ten days, but antibodies to cardiac myosin were evident.

Treatment and Outcome

Until recently, the only treatments for myocarditis and DCM have been supportive therapies, such as bed rest and treatment of heart failure, arrhythmias, and embolic events if present. In many centers, cardiac transplantation has become the eventual treatment of choice in patients with refractory heart failure. The role of immunosuppressive therapy in myocarditis remains controversial. Numerous reported studies on relatively small numbers of patients have generally found that, while some individuals respond well to immunosuppression (prednisone and cyclosporine), others fail to respond or even have serious adverse reactions that preclude continued treatment. The major problem at present is the difficulty in distinguishing immune-mediated cardiac disease from infectious, genetic, or toxic forms of the disease. Obviously, until there are reliable biomarkers to distinguish autoimmune myocarditis/DCM, treatment cannot be rational or capable of evaluation.

Future Directions for Research

At this time, the treatment of both myocarditis and DCM is problematic. In the case of myocarditis, the distinction between viral disease and autoimmune myocarditis remains uncertain. The appropriate treatment of DCM presents an even greater challenge. The disease process ends essentially in an enlarged, fibrotic, nonfunctioning heart. Although the idea of replacing the fibrous connective tissue with functioning myocytes using stem cells is attractive, the obstacles remain well beyond our present capabilities. We are left, therefore, with the difficult alternatives of supportive treatment or cardiac transplantation. The latter course of treatment raises its own series of problems, especially because it entails lifelong treatment with anti-inflammatory and immune-suppressive agents.

In considering future treatments for myocarditis or DCM, the most feasible strategy available to us at this time is prevention. The initial goal is to identify patients with viral myocarditis who are likely to progress to an autoimmune disorder. Although the task is daunting, some information from experimental studies gives hope that the goal is not out of reach. In the first instance, the genetic constitution of the host determines the transition from viral to autoimmune myocarditis. In mice, the MHC plays a role, but additional immunoregulatory genes are even more prominent. For example, in the BALB/c mice,

susceptibility genes have been identified on chromosome 1 and chromosome 6. On the basis of preliminary evidence, both of these genes may act through modulation of apoptosis in T cells. Obviously, any genetic trait that impairs T-cell apoptosis following antigen stimulation increases the probability of a later autoimmune consequence. If similar genes operate in humans, their presence in the form of specific alleles would provide important initial information on the risk of autoimmune progression. A second clue comes from detailed studies of the early innate immune response to the virus. Susceptible strains of mice produce somewhat higher levels of certain key cytokines such as IL-1β and TNF-α. Early elevation in these or similar key cytokines may provide useful biomarkers for subsequent autoimmune disease.

The second goal is to identify patients with autoimmune myocarditis who are most likely to progress to irreversible DCM. Again, studies of the experimental disease in mice provide some clues. Early data suggest that two key cytokines, IFN-γ and IL-13, exert important protective effects during autoimmune myocarditis. Consequently, mice deficient in either of these cytokine markers are likely to progress to a severe form of dilated cardiopathy. If these findings can be replicated in humans, valuable information can be gleaned about the risk of DCM.

Prediction of oncoming disease is only half of the story since that information must be coupled to some useful interventions. Turning again to experimental models, evidence shows that inhibiting some critical cytokines at the earliest stages of pathogenesis can avoid the autoimmune sequelae of viral infection. For example, administration of either the IL-1β receptor antagonist or monoclonal antibody to TNF-α prevents the development of autoimmune myocarditis, even in the most susceptible strains of mice. The use of such anti-inflammatory treatment has already proven to be beneficial in a number of other autoimmune disorders. A second, and even more targeted, approach is to focus on the responsible antigen. In the case of myocarditis, it seems that cardiac myosin is an important, if not the only, etiologic antigen. If that is the case in human disease, many strategies can be mobilized to induce antigen-specific tolerance. Nasal administration of myosin prevents development of autoimmune myocarditis. Recently published evidence suggests that a conjugate vaccine prepared with the myocarditic peptide can prevent the development of autoimmune myocarditis and even reverse the process if given during the early stages of immunization. Of course, the possible prophylactic and therapeutic use of such altered peptide vaccines has proved to be a double-edged sword in the past because these preparations can induce detrimental or even fatal immunological consequences. A careful study of the immunological events surrounding such peptide-based vaccines should provide the understanding necessary to avoid these unfortunate effects.

There are many reasons to believe that the future treatment of autoimmune disease in general depends on early prediction and appropriate prevention. The autoimmune diseases of the heart, myocarditis, and DCM are ideal candidates in which to develop feasible strategies to attain this long-range goal.

SUMMARY

The three major cardiac diseases described in this chapter exemplify the broad range of cardiovascular disorders with which autoimmune responses have been implicated. Until recently, the role of autoimmunity in cardiovascular diseases had been rather neglected. Yet before the early 1960s, rheumatic fever was a major topic of investigation. Although the decline of rheumatic fever in the 1960s in developed (but not in developing) countries accounted for a loss of interest in this topic, one must recognize that the studies of rheumatic fever were the stimulus for many current concepts of autoimmunity and autoimmune disease. Efforts to understand the role of autoimmunity in Chagas' disease and the viral myocardiopathies spearheaded the renaissance in cardiovascular immunology. There is now a substantial challenge in developing reliable and robust in vitro assays that define autoimmune heart disorders with the same sensitivity and specificity available to autoimmune disorders affecting other major organs. These studies have also served as the impetus to delineate the contribution of autoimmunity to other enigmatic cardiovascular diseases such as atherosclerosis. Further, they have served as a general model for studies relating infection to the onset of autoimmune disease.

BIBLIOGRAPHY – RHEUMATIC FEVER

REVIEWS

Cunningham MW. Molecular mimicry between Group A streptococci and myosin in the pathogenesis of rheumatic fever. In: Narula J, Vermani R, Ruddy KS, Tandon, R, eds. *Rheumatic Fever*. Washington, DC: American Registry of Pathology, Armed Forces Institute of Pathology; 1999:Chapter 7.

Gibofsky A, Zabriskie JB. Rheumatic fever: new insights into an old disease. *Bull Rheum Dis*. 1994;42(7):5–7.

Gibofsky A, Zabriskie J. Acute rheumatic fever and post-streptococcal arthritis. In: Harris E Jr, Budd RC, Firestein GS, et al. *Kelley's Textbook of Rheumatology*. Elsevier Sanders; 2005:1684–1696.

SUGGESTED ARTICLES

Dale JB, Simmons M, et al. Recombinant, octavalent group A streptococcal M protein vaccine. *Vaccine*. 1996;14(10): 944–948.

Fischetti VA. Streptococcal M protein: molecular design and biological behavior. *Clin Microbiol Rev*. 1989;2:285–314.

Guilherme L, Kalil J. Rheumatic fever: the T cell response leading to autoimmune aggression in the heart. *Autoimmun Rev*. 2002;1:261–266.

Husby G, van de Rijn I, Zabriskie JB, Abdin ZH, Williams RC Jr. Antibodies reacting with cytoplasm of subthalmic and caudate nuclei neurons in chorea and acute rheumatic fever. *J Exp Med* 1976;144:1094–1110.

Kemeny E, Grieve T, Marcus R, Sareli P, Zabriskie JB. Identification of mononuclear cells and T cell subsets in rheumatic valvulitis. *Clin Immunol Immunopathol*. 1989;52:225–237.

Khanna AK, Buskirk DR, Williams RC Jr, Gibofsky A, Crow MK, Menon A. Presence of a non HLA B cell antigen in rheumatic fever patients and their families as defined by a monoclonal antibody. *J Clin Invest*. 1989;83:1710–1716.

Krishna G, Iyer RR. Animal models of rheumatic fever. In: Narula J, Vermani R, Ruddy KS, Tandon R, eds. *Rheumatic Fever*. Washington, DC: American Registry of Pathology, Armed Forces Institute of Pathology; 1999:Chapter 10.

Li Y, Heuser JS, Kosanke SD, Hemric M, Cunningham MW. Cryptic epitope identified in rat and human cardiac myosin S2 region induces myocarditis in the Lewis rat. *J Immunol*. 2004; 172(5):3225–3234.

Murphy TK Goodman WK, Fudge MW, et al. B lymphocyte antigen D8/17: a peripheral marker for childhood-onset obsessive compulsive disorder and Tourette's syndrome? *Am J Psychiatry*. 1997;154:402–407.

Swedo SE, Leonard HL, Mittleman BB, et al. Children with PANDAS (Pediatric autoimmune neuropsychiatric disorders associated with strep. infections) are identified by a marker associated with rheumatic fever. *Am J Psychiatry*. 1997;154:110–112.

Veasy LG, Wiedmeier SE, Orsmond GS, et al. Resurgence of acute rheumatic fever in the intermountain area of the United States. *N Engl J Med*. 1987;316:421–427.

Welcher BC, Carra JH, Dasilva L, Hanson J, David CS, Bavari S. Lethal shock induced by streptococcal pyrogenic exotoxin A in mice transgenic for human leukocyte antigen-DQ8 and human CD4 receptors: implications for development of vaccines and therapeutics. *J Infect Dis*. 2002;186(4):501–510.

BIBLIOGRAPHY – CHAGAS' DISEASE

REVIEWS

Dutra WO, Rocha MO, Teixeira MM. The clinical immunology of human Chagas disease. *Trends Parasitol*. 2005;21(12):581–587.

Girones N, Cuervo H, Fresno M. *Trypanosoma cruzi*-induced molecular mimicry and Chagas' disease. *Curr Top Microbiol Immunol*. 2005;296:89–123.

SUGGESTED ARTICLES

Chagas C. (Nova tripanosomiase humana: estudos sobre a morfolojia e o ciclo evolutivo do *Schizotrypanum cruzi* n.g., n.s.p., ajente etiolojico de nova entidade morbida no homen. *Mem Inst/Oswaldo Cruz.* 1909;1:159–218.

Cunha-Neto E, Coelho V, Guileherme L, Fiorelli A, Stolf N, Kalil J. Autoimmunity in Chagas' disease: identification of cardiac myosin-B13 *Trypanosoma cruzi* protein cross-reactive T cell clones in heart lesions of a chronic Chagas' disease cardiomyopathy patient. *J Clin Invest.* 1996;98:1709–1712.

dos Santos RR, Rossi MA, Laus JL, Silva JS, Savino W, Mengel J. Anti-CD4 abrogates rejection and reestablishes long-term tolerance to syngeneic newborn hearts grafted in mice chronically infected with *Trypanosoma cruzi. J Exp Med.* 1992;175:29–39.

Jones EM, Colley DG, Tostes S, Reis Lopes E, Vnencak-Jones CL, McCurley TL. Amplification of a *Trypanosoma cruzi* DNA sequence from inflammatory lesions in human Chagasic cardiomyopathy. *Am J Trop Med Hyg.* 1993;48: 348–357.

Krettli AU, Brenner Z. Protective effects of specific antibodies in *Trypanosoma cruzi* infection. *J Immunol.* 1976;116: 755–760.

Noguiera N, Cohn Z. *Trypanosoma cruzi*: mechanism of entry and intracellular fate in mammalian cells. *J Exp Med.* 1976;143:1402–1420.

Reed SG. 1980. Adoptive transfer of resistance to acute *Trypanosoma cruzi* infection with T lymphocyte-enriched spleen cells. *Infect Immun.* 28:404–410.

Santos-Busch CA, Acosta AM, Zweerink HJ, et al. Primary muscle disease: definition of a 25-kDa polypeptide myopathic specific Chagas antigen. *Clin Immunol Immunopathol.* 1985;37:334–350.

Tarleton RL, Zhang L, Downs MO. "Autoimmune rejection" of neonatal heart transplants in experimental Chagas disease is a parasite-specific response to infected host tissue. *Proc Natl Acad Sci USA.* 1997; 94:3932–3937.

Van Voorhis, WC Eisen H. FL-160: a surface antigen of *Trypanosoma cruzi* that mimics mammalian nervous tissue. J Exp Med. 1989;169:641–652.

Viotti R, Vigliano C, Armenti H, Segura E. Treatment of chronic Chagas' disease with benznidazole: clinical and serological evolution of patients with long-term followup. *Am Heart J.* 1994;127: 151–162.

Viotta R, Vigliano C, Lococo B, et al. Long-term cardiac outcomes of treating chronic Chagas disease with benznidazole versus no treatment: a non-randomized trial. *Ann Int Med.* 2006;144:722–734.

BIBLIOGRAPHY – IMMUNE-MEDIATED MYOCARDIAL DISEASES

REVIEWS

Afanasyeva M, Rose NR. Viral infection and heart disease: autoimmune mechanisms. In: Shoenfeld Y, Rose NR, eds. *Infection and Autoimmunity.* Amsterdam: Elsevier; 2004:299–318.

Rose NR, Baughman KL. *Immune Mediated Cardiovascular Diseases in Autoimmune Diseases IV*, Rose NR and Mckay IR, eds. London: Elsevier/Academic Press.

SUGGESTED ARTICLES

Fairweather DL, Rose NR. Inflammatory heart disease: a role for cytokines. *Lupus.* 2005;14:1–6.

Fairweather D, Kaya Z, Shellam GR, Lawson CM, Rose NR. From infection to autoimmunity. *J Autoimmun.* 2001;16: 175–186.

Lane JR, Neumann DA, Lafond-Walker A, Herskowitz A, Rose NR. Interleukin 1 or tumor necrosis factor can promote Coxsackie B3-induced myocarditis in resistant B10.A mice. *J Exp Med.* 1992;175:1123–1129.

Neu N, Rose NR, Beisel KW, Herskowitz A, Gurri-Glass G, Craig SW. Cardiac myosin induces myocarditis in genetically predisposed mice. *J Immunol.* 1987;139: 3630–3636.

Rose NR, Beisel KW, Herskowitz A, et al. Cardiac myosin and autoimmune myocarditis. In: Evered D, Whelan J, eds. *Autoimmunity and Autoimmune Disease.* Ciba Foundation Symposium 129. Chichester, UK: John Wiley & Sons; 1987:3–24.

Rose NR, Neumann DA, Herskowitz A, Traystman MD, Beisel KW. Genetics of susceptibility to viral myocarditis in mice. *Pathol Immunopathol Res.* 1988;7:266–278.

13. Immunological Aspects of Chest Diseases: The Case of Tuberculosis

Ernesto Muñoz-Elías, Ph.D., and Robert J. Wilkinson Ph.D., FRCP

INTRODUCTION

The respiratory tract is one of the first portals of entry for many viral and bacterial microorganisms. The local defense systems are generally sufficient to handle most invading microorganisms in healthy individuals but if the lung is damaged by bronchiectasis or fibrosis, the infecting microorganisms are able to establish an infection, cross the epithelial layer, and cause invasive disease.

The respiratory tract has two main compartments. The first is the airways, which extend from the nose to the terminal bronchioli. The second area is the alveoli in the lung tissue. The airways' defenses include many features such as ciliary movement, mucus, antimicrobial proteins, and rapid arrival of neutrophils whose combined action make it difficult for organisms to establish an infection. The access to the alveoli is also generally limited to very small inhaled particles. In the alveoli, invading microorganisms encounter resident alveolar macrophages that play a major role in engulfing and killing invaders.

The lung has its own immune system, which is known as bronchus-associated lymphoid tissue. Antigen-specific immune responses are generated at these sites, which, similarly to the Peyer's patches in the intestine, contain dendritic cells (DCs), which are the main antigen-presenting cells, as well as T and B cells, the latter

organized into B-cell follicles, as well as macrophages. Immune responses occur in response to infections or injury to the tract. The main antibodies found in respiratory tract secretions are IgA and IgG. However, B cells producing IgE and IgG are also found in the lung. Why IgE is present in this tissue is unclear but IgE may have a role in controlling parasites that reach the lung as it does in the intestines. IgE plays a major role in hypersensitivity reactions that occur in the respiratory tract, such as asthma and hay fever.

There are a variety of respiratory diseases including infectious diseases, interstitial lung disease, and allergic diseases. However, we will concentrate on tuberculosis (TB), one of the most important global granulomatous diseases in the world today.

TB is arguably the single most successful pathogen humankind has ever known. The unparalleled penetrance of TB in the human population reflects the extraordinary ability of *Mycobacterium tuberculosis* to cause a lifelong persistent infection, a peculiarity that is likely the result of a long dynamic interaction with its host. Although microbial infections, including those caused by highly pathogenic bacteria, tend to run an acute course, with infectious cycles of a few weeks, mycobacterial infections such as leprosy and TB are unusually protracted due to these pathogens' proclivity to persist in their hosts.

Table 13.1 Genetic Immunodeficiency Syndromes that Predispose to Mycobacterial Infection

Molecule	Phenotype	Mutation
IFN-γ receptor I	Severe atypical mycobacterial infection	Point mutation at nucleotide 395 that introduces a stop codon
IFN-γ receptor II	*Mycobacterium fortuitum* and M. *avium* infection	Homozygous dinucleotide deletion at nucleotides 278 and 279, resulting in premature stop codon
IL-12p40	BCG and *S. enteritidis* infection	Large homozygous deletion
IL-12β1 receptor	Severe mycobacterial and salmonella infection	A variety of missense subunit and deletion mutations
Stat 1	Disseminated BCG or *M. avium* infection	Point mutation at nucleotide position 2116

Persistence by *M. tuberculosis* can occur in the form of chronic active disease or latent infection; in either form, the biology of *M. tuberculosis'* persistence is poorly understood. Because available antibiotics are inefficient in eradicating persistent bacteria, treatment must be extended, and often lasts between six and nine months. Despite the inherent difficulties in implementing these sorts of regimens, antibiotics have effectively reduced TB in most of the industrialized world. However, they have had less impact in the rest of the world, where lack of resources make implementing such cumbersome drug treatments considerably more difficult. Most people live in the developing world, and it is there – where poverty is extreme, public health deplorable, and malnutrition and overpopulation widespread – where TB relentlessly and inexorably continues to exact its deadly toll. Although it is clear that combating the current TB epidemic would be greatly facilitated by the development of new and more efficient drugs and vaccines, the major obstacle in dealing with TB and other major infectious diseases such as malaria and HIV is the uwillingness of the industrialized world to make the investments needed to facilitate the efficient distribution of already available drugs, as well as the discovery of new ones.

EPIDEMIOLOGY

Despite improvements in the prognosis of TB in affluent nations, the disease continues to be the leading cause of death among bacterial infections worldwide. Furthermore, about 2 billion people harbor latent *M. tuberculosis*, constituting a reservoir that has been estimated will result in about 100 million cases of reactivation TB. The World Health Organization (WHO) estimates that of about 50 million deaths occurring each year, about 2 million are from TB and over 95 percent of those deaths occur in the developing world. TB epidemics are extremely slow, typically expanding over centuries. Although the incidence of TB worldwide was in a downtrend since the 1950s, this has changed considerably in recent times: from 1985 to 1992 the incidence of TB rose by 20 percent in the United States, and a considerable percentage of the cases were drug-resistant. Among the most important reasons for such reversal were the AIDS pandemic, reduction in public health resources in inner cities, and continued immigration from areas of high TB prevalence.

TB and AIDS

AIDS in HIV-infected individuals (e.g., low $CD4^+$ T cells) is one of the most important contributors to the development of TB in co-infected individuals in many parts of the world, including the United States. The low $CD4^+$ T cell counts translate into suboptimal macrophage activation and an inability to mount a protective response. HIV-co-infection is the greatest single risk factor for progression from *M. tuberculosis* infection to disease. The risk of developing disease after infection with *M. tuberculosis* in an HIV-co-infected person is about 5 to 15 percent per year, compared with a lifetime risk of developing active TB after infection of about 10 percent in immunocompetent individuals. Furthermore, the inability to mount an effective adaptive immune response leads to a more progressive course of TB in HIV-infected individuals. Miliary TB, a highly disseminated form of TB that can affect multiple organs, is also more frequent in AIDS patients. Furthermore, some evidence suggests that the interaction might be reciprocal, since active TB might stimulate viral replication, thereby accelerating the onset of AIDS, perhaps through tumor necrosis factor-alpha (TNF-α,) which induces viral transcription, and/or activation of the $CD4^+$ T cells that support viral replication. Current estimates indicate that there are about 11 million individuals co-infected with HIV and *M. tuberculosis* worldwide. A recent study found that of an estimated 1.8 million deaths from TB, 12 percent were attributable to HIV, and similarly, TB was responsible for 11 percent of all deaths due to AIDS.

The emergence of drug-resistant strains of *M. tuberculosis* is another important factor modifying the current TB epidemic. A strain is considered multidrug resistant (MDR) if it is resistant to at least isoniazid and rifampicin, the two most effective drugs for TB. Rapidly spreading MDR *M. tuberculosis* strains, that are resistant to all four first-line TB drugs, including isoniazid, rifampin, pyrazinamide, and ethambutol, have already emerged. According to WHO estimates, around 5 percent of all active TB cases worldwide are caused by MDR strains.

The Tubercle Bacillus

Mycobacterium tuberculosis belongs to the class Actinobacteria, order Actinomycetales, suborder Corynebacterineae, family Mycobacteriaceae. The suborder Corynebacterineae encompasses other high G+C gram-positive bacteria including members of the Nocardia, Rhodococcus, and Corynebacterium families. *M. tuberculosis* bacilli are nonmotile rod-shaped bacteria with general dimensions ranging from 1 to 4 µm in length and 0.3 to 0.6 µm in diameter. Though *M. tuberculosis* requires oxygen for growth, it can grow at low oxygen tensions and even survive complete oxygen deprivation.

Mycobacteria are notorious for being very slow growers. *M. smegmatis*, a fast-growing innocuous mycobacterial saprophyte used as a surrogate to study *M. tuberculosis*, has a division time of about 3 hours in axenic culture and takes 3–4 days to form a colony on agar. *M. tuberculosis* has a doubling time of about 20 hours in culture and formation of a colony on agar requires 18–21 days. One of the most striking features of mycobacterial cells is their tremendously complex lipid-rich envelope, which comprises half of the cell's dry weight. This property causes mycobacterial cells to aggregate into clumps in culture, making their experimental manipulation difficult. Limited studies suggest that mycobacterial cells might be relatively less permeable to hydrophilic substrates due to the presence of mycolic acids and mycosides; this impermeability could prevent transport of hydrophilic substrates into the cell. This lipid "shield," which causes *M. tuberculosis* to retain carbol fuchsin dye despite acid treatment ("acid fastness"), plays an important protective function from physical and chemical stress, and accumulating evidence indicates that its components mediate complex interactions with the host immune response. These properties might also limit the ability of certain drugs to efficiently enter the cell.

In 1998, Cole and colleagues were the first to sequence an *M. tuberculosis* genome – that of virulent laboratory strain H37Rv. A recent clinical isolate, termed *CDC1551*, was sequenced shortly after, and a third clinical isolate (strain 210) has also been completed. This wealth of information has uncovered unique aspects about mycobacterial biology. The constant G+C content of around 65 percent throughout mycobacterial genomes suggests the absence of horizontally acquired pathogenicity islands, which are widespread in other pathogenic bacteria. The most salient characteristic of the *M. tuberculosis* and other mycobacterial genomes is the presence of lots of genes dedicated to lipid metabolism (more than 8 percent of the *M. tuberculosis* genome); considering that nearly 40 percent of the dry weight of the mycobacterial cell wall is made up of lipids, it is reasonable to

conclude that lipid metabolism plays a major role in the biology of mycobacteria.

CLINICAL TUBERCULOSIS

M. tuberculosis contagion occurs when a susceptible person inhales bacilli-containing infectious droplets that have been expelled from the lungs of a tuberculous individual by sneezing, coughing, or simply talking. Of those infected, only a minority (around 10 percent) will develop disease; about half will do so within a few months to a couple of years immediately following infection (primary TB), while the other half will do so only after an indeterminately long period of latency (postprimary TB).

Primary TB

After reaching the alveoli, phagocytosis of the bacilli by resident macrophages is followed by unrestricted bacterial and exponential intracellular growth. Uptake of bacteria by DCs and migration of infected DCs to the draining lymph nodes for antigen presentation likely contribute to the lymphohematogenous dissemination of bacteria to extrapulmonary organs and uninfected parts of the lung, leading to the formation of secondary lesions. Exponential bacillary growth is thought to continue in primary and secondary lesions until a specific T-cell response is generated around each lesion, curtailing bacillary growth and likely killing some of the bacteria within macrophages as these bacteria become mycobacteriostatic or mycobacteriocidal after activation. The caseous centers of newly formed lesions are surrounded by activated macrophages. Presumably, bacterial antigens being released by the bacteria or captured from them are constantly being processed and presented to surrounding T cells in the context of IL-12 and other cytokines that induce a type of immune response. Constant presence of antigen likely contributes to expansion of the T-cell populations and continued activation of macrophages, which avidly ingest and inhibit or kill bacilli accumulated during the acute phase of the infection. In a lesion where the bacteria are effectively controlled by cell-mediated immunity, the caseous center becomes surrounded by a capsule, forming a protective granuloma. Over time, the number of viable bacilli in these granulomas likely diminishes. Old caseous foci of this sort contain little to no bacilli, and some of the old lesions can ossify and be reabsorbed as Opie and Aronson demonstrated in 1927. The interactions just described result in control of the infection in most infected individuals.

For reasons poorly understood, some individuals fail to generate the protective type of immune response just described. In these cases, bacteria continue to replicate and the granulomas become increasingly necrotic. Part of the tissue damage that occurs is the result of immunopathology, that is, an excessive host-mediated inflammatory response to bacterial antigens. When the centers of granulomas undergo caseating necrosis, the sheaths of monocytes and T cells that normally suppress the intracellular growth of the bacilli can also become necrotic; as the bacteria continue to replicate in nonactivated macrophages at the periphery of the lesion, progressive destruction of lung tissue ensues, ultimately leading to the death of the host. Massive inflammation and tissue damage can also be caused directly by some components of the bacterial cell wall as well as by secreted lipids and proteins;

lipoarabinomannan, for instance, triggers TNF-α secretion by macrophages, while some secreted lipids lead to secretion of proinflammatory IL-6.

Although *M. tuberculosis* is not an obligate intracellular pathogen, whether it is capable of extracellular growth in the acellular necrotic centers of caseous lesions is unclear. In contrast, solid caseum that has undergone liquefaction is believed to be permissive for bacillary replication. The coughing up of this highly infectious material is in fact responsible for the transmission of the bacilli. These observations illustrate how pathology is a necessary step in the life cycle of *M. tuberculosis* infection in humans.

Latent TB Infection and Reactivation

Little is known about the factors that determine whether an individual that is exposed to *M. tuberculosis* will go on to develop primary TB or become latently infected. That the immune status of the host is involved in both the establishment and maintenance of latency can be inferred from the observation that HIV–*M. tuberculosis* co-infected individuals have a much higher risk of developing TB after infection. The only sign of infection in individuals with latent TB infection (LTBI) is the appearance (between two and six weeks postexposure) of a detectable delayed-type hypersensitivity (DTH) reaction to a mycobacterial purified protein derivative (tuberculin). By taking necropsy specimens of lung lesions from immune-competent individuals who had died of causes other than TB and inoculating necropsy speciments into guinea pigs to determine the presence of infectious bacilli, Opie and Aronson (1927) showed that some individuals can harbor viable tubercle bacilli for many years without showing any symptoms of disease. In this and other early studies, it was found that while specimens from encapsulated or calcified lesions rarely were infectious, those isolated from caseous lesions in the lung's apex generally were. Unexpectedly, apparently healthy tissues were also often infectious. Recently, Gomez and McKinney (2004) have reviewed several other studies from the pre-antibiotic era that indicated that lung lesions from asymptomatic individuals can harbor viable bacilli to different degrees. Recent molecular evidence of potential LTBI in normal human lung tissue was provided by the finding that about 30 to 50 percent of samples from individuals from endemic regions (Mexico and Ethiopia) could harbor *M. tuberculosis* DNA.

Perhaps the most compelling evidence for the prevalence of LTBI has come from the observed increased rates of TB in AIDS patients, as well as the high reactivation TB associated with the intake of TNF-α inhibitors prescribed for rheumatoid arthritis. These observations indicate that many individuals with LTBI accomplish lifelong suppression of the bacillus, but never actually achieve sterilization. Reactivation TB usually presents clinically as a slowly progressive, chronic condition; individuals with chronic subacute TB may infect scores of contacts without realizing that they have the disease. Patients with cavitary TB are particularly infectious because they shed enormous numbers of tubercle bacilli in their sputa. Cavitation is caused by the liquefaction of necrotic tuberculous tissue and its expulsion through the airways; liquefaction is linked to a strong DTH response and is an important example of immunopathology in TB. The molecular basis of cavity formation has not been determined, nor is it clear whether the immune mechanisms

responsible for pathogenesis and protection are the same.

EXPERIMENTAL STUDIES OF TUBERCULOSIS

The Mouse Model of Chronic Tuberculosis

Animals infected with *M. tuberculosis* – mice, guinea pigs, or rabbits – typically develop a chronic, progressive form of the disease that varies in severity depending on the species, the guinea pig being the most susceptible, the rabbit the most resistant, and the mouse somewhere in between.

The mouse has become the animal of choice in the study of TB. In fact, Robert Koch himself employed mice in his pioneering experiments over 100 years ago. A chronic infection in mice can be established by inoculation of bacilli by intravenous injection or by aerosol exposure. The bacilli multiply logarithmically during the first two to four weeks postinfection and then stop increasing in numbers in the lung and start to slowly decline in numbers in the liver and spleen. Depending on the titer of the initial inoculum, the chronic infection can last from months to over a year. The model is useful in that it allows host–*M. tuberculosis* interactions to be studied in the context of a prolonged persistent infection. The maintenance of a relatively high bacterial load, accompanied by accumulating pathology, might pertain to human active TB, while the apparent lack of bacterial replication might be relevant to both active TB and LTBI. Among the limitations of the mouse model are differences in the composition and organization of the granulomatous structures compared with those formed in human lungs, and in the location of the bacilli in the infected lungs – almost exclusively intracellular in mice, considerably more extracellular in humans.

Spontaneous *M. tuberculosis* latency in animals only occurs in nonhuman primates. A drug-induced model of latency known as the Cornell model, in which *M. tuberculosis*–infected mice are sterilized by drug treatment, and then allowed to reactivate spontaneously or by immunesuppression, was developed in the 1950s by McCune and Tompsett. This model allows host–pathogen interactions to be studied in the context of an infection where very low numbers of bacteria are present and has been used to study host factors involved in establishing and maintaining this type of "latency." However, the relevance of the model to true latency awaits validation.

Host–Pathogen Interactions in TB

Upon entering the respiratory tract, bacilli reaching the lung alveoli are phagocytosed by resident macrophages through mannose, complement, and Fc receptors (in differentiated macrophages). As demonstrated more than three decades ago by Armstrong and Hart (1975), bacterial uptake through Fc receptors increases phagolysosomal fusion, triggers the oxidative burst, and leads to bacterial killing in human macrophages ex vivo. Regardless of the receptor involved, uptake apparently requires recruitment of cholesterol to the nascent phagosome. Uptake by resident DCs is believed to occur through DC-SIGN adhesion.

CELLULAR INTERACTIONS LEADING TO A PROTECTIVE IMMUNE RESPONSE

A protective immune reponse to *M. tuberculosis* involves mainly the T-cell-mediated branch of adaptive immunity.

As early as one week postinfection, bacteria-specific CD4$^+$ and CD8$^+$ T cells migrate to the lung, where they peak in numbers at around four weeks postinfection, Studies in immune-deficient mice have established that IFN-γ, TNF-α, and IL-12 are the main cytokines involved in orchestrating a protective immune response after *M. tuberculosis* infection. The relevance of IFN-γ and IL-12 in antimycobacterial immunity is supported by human genetic data; the recent association between administration of TNF-α inhibitors used to treat rheumatoid arthritis and the reactivation of LTBI has underscored the protective role of this cytokine in control of *M. tuberculosis* in humans.

The initiation of the immune response occurs through presentation of *M. tuberculosis* antigens, presumably by DCs, on MHC class I and II molecules to naïve T cells, which in the context of IL-12 and IL-23 produced by infected macrophages and DCs themselves, are instructed to differentiate into IFN-γ-secreting cells (helper T type 1, T_H1) cells (see Figure 1). Both CD4$^+$ and CD8$^+$ T cells contribute to the activation of infected macrophages through IFN-γ secretion, while CD8$^+$ T cells might additionally contribute to protection by causing apoptosis of infected macrophages through the Fas-FasL pathway, as well as through secretion of granulysin and other microbicidal molecules. However, the relative contribution of CD8$^+$ T cells to the overall protective cell-mediated immunity might not be as significant as that by CD4$^+$ T cells because *M. tuberculosis*–infected mice deficient in the former live almost as long as infected wild-type mice, while those deficient in the latter are significantly more susceptible.

Mice lacking CD4$^+$ T cells exhibit reduced macrophage activation, which is associated with lower IFN-γ production,

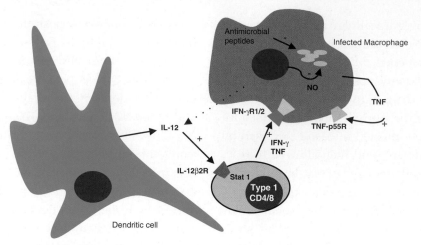

Figure 13.1 Cellular immune responses to *M. tuberculosis* infection. Some aspects of the innate and adaptive cellular immune responses to infection by *M. tuberculosis* are shown as inferred from studies using ex vivo and in vivo models of tuberculosis. Bacteria are assumed to reside mostly inside vacuoles in macrophages. Not shown are CTL- and gamma-, delta-T-cell-mediated proposed mechanisms of protection.

and are therefore highly susceptible to *M. tuberculosis* infection. Even though CD8+ T-cell production of IFN-γ can compensate and restore the concentrations of IFN-γ back to normal levels in CD4+ T-deficient mice, the latter still succumb to the infection earlier than wild-type mice, suggesting that CD4+ T-cell-derived IFN-γ production early in the infection, or an IFN-γ-independent mechanism might be important for control of the infection. An IFN-γ-independent CD4+ T-cell-mediated mechanism dependent on NOS2 has recently been shown in vitro and suggested to be important in vivo by the demonstration that IFN-γ-deficient mice can be effectively protected by BCG vaccination in a CD4+ T-cell-dependent manner.

Cell-mediated immunity to *M. tuberculosis* promotes the formation of granulomas – infected macrophages surrounded by antigen-specific lymphocytes, multinucleated giant cells, and a ring of fibrous deposition. Granulomas typically encompass the entire infection foci and effectively isolate the bacilli from the rest of the lung. Granuloma formation depends largely on TNF-α and GM-CSF, which are produced by infected macrophages, T cells, and other hemaetopoetic cells, and which drive tissue-resident stromal cells to produce macrophage-inflammatory protein-1β (MIP-1β), MIP-1α, and other chemokines needed to recruit neutrophils, lymphocytes, and monocytes to the site of infection. TNF-α$^{-/-}$ mice infected with *M. tuberculosis* fail to form organized granulomas, are incapable of controlling *M. tuberculosis* replication, and succumb to *M. tuberculosis* within 20 to 30 days of infection. Importantly, the levels of TNF-α must be tightly regulated because overproduction can lead to excessive pathology.

SURVIVAL OF *M. TUBERCULOSIS* IN THE MACROPHAGE

Pathogenic mycobacteria reside and readily replicate within tight vacuoles of non-immune-activated macrophages. Pioneering studies by Rees and Hart (1961) showed that tubercle bacilli prevent the fusion of lysosomes to *M. tuberculosis*–containing vacuoles, thus preventing the vacuoles' normal acidification and facilitating bacterial survival and replication. Vacuoles containing live virulent *Mycobacterium avium* have a relatively high pH (6.3–6.5), which correlates with a lower density of vesicular H^+ ATPase pumps on their membranes. Mycobacterial vacuoles reside within the recycling and sorting endosomal compartment – markers of early endosomes (Rab5) are retained, markers of late endosomes (Rab7) and lysosomes (LAMP1-1 and LAMP-2) are largely excluded; communication with the cytoplasmic membrane appears to be maintained, as suggested by the cycling of transferrin in and out of the vacuoles. Diversion of the mycobacterial phagosome from the normal maturation pathway correlates with retention of the actin-binding coronin TACO on the phagosomal membrane. Active evasion of phagolysosomal fusion by *M. tuberculosis* involves bacterial effectors such mannose-capped lipoarabinomannan (ManLAM), which interferes with phagolysosomal fusion by blocking the acquisition of the lysosomal cargo and syntaxin 6 from the trans-Golgi network. LAM alone can specifically block the cytosolic Ca^{2+} increase necessary for a signaling cascade involving phosphatidylinositol (PI) 3 kinase hVPS34, which is needed for production of PI 3 phosphate (PI3P) on phagosomes.

The importance of type 1 cytokines in human immunity to *M. tuberculosis* infection has been confirmed by studies of naturally occurring polymorphisms in the genes encoding type 1 cytokines and their receptors in humans. The principal role of type 1 cytokines in anti-TB immunity is to activate the antimicrobial functions of macrophages. IFN-γ activation and infection of murine macrophages with *M. tuberculosis* results in the differential expression of some 40 percent of the macrophage genes, an indication of just how dynamic the host–*M. tuberculosis* interaction is. Many of these differentially expressed genes likely encode functions involved in the curtailment of growth and killing of the intracellular bacilli.

EFFECTOR MECHANISMS OF THE IMMUNE-ACTIVATED MACROPHAGE

Schaible and colleagues (1998) found that upon activation of *M. avium*–infected macrophages with IFN-γ and lipopolysaccharide (LPS), the mycobacterial vacuoles fuse to each other, become more acidic (pH 5.3), and as a result of fusion with lysosomes accumulate hydrolases. These and other changes in the intracellular milieu lead to stasis and killing of the bacilli.

MacMicking and colleagues (2003) indicate that LRG47, a member of a family of IFN-γ–dependent GTPases that mediate fusion events in endosomal networks, is one of the facilitators of phagolysosomal fusion and acidification downstream of IFN-γ and is essential for protection. These GTPases play different functions in response to infection by different pathogens as suggested by the findings that IGTP$^{-/-}$ and IRG-47$^{-/-}$ mice, which are susceptible to infection by viral, bacterial, and eukaryotic pathogens are resistant to infection by *M. tuberculosis*. In contrast, LRG47$^{-/-}$ mice succumb to infection by *M. tuberculosis* with kinetics similar to those of NOS2$^{-/-}$ mice, the other major pathway of antimycobacterial immunity.

Work from the laboratories of Carl Nathan and Ferric Fang over the years has demonstrated that the immune system relies on chemically reactive micromolecules to neutralize and eliminate invading pathogens and their products. Some of the most efficient of these reactive molecules in killing and controlling *M. tuberculosis* include the reactive nitrogen intermediates derived from nitric oxide (NO) produced by NO synthase 2. *M. tuberculosis* is killed by murine peritoneal macrophages and cell lines activated with IFN-γ and either LPS or TNF-α through reactive nitrogen intermediate (RNI) production, and IFN-γ and TNF-α synergistically increase NO synthesis by macrophages. The demonstration that NOS2$^{-/-}$ mice are highly susceptible to *M. tuberculosis* infection provides clear functional genetic evidence that NOS2 is essential for the protective immune response against *M. tuberculosis.*

Even though macrophage activation and resulting RNI production result in bacteriostasis, *M. tuberculosis* is nonetheless able to resist eradication in mouse lungs and in activated macrophages in tissue culture, despite the fact that in vitro reagent NO is a potent mycobactericidal. Having evolved to infect the mammalian lung, *M. tuberculosis* appearently has ways of countering the nossive effects of NO and related RNI. One such mechanism involves the product of the *mpa* gene, which forms hexamers that have ATPase activity, and is believed to be associated with a mycobacterial proteasome. Δmpa *M. tuberculosis* bacteria are attenuated in wild-type mice and show some reversion to virulence in NOS2$^{-/-}$. It remains to be shown whether Δmpa *M. tuberculosis* bacteria have defects in protein degradation through this presumptive proteasome, and whether this proposed function is involved in protecting the bacteria from RNI. An additional strategy adopted by *M. tuberculosis* to deal with RNI appears to be simple avoidance of NOS2. Recent microscopy studies indicate that *M. tuberculosis* might be able to prevent NOS2 from being recruited to bacteria-containing phagosomes.

The role of NO in protection against *M. tuberculosis* in humans is somewhat controversial. While some investigators have reported NOS2 protein induction, NO, which is measured by determining the concentration of its breakdown products nitrate (NO_3) and nitrite (NO_2), cannot be consistently detected in *M. tuberculosis*–infected cultures of human monocytes/macrophages. Furthermore, no mutations in *nos2* in humans have been associated with susceptibility to *M. tuberculosis*. However, patients with active TB apparently exhale high levels of NO, which correlate with high expression of NOS2 and spontaneous production of nitrite by alveolar macrophages.

Another reactive micromolecule that is a potent antimicrobial effector of the immune response is the nicotinamide adenine dinucleotide phosphate (NADPH) oxidase (PHOX)-mediated production of reactive oxygen intermediates (ROIs) including reduction products of O_2 such as superoxide, hydrogen peroxide, and hydroxyl radical. ROI generation is an effective antimicrobial defense against many bacterial pathogens including *Salmonella* and *Burkholderia cepacia*. However, recent work from John McKinney's laboratory indicates that the protective role of ROI in TB appears to be less prominent than during *Salmonella* infections. Chronic granulomatous disease (CGD) patients that lack phagocyte oxidase have not been reported to be more susceptible to *M. tuberculosis* infection. Furthermore, gp91$^{(phox-/-)}$ mutant mice, which lack a functional phagocyte oxidase, are not more susceptible to *M. tuberculosis* than wild-type mice, while mice lacking the gp47 subunit of PHOX are less able to control *M. tuberculosis* replication only transiently. Furthermore, *M. tuberculosis* appears to be able to effectively counteract the damaging effects of ROIs. ROI detoxification mediated by the *KatG* catalase is essential for bacterial persistence in mice following induction of adaptive immunity, and an *M. tuberculosis* mutant of *katG* is attenuated in wild-type mice, but reverts to wild-type levels of virulence in mice lacking PHOX. The product of *katG* is also a peroxynitritetase, thus it may protect *M. tuberculosis* from both RNI and ROI. At least one of the superoxide dismutases of *M. tuberculosis* contributes to intracellular survival.

IMMUNITY DURING *M. TUBERCULOSIS* CHRONIC INFECTION

Several of the components that are important for generating a protective immune response to *M. tuberculosis* infection are also important for maintaining the equilibrium between host and pathogen during the chronic phase of the infection. As expected, T_H1 maintenance is important for controlling *M. tuberculosis* during the chronic phase of the infection, and sustaining this type of response requires IL-12. Neutralization of TNF-α by antibodies or by infection with an adenovirus expressing a soluble TNF-α receptor resulted in marked increases in bacterial loads and exacerbation of disease in the mouse model of chronic TB and in a variation of the Cornell model of drug-induced latency. Work from the laboratories of John Chan and Joan Flynn using the Cornell model of TB, has demonstrated that IFN-γ is involved in preventing reactivation. Similarly, chemical inhibition of NOS2 in chronically infected mice resulted in rapid increases in lung bacterial loads. NOS2-inhibiton also reactivated *M. tuberculosis* in variations of the Cornell model of latency.

EXTRACELLULAR PERSISTENCE OF *M. TUBERCULOSIS* IN VIVO

In the human lung, *M. tuberculosis* is thought to reside both intracellularly and extracellularly, depending on the type of lesion. Pioneering work by Lurie (1964) and continued by Dannenberg using the rabbit model showed the existence of extracellular *M. tuberculosis* in caseous necrotic lesions. Because immunity to TB was thought to be mainly mediated by activated phagocytes that kill intracellular bacteria, it was suspected that the extracellular milieu represented a safe heaven for bacterial replication and persistence. In order to study this population of bacteria directly back in 1939, Lurie devised a very ingenious method of cultivating bacteria extracellularly in vivo: Parlodion-film–encased silk bags that were impervious to host cells, but not to plasma, were inoculated with bacilli and then implanted subcutaneously in rabbits. These extracellular bacteria replicated unhindered during the first two weeks of infection, but then leveled off at around two weeks postinfection. When immunized animals were studied, bacteria stopped growing earlier and were killed more efficiently than in naïve counterparts, strongly implicating acquired immunity in controlling the growth of extracellular bacteria. Because control of growth correlated with a more rapid mobilization of mononuclear cells toward the encased focus of infection, it was proposed that factors secreted by activated macrophages rendered the fluids entering the infection foci inimical to bacterial replication.

Recently, work in William Bishai's laboratory adapted Lurie's strategy to the widely used model of murine TB: *M. tuberculosis* was encapsulated in cell-impermeable hollow fibers, and these were implanted subcutaneously into mice for in vivo cultivation. As expected, an initial period of bacterial replication was followed by curtailment of growth, followed by a considerable decline in numbers, and, interestingly, an eventual stabilization of the counts. These stationary-state colony forming unit (CFU) counts, similarly to those in the equilibrium that characterized the chronic phase of infection in the mouse model of chronic TB as described by Rees and Hart in 1965, represented a somewhat static scenario: they found that about half of the encapsulated bacilli were alive by differential staining; a highly dynamic equilibrium would have resulted in a large accumulation of dead bacteria and a decreasing proportion of live ones. Furthermore, indirect analysis – comparison of ATP utilization and CFU at corresponding time points – indicated that soon after implantation, bacteria decreased their metabolism. The rapid cessation of multiplication and rather swift reduction in metabolic activity suggest that innate defenses or perhaps immune-independent mechanisms prompt these adaptations. These adaptations were also suggested by Lurie's studies using vaccinated animals, which implicated an unknown plasma factor in bacterial growth inhibition. This factor could be nitric oxide, which is known to block *M. tuberculosis* replication in vitro by inhibiting bacterial respiration. Careful analysis of the hollow fiber's contents in this extracellular model of persistence in vivo, including concentrations of NO, oxygen, essential elements, and nutrients, might be of value.

VACCINATION STRATEGIES FOR TUBERCULOSIS

This section is not meant to be a complete description of the whole vaccination program against TB but rather a brief summary of where the field is headed. A review by Wilkinson and Young (2004) gives a much more comprehensive summation of the field. Within recent years the approach to controlling and/or preventing TB infections has undergone a remarkable transformation. This transformation is certainly in part because we now know the entire genome sequence of *M. tuberculosis*. It is further aided by the completion of the Human Genome Project. Novel analytical techniques now allow us to study the organism from varying sources under differing conditions. It is also now possible to achieve genetic recombination in *M. tuberculosis*. This has shifted the emphasis from purely microbiological characterization of recombinant strains to their cellular characterization in model systems. Indeed TB was one of the first diseases to be shown to be potentially preventable by DNA vaccines.

With the advent of HIV coexisting with TB coupled with MDR strains emerging, there is now a greater need for new approaches to improved or additional vaccines against TB. We will now discuss a number of these potential candidates.

Bacille Calmette-Guérin (BCG)

For some time a safe, inexpensive TB vaccine has been effective in humans and animals. It has been used in more than 100 million newborn children each year but the efficacy of this vaccine has been under continuous debate.

The vaccine was originally made by Calmette and Guérin by continuous laboratory passage of a virulent strain of *Mycobacterium bovis* on deficient media for thirteen years. The resulting isolate was tested in mice, guinea pigs, and humans and was found to be effective as an experimental vaccine in animals.

The situation in humans appears to be more controversial. Several studies such as the one in the United Kingdom by Hart and Sutherland (1977) have shown that the incidence of TB decreased by 77 percent when compared with a control group. In contrast, other studies, most notably in South India, indicated close to zero protection. The difference is mainly in the vaccine's inability to protect adults from pulmonary TB because the vaccine has consistently been effective against the disseminated forms of TB that are a major cause of childhood mortality. In addition, a small amount of limited data indicates that the efficacy of BCG may wane over time.

What are the possible reasons for this variation in vaccination studies? One view is that, with continuous passage over the years, the BCG organism has changed genetically and is not like the original strain. In fact, many of these trials were carried out with six different BCG strains. Thus, using the H37Rv genome of *M. tuberculosis* as a template, it is not surprising that identifying genetic regions that are missing in the various substrains of the original BCG vaccine has been possible. Furthermore, five regions encompassing thirty-eight open reading frames are also deleted in some or all BCG substrains. Calmette maintained that isolates of BCG that caused extreme scar formation and regional lymphadenopathy were better vaccines.

Other factors that could influence the success of BCG are that strains may differ in their immunogenicity. The route, administration, and the efficacy of the immunizing technique must also be considered. Finally, a favored hypothesis (see Black et al. 2001) is that saphophytic mycobacteria seen more commonly in warmer climates may influence the results of the trials. Thus, sensitization by environmental mycobacteria could reverse the immunological benefits conferred by BCG vaccination since all individuals had already been sensitized by saphophytic organisms.

Finally, the comorbidity of HIV infections coupled with the recrudescence of latent TB or just HIV infection has raised the possibility that administration of BCG (attenuated strain) in an immunocomprised host may allow the BCG strain to multiply rapidly in the host and not prevent disease. These caveats, coupled with the emergence of MDR strains of the TB organism and present poor adherence in taking the medicines (long-lasting regimens), have only served to emphasize the urgency for an effective and safe vaccine to control the current TB pandemic. In the following section, we will discuss the merits and drawbacks of these various vaccine candidates. Before that, however, some understanding of the various immune responses to this organism needs to be discussed.

The Framework for Vaccine Development and Evaluation

Although most vaccines are produced by large pharmaceutical companies, vaccines for the prevention of TB may not interest the pharmaceutical industry because such a vaccine would be primarily used in resource-poor countries. Thus, the major impetus for vaccine development may have to come from the public, not the private, sector.

Considerable momentum toward testing and developing novel vaccines has built up in the past few years and the National Institutes of Health after consultations with many worldwide organizations has issued a blueprint for TB vaccine development. A specific commitment to evaluate novel vaccines in aerosol-infected mice and guinea pigs was made, and many candidates and combinations thereof have been tested. The European community has also recognized the need for a wide pre-clinical research approach and includes a primate model for testing novel vaccines. Another important area has been to identify high-incidence areas of infection for future efficacy trials and the establishment of long-term clinical and epidemiological support for such ventures. Even in high-incidence areas, phase III trials may involve thousands of individuals because the efficacy of BCG is known to vary by geographical region and thus parallel trials may need to be established in different parts of the world.

Vaccine Candidates

Many new vaccine candidates have been produced, and there is no clear rationale for the design of the optimal TB vaccine. However, BCG provides a precedent that a live mycobacterium can confer protection. However, the coexistence of HIV infection in many areas of the world favors a nonreplicating subunit formulation. This approach, however, does require identification of relevant antigens and the selection of appropriate delivery systems.

LIVE VACCINES

Experience with BCG does prove that a live attenuated vaccine does confer protection, and the improvement of the existing BCG vaccine represents one general approach to the question of new vaccine candidates. In view of the complete dissection of the genome for the organism, new tools for the genetic manipulation of myco-

bacterial antigens allow us to refine the live vaccine strategy of Calmette and Guérin by either addition of genes to BCG or targeted removal of genes from an initially virulent *M. tuberculosis* strain.

1. *Modified BCG Strains.* BCG has now been engineered to express recombinant mammalian cytokines designed to augment immunogenicity or decrease immunopathology. The addition of the listerolysin gene has been shown to enhance the ability of BCG antigens to traffic into the cytoplasm, thereby inducing a CD8+ T-cell response. Another approach has been the overexpression of antigen 85B carried on a multicopy episomal plasmid in recombinant BCG.

Another possible reason for the incomplete efficacy of BCG is that it lacks "protective" antigens present in the original *M. tuberculosis*. For example, comparison of these two genomes showed that a 9.5-kb region called *RD1* is missing from all strains of BCG. The RD1 encodes two antigens (ESAT-6 and CFP-10) that are highly immunogenic and prominent immune targets in *M. tuberculosis* infected humans. Obviously, reintroduction of the ESAT-6 and CFP-10 is an attractive concept but one must be sure this reintroduction does not increase virulence.

2. *Attenuation of M. tuberculosis.* A number of novel attenuated strains have been developed and three strategies have evolved: (1) The first involves auxotrophic mutations that render the bacteria dependent on exogenous growth factors that are in limited supply. For example, the derivation of attenuated strains dependent on leucine and tryptophan has been successful. (2) A second

approach is to inactivate *M. tuberculosis* analogously to those involved in virulence in other bacterial pathogens. A recent example is the generation of a *phoP* attenuated mutant, based on the knowledge of the key role of this regulator in pathogenic salmonella. (3) The third strategy exploits the technique of signature-tagged transposon mutagenesis. This involves screening of a library of transposon mutants to identify clones selectively lost during murine infection. Using this technique has identified mutants with defects in biosynthesis of cell wall lipids. Decreased persistence within tissues and altered patterns of tissue dissemination have been described for several attenuated variants of *M. tuberculosis*.

Whether any of these mutants could function as a vaccine candidate still needs further testing, and issues such as safety, the properties required for an improved live vaccine, interactions with antigen-presenting cells all need to be investigated further.

PROTEIN SUBUNIT VACCINES

Two criteria have been used to identify *M. tuberculosis* antigens for incorporation into programs for subunit vaccine development. The first is the ability to elicit a strong recall response in humans or experimental animals exposed to *M. tuberculosis* infection. The response is assessed primarily in terms of the release of IFN-γ from antigen-specific CD4$^+$ T cells. Although this represents a realistic strategy to identify antigens available for T-cell recognition, it will (like BCG) tend to reproduce rather than augment the natural immune response. Amplification of naturally subdominant responses represents a potentially interesting alternative

approach, particularly in the context of postexposure vaccination.

A second common criterion for antigen selection is its identification in the supernatant of in vitro cultures. This idea is supported by experiments from several laboratories demonstrating successful vaccination with culture filtrate preparations. However, live mycobacteria also require immunogenic proteins that are not secreted, such as the small heat-shock protein Acr or 16-kDa antigen.

Several purified protein antigens have been shown to induce protective immunity following immunization in appropriate adjuvants. The most extensively studied are antigen 85B (Ag85B) and ESAT-6. Ag85B is a member of an antigen complex, a set of three closely related proteins that function as mycolyl transferases and are the most abundant protein components in culture filtrate preparations. Because any single protein may be insufficiently immunogenic, the use of fusion proteins could be important for future subunit vaccine development. Subunit vaccination with purified proteins requires delivery of the protein in adjuvant to generate a strong immune response. Unfortunately, the adjuvants currently licensed for use in humans generally optimize the antibody rather than the T-cell responses, although novel preparations such as the SBAS2 adjuvant or microspheres may be useful in moving mycobacterial protein subunit candidates into clinical trials.

DNA VACCINES

DNA vaccination against TB has proved effective in small animal models using some, but not all, antigens. Two examples from DNA vaccine studies highlight the potential importance of fine antigenic specificity in the protective response. First, Ag85A, but not Ag85B, is effective when administered as a DNA vaccine to mice. Interestingly, when antigen 85B is delivered to guinea pigs either as a subunit or overexpressed in a recombinant BCG, it is an effective vaccine, and protection has also been reported using an alternative Ag85B DNA formulation. Thus, the form of vaccination and host species are also crucial for any given antigen. The second instance, indicating a potential contribution of fine specificity to the immune response in TB, concerns the closely related Hsp60 molecules of *Mycobacterium leprae* and *M. tuberculosis*. DNA vaccination using Hsp60 of *M. leprae* is effective in mice both as a prophylactic and an immunotherapeutic vaccine. The vaccine efficacy could not be reproduced using a construct of the closely related Hsp60 of *M. tuberculosis*.

COMBINATION VACCINES

Vaccinia virus has been used as a delivery system for mycobacterial antigens. This live vector has the advantage of proven safety and efficacy in the context of the smallpox eradication program. The combination of three vaccinations of plasmid DNA containing MPT63 and ESAT-6 plus one "boost" with a recombinant *Vaccinia* construct expressing the same antigens induced protection against intraperitoneal infection of mice close to that conferred by BCG. However, there is at least one report of a theoretically elegant prime-boost strategy using ESAT-6 in which there was no enhancement above the protection provided by individual subunits. Perhaps of greatest interest is that sequential immunization with antigen AG85B-expressing DNA followed by BCG was more effective than BCG immunization alone. In this case, deple-

tion of the CD8$^+$ T cells in the immunized mice impaired protection in their spleens, indicating that this improved efficacy was partially mediated by CD8$^+$ T cells.

STRATEGIES FOR VACCINE EVALUATION

Although animal models have been helpful in designing new vaccine strategies for TB, there is no guarantee that success or failure in animal models will not necessarily produce similar behavior in humans. With respect to animal models, mice and guinea pigs have been used most extensively. However, other larger models such as rabbits, cattle, and nonhuman primates are available for further characterization of a given vaccine candidate. A consensus exists that nonhuman primate studies are necessary before phase I studies of novel anti-TB vaccines in humans.

1. *Mouse*: This is the least costly model and has been a valuable model for investigating genetics and immunology of the host response to TB. Yet, they are relatively resistant to the disease, the skin test reactivity is not very good, and pathological examination of tissues does not show the caseation and fibrosis of the lungs so commonly seen in human TB.
2. *Guinea pig*: These animals are quite susceptible to low-dose infection with virulent *M. tuberculosis* and exhibit some of the necrotic pathology seen in humans. Their exquisite sensitivity to TB provides an experimental window of sufficient width to allow the ranking of different vaccines according to their individual protective efficacies.
3. *Rabbit*: Perhaps the most striking feature of this model is not rabbits' response to *M. tuberculosis* but rather to *M. bovis* strains. Infection with these

strains produces cavities in the lungs by caseation, and the extracellular multiplication of bacilli are very similar to that of humans.

4. *Cattle*: TB in cattle and farmed deer is of considerable economic significance, and efforts to develop a new vaccine against human TB are paralleled by attempts to develop diagnostic agents and vaccine control strategies for bovine TB. Given the relationship between the respective infectious agents, *M. tuberculosis* and *M. bovis*, it may be that the prevention of human and bovine TB can be achieved using similar vaccines. Therefore, vaccine trials in cattle can be considered a relevant animal model for human TB, given that the endpoint of this model will be the reduction of transmission in a naturally susceptible host system.

5. *Nonhuman primates*: Establishment of experimental TB in nonhuman primates provides an opportunity to study protective and pathological mechanisms with close resemblance to those in humans. BC6 vaccination has been characterized in rhesus and cynomolgus monkeys, and studies have been initiated with new candidates. Nonhuman primate models are relatively poorly standardized, however, and ethical and financial aspects of such research dictate that it should be reserved for the end stages of preclinical evaluation.

Summary

In each of these model systems, challenge with virulent mycobacteria can be by parenteral infection or, in an attempt to mimic the natural route of infection, by aerosol infection. Measuring the reduction of bacterial load in target tissues, particularly in the lung and spleen, at a specific time after challenge is the most widely accepted system to assess protection in the above animal models, although there is increasing recognition that the effect of vaccination on longer-term pathological changes is important in the comprehensive analysis of a new candidate. Typically, BCG vaccination results in a reduction of approximately tenfold in bacterial numbers in mice and up to 5-log reduction in guinea pigs. The slow growth rate of mycobacteria makes the standard determination of CFUs both labor intensive and time-consuming. Recently, reporter gene technology has been applied to mycobacteria with luciferase-expressing mycobacteria allowing the measurement of luminescence in organ homogenates as a rapid endpoint for vaccine evaluation. Extension of the use of such bacteria into simple whole-blood-based assays in humans also has considerable potential as a surrogate of protective immunity that makes no assumptions of the detailed nature of this response.

Clinical Trials in Humans

General logistic and ethical issues related to TB vaccine trials will determine the type of vaccine that can be tested and may therefore have an important influence on more immediate research strategies. These issues should be addressed now, rather than waiting until vaccine candidates have already reached the stage of field evaluation.

1. *Preinfection trials:* In designing new trials for novel TB vaccines designed to replace BCG, one runs into an immediate ethical problem – to use a novel untested vaccine candidate side by side with a proven BCG effect, namely, the prevention of childhood forms

of TB, particularly the miliary form. A comparative trial may be impossible in children from developing countries, the most important group of future users of a new TB vaccine. A second problem is the length of the trials. Even in high-incidence areas, TB case rates rarely exceed 250/100,000, so huge numbers of individuals will have to be followed for twenty years before a known end-point (adulthood) is reached.

2. *Postinfection trials:* An anti-reactivation trial may be simpler to evaluate. By administration to a high-risk young adult cohort, a trial period of several years might be sufficient. Evaluation of a transmission-blocking vaccine (i.e., reduction in smear-positive cases) will require the development of improved diagnostic tools for smear-negative TB. In the absence of an understanding of the factors responsible for variable results with BCG, a series of trials in different populations of BCG will be necessary.

3. *Immunotherapeutic vaccination:* Control of TB by immunomodulation has been a longstanding scientific goal. After the discovery of the tubercle bacillus in 1882, Robert Koch devoted his efforts to developing an immunotherapeutic vaccine. In some patients, the results were disastrous, with the induction of pathogenic responses leading to death, dramatically illustrating that the immune response also mediates the pathology of TB. However, one new TB vaccine has already undergone clinical trials. *Mycobacterium vaccae* is an environmental mycobacterium, which in some trials showed dramatic effects, including prolonged survival of HIV-positive TB patients. However, the initial promise of *M. vaccae* as an immunotherapeutic vaccine has not been upheld by more recent randomized clinical trials.

CONCLUSION

The goal of TB vaccine development has frustrated several generations of enthusiastic research. Nevertheless, there has been considerable progress and phase I and II trials in humans can be anticipated in the near future. In the meantime, the availability of genetic tools for mycobacteria and the development of novel immunization strategies remain to be important objectives. The magnitude of the public health problem requires international coordination of translational effort and is a problem that cannot be put aside. *M. tuberculosis* is arguably the single most successful pathogen humankind has ever known. As Koch (1882) put it in The Etiology of Tuberculosis: "If the number of victims is a measure of the significance of a disease, then all disease, even the most dreaded infectious diseases, such as plague or cholera, must rank far behind tuberculosis." Today, 120 years later, President Mandela tells us: "We cannot cure AIDS without curing TB."

REFERENCES

ORIGINAL PAPERS

Armstrong JA, PD Hart. Phagosome-lysosome interactions in cultured macrophages infected with virulent tubercle bacilli. *J Exp Med.* 1975;142:1–16.

Black FL. Infectious diseases in primitive societies. *Science* 1975;187:515–518.

Cole ST, Brosch R, Parkhill J, et al. Deciphering the biology of *Mycobacterium tuberculosis* from the complete genome sequence. *Nature* 1998;393:537–544.

Dannenberg AM Jr, Rook GAW. Rabbit model of tuberculosis. In: Bloom BR, ed. *Tuberculosis, Pathogenesis, Protection and Control.* Washington, DC: ASM Press; 1994:149–156.

Hart PD, Sutherland I. BCG and vole bacillus vaccines in the prevention of tuberculosis in adolescence and early adult life. *Br Med J.* 1977;2:293–295.

Lurie MB. Studies on the mechanism of immunity in TB: the role of extracellular factors and local immunity in the fixation and inhibition of growth of tubercle bacilli. *J Exp Med.* 1939;69:555–578.

MacMicking JD, North RJ, LaCourse R, Mudgett JS, Shah SK, Nathan CF. Identification of nitric oxide synthase as a protective locus against TB. *Proc Natl Acad Sci USA,* 1997;94:5243–5248.

McCune RM, Feldmann FM, Lambert HP, McDermott W. Microbial persistence. The capacity of tubercle bacilli to survive sterilization in mouse tissues. *J Exp Med.* 1966;123:445–468.

Opie EL, Aronson JD. Tubercle bacilli in latent tuberculous lesions and in lung tissue without tuberculous lesions. *Arch of Pathol.* 1927;4:1–21.

Raviglione MC, Snider DE Jr., Kochi A. Global epidemiology of tuberculosis. Morbidity and mortality of a worldwide epidemic. *JAMA* 1995;273:220–226.

Rees R, Arcy Hart, PD. Analysis of the host-parasite equilibrium in chronic murine tuberculosis by total and viable bacillary counts. *Brit J Exp Pathol.* 1961;42:83–88.

Sambandamurthy VK, Wang X, Chen B, et al. A pantothenate auxotroph of *Mycobacterium tuberculosis* is highly attenuated and protects mice against tuberculosis. *Nat Med.* 2002;8(10):1171–1174.

Schaible UE, Sturgill-Koszycki, S, Schlesinger PH, Russell DG. Cytokine activation leads to acidification and increases maturation of mycobacterium avium-containing phagosomes in murine macrophages. *J Immunol.* 1998;160:1290–1296.

Sturgill-Koszycki S, Schlesinger, PH, Chakraborty P, et al. Lack of acidification in *Mycobacterium* phagosomes produced by exclusion of the vesicular proton-ATPase. *Science* 1994;263:678–681; erratum. 1994;263:1359.

REVIEWS

Bloom BR, Murray CJ. Tuberculosis: commentary on a reemergent killer. *Science* 1992;257:1055–1064.

Bloom BR, Fine PEM. The BCG experience: implications for future vaccines against tuberculosis. In: Bloom BR, ed. Tuberculosis: Pathogenesis Protection and Control. Washington DC: ASM; 531–557.

Flynn, JL. Immunology of Tuberculosis and implications in vaccine development. *Tuberculosis* 2004;84:93–101.

Gomez JE, McKinney JD. *M. tuberculosis* persistence, latency, and drug tolerance. *Tuberculosis* 2004;84:29–44.

Farmer P. Social inequalities and emerging infectious diseases. *Emerg Infect Dis* 1996;2:259–269.

Gormus BJ, Meyers WM. Under-explored experimental topics related to integral mycobacterial vaccines for leprosy. *Expert Rev of Vaccines.* 2003;2(6): 791–804.

Lurie MB. *Resistance to Tuberculosis: Experimental Studies in Native and Acquired Defensive Mechanisms.* Cambridge, MA: Harvard University Press; 1964.

Nathan C. Antibiotics at the crossroads. *Nature* 2004;431:899–902.

Nicod LP. Immunology of tuberculosis *Swiss Med Weekly.* 2007;1137:357–362.

North RJ, Jung YJ. Immunity to TB. *Annu. Rev. Immunol.* 2004;22:599–623.

Wayne LG, Sohaskey CD. Nonreplicating persistence of *Mycobacterium tuberculosis*. *Annu Rev Microbiol* 2001;55: 139–163.

Wilkinson RJ, Young DB. Novel vaccines against tuberculosis. In: Levine MM, Kaper JB, Rappuoli R, Liu MA, Good MF, eds. *New Generation Vaccines*. 3rd ed. New York: Marcel Dekker; 2004:519–535.

Young, DB, Duncan K. Prospects for new interventions in the treatment and prevention of mycobacterial disease. *Annu Rev Microbiol*. 1995;49:641–673.

14. Immunological Aspects of Gastrointestinal and Liver Disease

Christine Moung, M.D., and Lloyd Mayer, M.D.

MUCOSAL IMMUNITY

The mucosal immune system is distinct from its systemic counterpart. The peripheral immune system is characterized primarily by its ability to eradicate foreign antigens and functions in a relatively antigen-free environment. In contrast, the mucosal immune system is in constant juxtaposition with luminal flora and dietary proteins. Therefore, instead of mounting active immune responses, which would result in devastating consequences to the host, the general immune response of the gut is suppression. These responses are supported by several phenomena that have been observed in the gut, including oral tolerance and controlled or physiological inflammation. Suppression appears to be a selective process, as it does not preclude the ability of the gut to mount appropriate responses to pathogens (e.g., secretory IgA response). This emphasizes the dynamic ability of the mucosal immune system to adapt to environmental stimuli in a way that best suits the needs of the host. Aberrations in this balance result in inflammatory diseases of the bowel and food allergy.

The alternative pathways of immune regulation observed in the mucosal immune system are most likely explained by the distinct organization of the lymphoid structures and lymphocyte populations that are present. At this point,

study of the anatomy and components of the mucosal immune system will facilitate understanding of the mechanisms involved in both health and disease of the gastrointestinal (GI) tract.

Anatomy of the Gut-Associated Lymphoid Tissue

Anatomically, the gut-associated lymphoid tissue (GALT) is composed of a single layer of epithelial cells separating the external environment from the underlying loose connective tissue, the lamina propria (LP) (Figure 14.1). Two general categories of defenses that serve to protect the mucosa are innate and adaptive (Figure 14.2). Innate defenses include both physical and chemical barriers. The first line of defense includes the glycocalyx and mucous coat, which cover the epithelium. Bacteria and viral particles are trapped in the mucous, and these are subsequently expelled from the body through rectal, vaginal, and nasal secretions. The epithelium also prevents the entry of microorganisms into the LP. Breeches in the epithelium are rapidly restored by intestinal trefoil factors. Some pathogens are capable of invading the host through penetration of the epithelium, but the tight junctions that join the epithelial cells are virtually impermeable to foreign particles. The crypt epithelium in the small intestine (Paneth cells) produces defensins that inhibit bacterial growth. In addition,

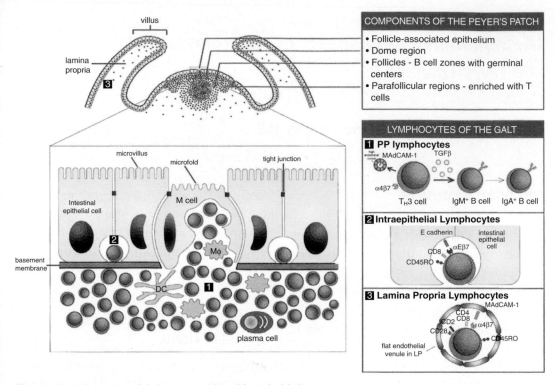

Figure 14.1 Anatomy of the gut-associated lymphoid tissue.

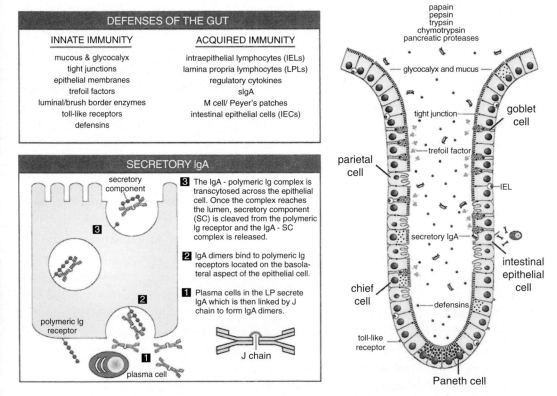

Figure 14.2 Immune defenses of the gastrointestinal tract.

Immunological Aspects of Gastrointestinal and Liver Disease

enzymes such as papain, pepsin, trypsin, chymotrypsin, and pancreatic proteases allow for the destruction and degradation of antigens to nonimmunogenic di- and tripeptides.

Within the GALT, lymphocytes are found at three sites in the mucosa (Figure 14.1). These lymphocytes, in addition to secretory IgA (SIgA) make up the adaptive arm of mucosal immunity. Lymphocytes are found in the Peyer's patch (PP) – the main organized lymphoid tissue of the GALT, in the epithelial layer, and in the LP. Each group has demonstrated special characteristics, which will be discussed in detail later.

The GALT also contains cells that may be indirectly responsible for the initiation or down-regulation of immune responses through their role as antigen-sampling cells. One such cell is the M (microfold) cell or follicle-associated epithelium, which overlies the PP. These cells lack a glycocalyx or microvilli. They allow for the uptake and transport of particulate antigens to the underlying PP, which ultimately results in an active immune response. Intestinal epithelial cells (IECs), which make up the majority of the epithelial layer, are capable of sampling soluble antigens and have been observed to stimulate regulatory $CD8^+$ T-cell populations, suggesting their role in the pathways involved in down-regulation of the immune response.

Lymphocyte Populations of the GALT

INTRAEPITHELIAL LYMPHOCYTES

Intraepithelial lymphocytes (IELs) are predominantly $CD8^+$ T cells situated between epithelial cells of the mucosa, on the basement membrane. These cells express a variety of activation markers including $CD45RO^+$, which is characteristic of memory cells. The function of these cells is uncertain as they demonstrate little proliferation when activated through their T-cell receptor (TCR). Some studies suggest that they may be cytotoxic and involved in maintaining the health of the epithelium. They do not appear to move in and out of the epithelium as epithelial cells generally grow over them. IELs express the surface molecule, $\alpha E\beta 7$, which recognizes the ligand E-cadherin on epithelial cells. Unlike $\alpha 4\beta 7$ (a mucosal addressin discussed with lamina propria lymphocytes $T_H 3$ cells), $\alpha E\beta 7$ does not appear to be a homing molecule because the number of IELs is not significantly decreased when this integrin is knocked out by targeted gene deletion. Transforming growth factor β (TGF-β) induces the expression of this integrin.

LAMINA PROPRIA LYMPHOCYTES

Unlike IELs, which are predominantly T cells, lamina propria lymphocytes (LPLs) represent a heterogeneous mix of IgA plasma cells, T cells, B cells, macrophages, and dendritic cells. Similar to IELs, LPLs express an activated memory phenotype. They express the mucosal addressin $\alpha 4\beta 7$ and up to 40 percent express $\alpha E\beta 7$. Similar to IELs, they do not respond to signals mediated through TCRs but rather can be activated through alternate pathways such as CD2 and CD28. This down-regulated response to TCR activation in both LPLs and IELs suggests this mechanism may be a means by which the mucosal immune system dampens the response to luminal flora and diet.

$T_H 3$ CELLS

Particulate antigens taken up by the M cells are ultimately presented to the lymphocyte populations in the PP through macrophages and dendritic cells. One such lymphocyte population, commonly referred to as T$_H$3 cells, secretes a key suppressor cytokine, TGF-β. The significance of TGF-β will become evident with the discussion of secretory IgA and oral tolerance. These lymphocytes can migrate systemically from the PP to other mucosal sites, which comprise the common mucosal immune system (described later). These activated cells express surface molecules, α4β7, which provide a homing signal for mucosal sites through the ligand MAdCAM-1. Specifically in the gut, they can home to the LP where they are terminally differentiated (e.g., into plasma cells for B cells).

Common Mucosal Immune System

Evidence suggests that the various mucosa-associated lymphoid tissues (MALT) throughout the body are part of a common mucosal immune system. One study introduced labeled PP lymphocytes in mice by injection and observed the pathway they appeared to migrate from the PP to the mesenteric lymph nodes, the thoracic duct, the inferior vena cava, the systemic circulation, and finally to the LP. These labeled lymphocytes could also be found in the LP throughout the remainder of the GI tract, in the mammary gland, and the lung and genitourinary tract. More recent studies suggest there is compartmentalization in the MALT; in other words, immunizing at one site induces lymphocytes with a preference for migration to certain MALT sites over others. For instance, GI tract immunization provides effector cells throughout the gut and mammary gland as demonstrated by SIgA in breast milk, while nasal and intratracheal immunization results in lymphocytes in the lung, genitourinary tract, and rectum. The important implication is that immunization at one site can confer protection at another.

Secretory IgA

Although IgG is the most abundant immunoglobulin in the serum, secretory IgA (SIgA) is the most abundant immunoglobulin in secretions. Serum IgA is a monomer, whereas SIgA exists as a dimer bound together by J (joining) chain (Figure 14.2). TGF-β initiates class switching of B cells within the PP from production of IgM to IgA. The basolateral surface of the epithelial cell expresses the polymeric immunoglobulin receptor (pIgR), which serves as a site of attachment for SIgA produced by LP plasma cells. Once bound to the pIgR, the SIgA–pIgR complex is endocytosed within vesicles and transported to the apical surface where proteolysis of the pIgR occurs. The proteolytic fragment of the pIgR is called the secretory component (SC), and it remains complexed to SIgA following secretion into the lumen of the gut. SC, a 55-kDa fragment, protects IgA against enzymatic (papain, pepsin) degradation by wrapping itself around the Fc portion of the dimeric antibody. The SIgA–SC complex remains situated in the mucous coat where it binds up bacterial and viral particles, preventing their attachment to the epithelium.

Secretory IgA complexed with antigens in the lumen is recycled through the enterohepatic circulation. After the SIgA-antigen complex is absorbed in the distal small intestine, it travels to the liver sinusoids through the portal vein, where Kupffer cells take up the complex, destroy the microorganism, and release free SIgA. The pIgR seen on the gut epithelial cells is also expressed on the basal surface of bile duct epithelium. This epithelium takes up the free SIgA and transports it into the bile duct. Bile containing SIgA then flows to the duodenum to be reused in the gut lumen.

Antigen Sampling

M cells sample particulate antigens such as intact bacteria, viruses, and parasites. This process ultimately leads to an immune response to clear these potentially harmful and infectious agents. IECs, however, have been found to sample soluble antigens. Studies have demonstrated that IECs, a type of nonclassical antigen-presenting cell, express class I and class II major histocompatibility complex (MHC) molecules constitutively. However, they have been shown to activate $CD8^+$ T cells through expression of the nonclassical MHC class I molecule CD1d. This restriction element interacts with gp180, a member of the carcinoembryonic antigen family, which binds to CD8.

Oral Tolerance

There are several phenomena that support the idea that suppression is the general response of the gut. One of these is oral tolerance (OT), which is defined as the active nonresponse to a soluble antigen that is administered through the oral route. H. G. Wells carried out one of the first documented experiments demonstrating this phenomenon in guinea pigs. By feeding them ovalbumin (OVA), he was subsequently unable to elicit an allergic/anaphylactic response when OVA was introduced systemically. This tolerant state has been determined to be active as it can be transferred to a naïve recipient by T cells.

Multiple mechanisms are involved in the induction of OT. Low-dose tolerance is mediated by the $CD4^+$ cells secreting the cytokines TGF-β, IL-10, and IL-4. Higher doses of fed antigens can induce anergy or deletion. Antigen-specific $CD8^+$ suppressor T cells may also play a role in this process. Loss of OT may be the mechanism responsible for the immune response to commensal flora and dietary antigens, leading to food allergies and possibly inflammatory bowel disease (IBD).

Oral tolerance has recently gained much interest as it proposes a mechanism by which to generate suppression to specific antigens. Several groups have suggested its use in the treatment of autoimmune/inflammatory disorders. Autoantigen can be fed to hosts, which would then result in the stimulation of regulatory T cells to these same antigens. Although induction of OT is specific for a given antigen, the effector response is not. This induction is potentially due to the effects of suppressive cytokines such as TGF-β; that is, by feeding an antigen situated in close proximity to the autoantigen of interest, you can suppress an immune response to both antigens. Thus, you do not necessarily need to feed the antigen to which the autoreactive response is targeted. This process has been termed *bystander suppression*.

IMMUNE-MEDIATED DISEASES OF THE GASTROINTESTINAL TRACT

Pernicious Anemia

Pernicious anemia (PA) is an organ-specific autoimmune disease characterized by chronic inflammation of the stomach (gastritis) with subsequent loss of parietal cells. This loss of parietal cells results in decreased synthesis of intrinsic factor (IF), which is critical for the absorption of vitamin B12 (cobalamin) in the terminal ileum. Although there are many causes of B12 deficiency (not discussed here), it should be emphasized that the term PA is reserved for instances where a lack of B12 results specifically from a deficiency of IF in the stomach.

The stomach is divided into three regions: the body and fundus, which produce acid and pepsinogen through the parietal cells and chief cells, respectively, and the antrum where G cells produce gastrin (Figure 14.3). Chronic gastritis can be divided into two categories depending on the etiology. The gastritis associated with

PA is commonly referred to as type A or autoimmune gastritis and is characterized by autoantibodies that are targeted against gastric parietal cells and IF in the body and fundus. The antrum is spared. This process results in decreased levels of acid and pepsinogen, but increased levels of gastrin subsequent to a loss of negative feedback inhibition of G cells from achlorhydria.

On a histologic level, there is a chronic inflammatory infiltrate in the LP composed of mononuclear cells, plasma cells, T cells, and B cells. The plasma cells produce the autoantibodies directed against gastric parietal cells and IF. Persistent chronic inflammation with involvement of the mucosa results in the degeneration

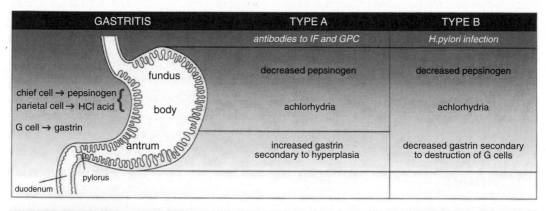

GASTRITIS	TYPE A _antibodies to IF and GPC_	TYPE B _H.pylori infection_
fundus	decreased pepsinogen	decreased pepsinogen
chief cell → pepsinogen parietal cell → HCl acid G cell → gastrin body	achlorhydria	achlorhydria
antrum pylorus duodenum	increased gastrin secondary to hyperplasia	decreased gastrin secondary to destruction of G cells

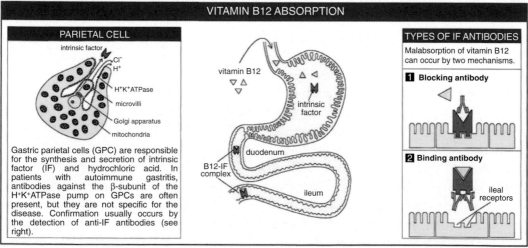

VITAMIN B12 ABSORPTION

PARIETAL CELL

intrinsic factor
Cl⁻
H⁺
H⁺K⁺ATPase
microvilli
Golgi apparatus
mitochondria

Gastric parietal cells (GPC) are responsible for the synthesis and secretion of intrinsic factor (IF) and hydrochloric acid. In patients with autoimmune gastritis, antibodies against the β-subunit of the H⁺K⁺ATPase pump on GPCs are often present, but they are not specific for the disease. Confirmation usually occurs by the detection of anti-IF antibodies (see right).

vitamin B12
intrinsic factor
duodenum
B12-IF complex
ileum

TYPES OF IF ANTIBODIES

Malabsorption of vitamin B12 can occur by two mechanisms.

1 Blocking antibody

2 Binding antibody

ileal receptors

Figure 14.3 Pernicious anemia.

of parietal and chief cells. In advanced lesions, there is replacement of these cells by mucus-secreting cells referred to as *intestinal metaplasia*. In contrast to type A gastritis, type B (or nonautoimmune) gastritis is the result of *Helicobacter pylori* infection that involves the entire stomach, including the antrum (gastrin levels are decreased).

PA is indolent in its course and may take as long as twenty to thirty years for the disease to progress from its histologic findings of gastritis to that of gastric atrophy and clinical anemia. As many as 2 percent of individuals greater than sixty years old have PA but go undiagnosed. At one time, PA was thought to be prevalent predominantly in northern European populations, but the disease has also been found to affect Latin American and black populations as well. Although no associations with specific haplotypes have been found, the disease tends to cluster in families, suggesting a genetic component. In addition, there is a predisposition of individuals who have PA to also have other autoimmune endocrinopathies such as autoimmune (Hashimoto's) thyroiditis, Addison's disease, and insulin-dependent diabetes mellitus.

Great progress in understanding PA was made with the discovery that the target of the gastric parietal cell (GPC) autoantibodies was H^+/K^+ ATPase, an enzyme present in the secretory canaliculi. In vitro, anti-GPC antibodies are capable of activating complement and lysing cells, but it is unlikely that these antibodies are the cause of PA, given their limited accessibility to the intracellularly situated H^+/K^+ ATPase. Instead, research suggests that the primary lesion is initiated by $CD4^+$ T cells that recognize the β subunit of H^+/K^+ ATPase. The best-characterized murine model in

the study of autoimmune gastritis is that of neonatal thymectomized mice that develop gastritis. However, when transgenic mice induced to express the β subunit of H^+/K^+ ATPase in the thymus are thymectomized, they do not develop gastritis. The implication here is that exposure to the β subunit of H^+/K^+ ATPase in the thymus early on in life may be critical in the induction of some regulatory cell population that is necessary to prevent gastritis or that autoreactive cells are deleted.

Diagnosis of vitamin B12 deficiency has traditionally been based on low serum vitamin B12 levels along with clinical evidence of disease (most commonly megaloblastic anemia). However, some studies have shown that increased levels of methylmalonic acid and homocysteine, key metabolites in the enzymatic reactions that require vitamin B12, are more sensitive for the diagnosis of vitamin B12 deficiency. The presence of anti-GPC autoantibodies is very sensitive but lacks specificity as they can occur in other autoimmune states. In contrast, antibodies to IF have 50 percent sensitivity, but are fairly specific.

Normally, upon intake, vitamin B12 forms a complex with IF in the duodenum and the B12–IF complex is subsequently taken up by receptors in the distal ileum for absorption. Two types of anti-IF autoantibodies – blocking and binding – have been found to interfere with this process in PA. Blocking antibodies prevent the attachment of B12 to IF while binding antibodies are thought to prevent the adhesion of the complex to ileal receptors.

Intramuscular injection of vitamin B12 has been the mainstay of treatment for PA. However, clinical trials now suggest that in individuals who do not show signs of neurologic involvement (even those individuals with IF deficiency), oral therapy may be considered as an alternative. This is supported by studies that demonstrate B12 absorption may also occur by a pathway independent of IF. Treatment is important to prevent anemia and neurologic sequelae.

Gluten-Sensitive Enteropathy

Gluten-sensitive enteropathy (GSE), also known as celiac disease or celiac sprue, is characterized by inflammatory injury to the mucosa of the small intestine after ingestion of gluten in genetically predisposed individuals. The inciting agent is gluten, a storage protein commonly found in wheat. More specifically, GSE is caused by T-cell-mediated recognition of gliadin, an alcohol-soluble fraction of gluten. Removal of gluten from the diet has been found to result in significant regression of the inflammatory lesion and symptoms seen with the disease.

For some time, GSE was thought to be rare, as its often nondescript clinical presentation masked its true prevalence. However, the advent of new serologic tests has allowed for more accurate diagnosis in the general population. Currently, it is thought to affect as many as 1 in 100 to 250 individuals worldwide – predominantly affecting Caucasians and people mainly in North America, Europe, and South America. GSE has also been observed among populations in North Africa, Iran, and India, which attests to the widespread occurrence of the disease.

Genetics plays a major role in the pathogenesis of GSE. Individuals expressing the MHC haplotypes -DR3, -DR5, -DR7, and, more importantly, -DQ2 or -DQ8 are at increased risk of developing GSE. The disease tends to cluster in families, and the monozygotic twin concordance rate of 75 percent further emphasizes the strong genetic component. Less is known about the involvement of non-HLA (human leucocyte antigen) genes, which can modify the clinical expression of the disease. GSE has been associated with a region on the long arm of chromosome 5 (5q31–33), which is where other candidate susceptibility genes that have been implicated in Crohn's disease and asthma are also located. It has been speculated that there is some involvement of the gene that encodes the negative co-stimulatory molecule, cytotoxic T-lymphocyte antigen-4 (CTLA-4).

The myriad of symptoms associated with GSE has made detection of disease especially difficult. It was once thought to occur only in childhood, but GSE can manifest at any age. Patients commonly present with malabsorption, steatorrhea, and weight loss relating to the flattening of proximal small intestinal villi. Diarrhea is not usually present unless the distal small bowel, in addition to the proximal portion, is affected. Some patients do not present with any gastrointestinal symptoms, but with effects secondary to malabsorption of vitamins such as iron, folate, and calcium. These patients may only present with anemia and osteoporosis, respectively. In addition, there is a strong association between GSE and autoimmune disease. Some individuals with GSE also present with dermatitis herpetiformis (DH), a pruritic vesicular rash that commonly presents on the extensor surfaces and the scalp. Most DH patients have GSE, whereas all individuals with GSE do not have DH. These lesions improve with the removal of gluten from the diet. Dapsone can help expedite the healing process.

Immune responses to gliadin occur in two places: the LP and the epithelium. At a low pH, tissue transglutaminase (tTG, a calcium-dependent enzyme), deamidates glutamine on gliadin, rendering these peptides more capable of binding HLA-DQ2 and HLA-DQ8. After CD4$^+$ LP T cells recognize the gliadin epitope presented by DQ2 and DQ8, they are thought to secrete interferon-γ (IFN-γ), which then causes the destructive lesions seen in GSE. The expansion of IELs (predominantly CD8$^+$) that occurs is more controversial and difficult to understand, but may relate to the reduction of IL-15 by IECs in the presence of gliadin. However, the development of lymphoma in individuals with refractory sprue has been shown to consist of a clonal expansion of CD8$^+$ T cells, implicating the IELs as a possible source. However, as gliadin-specific IELs have not been identified, this has led to the conclusion that expansion of CD8$^+$ T cells is secondary to the CD4$^+$ T-cell response to gliadin. But this same expansion of CD8$^+$ T cells does not occur in other inflammatory disorders of the GI tract such as IBD and autoimmune enteropathy, where CD4$^+$ T cells are also activated.

A mechanism to explain this inconsistency may involve the expression of nonclassical MHC class I molecules such as major histocompatibility class I chain related (MIC) and human leucocyte antigen E (HLA-E), which are induced by stress and IFN-γ. Natural killer receptors NKG2D and CD94 present on IELs are up-regulated by IL-15 and can recognize MIC and HLA-E on damaged cells. Up-regulation of IL-15 could cause the uncontrolled activation of IELs and villous atrophy. In this situation, IELs do not have to recognize gliadin peptides directly. These data have laid the groundwork for an alternate therapy for GSE, using antibodies against IL-15 in refractory sprue because IL-15 activates

IELs and promotes the development of lymphoma.

An ongoing controversy has been whether gliadin is acting as an immunologic trigger for an adaptive (CD4$^+$ T-cell) response or whether gliadin fractions are directly toxic to the epithelium, initiating the disease process. Several groups have shown that gliadin peptide can cause the lysis of certain epithelial cell lines. More recently, newer studies have supported both sides of the argument. A major gliadin fragment possesses two activities: (1) a T-cell epitope in the N terminus and (2) a fragment that is rapidly taken up by epithelium and subsequently subepithelial cells, inducing the production of IL-15 (an innate immune response). The combination of both activities accounts for the CD4$^+$ T-cell activation, CD8$^+$ IEL lymphocytosis, and IFN-γ secretion. The ability or inability to generate the complete response may account for some of the disease heterogeneity.

The gold standard for the diagnosis of GSE is a small-bowel biopsy. Histologically, GSE is characterized by a triad of villous atrophy, hyperplastic crypts, and intraepithelial lymphocytosis. Empiric therapy with a trial of gluten-free diet should be avoided as this will alter the small-bowel biopsy findings. In addition, serologic tests are useful for the diagnosis and management of GSE as they allow for a noninvasive means of monitoring adherence to diet and the identification of individuals who are at high risk for the disease who otherwise might not have been detected. IgA antibodies to endomysium, tTG, and gliadin are typically identified. Even though tTG is the autoantigen recognized by endomysial antibodies, there is not always concordance between antibodies against endomysium and tTG. Detection of GSE is optimized by looking for both antibodies. Interestingly, antibodies to tTG do not alter the function of this enzyme. The presence of antibodies against endomysium is 100 percent specific for the diagnosis of GSE. IgA deficiency occurs in about 1.7 percent to 2.6 percent of patients with GSE, a rate that is ten- to sixteenfold higher than the general population. In these instances, it is acceptable to look at IgG antibodies to endomysium, tTG, and gliadin instead of IgA. The detection of both IgA and IgG antibodies requires indirect immunofluorescence with either monkey esophagus or human umbilical cord as the substrate or tTG by enzyme-linked immunosorbent assay.

The only disease-controlling action is the removal of all gluten from the diet for life. The major limiting factor in healing is noncompliance especially in adolescents with GSE. In cases in which there is poor clinical improvement, continued ingestion of gluten is the most likely cause. Poor control is thought to be a major factor in the development of IEL lymphomas.

Inflammatory Bowel Disease

Crohn's disease (CD) and ulcerative colitis (UC) are chronic relapsing and remitting inflammatory disorders of the gastrointestinal tract, which together are referred to as IBD. Although clinical evidence suggests they are distinct entities, CD and UC are classified under the common name of IBD as they tend to occur in members of the same family and are thought to share genetic factors. While the exact pathogenetic mechanisms remain to be uncovered, the current hypothesis is that IBD results from an inappropriate mucosal immune response to commensal flora in genetically predisposed hosts.

Much of what is known about CD and UC is the result of extensive study of mouse models of intestinal inflammation that resemble IBD. The four general categories of such models are as follows: (1) spontaneous colitis due to a naturally occurring genetic abnormality; (2) spontaneous colitis in mice that have been genetically manipulated – knockout and transgenic mice; (3) colitis induced by exposure to a haptenating agent – an antigen that is immunogenic only upon being complexed with a carrier; and (4) adoptive transfer models that involve transfer of T-cell populations to a lymphopenic host such as mice with severe combined immunodeficiency (SCID).

Current research is focused on elucidating the complex interplay between genetic and environmental factors in the pathogenesis of IBD. Mouse models have allowed several broad conclusions to be made. The first, as demonstrated by the numerous murine models of colitis, is that different genetic defects can result in the same features of intestinal inflammation. The implication here is that there may be several mechanisms of IBD pathogenesis, which rely on a common pathway. Second, regardless of the genetic defect that is known to cause colitis, the host background can largely determine whether inflammation occurs. One example is that IL-10 knockout mice bred onto different backgrounds express varying clinical phenotypes. Careful study of these mice could provide insights about why some people develop IBD while others do not. Third, the normal luminal flora is an essential part of the development of colitis. Studies in several mouse models have demonstrated that colitis does not occur when mice are bred and maintained in a germ-free environment. However, once these mice are colonized by normal commensal flora, colitis rapidly ensues.

It is thought that IBD is the result of loss of tolerance to commensal flora and hence much interest is focused on uncovering the mechanisms that govern OT induction and the regulatory T-cell populations that are involved. By understanding OT, it may be possible to determine what defects occur in IBD, which would subsequently result in novel targets for immunotherapy.

CROHN'S DISEASE

In the United States, approximately 380,000 to 400,000 individuals are thought to be affected with CD. Even though it can occur at any age, a bimodal peak in the third and fifth decades of life has been observed. The incidence appears to be greater in whites than in blacks, and it has a predilection to affect the Ashkenazi-Jewish population.

There is a high concordance rate of 40–58 percent in monozygotic twins with CD. The use of microsatellite markers in genomewide screening of affected individuals and family members has reaped the greatest benefits in terms of identifying susceptibility loci and genes that predispose to the development of CD. There is a strong association with a single gene, *NOD2*, also referred to as *CARD15* (caspase activation and recruitment domain) located on chromosome 16 and referred to as *IBD1*. *NOD2* is an intracellular pattern recognition receptor involved in the binding of muramyl dipeptide, the product of peptidoglycan derived from Gram-positive organisms. Of the three major mutations in *NOD2* defined in CD, all result in the failure of muramyl dipeptide binding and loss of NFκB activation.

CD can involve any part of the GI tract, although it commonly affects the terminal ileum (30 percent), cecum and ileum (40 percent), perianal area (10 percent) and colon (20–30 percent). Endoscopy will often reveal diseased areas interspersed with normal areas of the bowel, called *skip lesions*. The nature of the inflammatory response leads to what is seen as a "cobblestone" appearance of the mucosa. This response is the result of linear ulcers intersecting with sections of normal tissue. Histologically, inflammation affects all the layers of the bowel wall (transmural). There is a dense infiltration of lymphocytes and macrophages and the presence of granulomas. Clinical features include abdominal pain, narrowing of the gut lumen (fibrosis) leading to strictures and bowel obstruction, abscess formation, fistulization to skin and internal organs, and if the colon is involved, diarrhea and bleeding (Figure 14.4).

Much evidence supports that CD is primarily a T_H1-mediated immune response. However, recent studies implicated T_H1 T-cells in the disease process. In mouse models, the introduction of the haptenating agent, trinitrobenzene sulfonic (TNBS) acid, results in increased secretion of the cytokines IL-12, IFN-γ, and TNF-α. Histologic findings reveal a transmural inflammation in these mice that resembles that seen in CD. Increased secretion of IL-12 both in vivo and ex vivo by macrophages and dendritic cells isolated from patients with CD has also been observed. In CD patients, STAT-4 (signal transducer and activator of transcription–4) is increased in the bowel. IL-12 signals through STAT-4 to up-regulate IFN-γ. Antibodies specific for the p40 chain of IL-12 have been shown to cause

CROHN'S DISEASE	IBD	ULCERATIVE COLITIS
abdominal pain obstruction fever	SIGNS & SYMPTOMS	bloody diarrhea urgency
mouth to anus (rectum spared)	GI INVOLVEMENT	colon and/or rectum
abscesses fistulas strictures granuloma formation transmural inflammation	PATHOLOGY	pseudopolyps toxic megacolon mucosal or submucosal inflammation
"string sign" on barium x-ray skip lesions "cobblestone" appearance on endoscopy	DIAGNOSIS	ulcerations, edema, & erythema of colonic mucosa negative stool cultures continuous disease
increased after 15 years	CANCER RISK	increased after 10 years
medical surgery not curative	MANAGEMENT & TREATMENT	medical surgery can be curative

Figure 14.4 Characteristics of Crohn's disease and ulcerative colitis (a and b). Courtesy of Jonathan B. Kruskal, MD - Beth Israel Deaconess Medical Center, Boston MA.

prompt resolution of inflammation in the TNBS model. Preliminary studies in man using humanized anti-IL-12 monoclonal antibodies demonstrate efficacy as well.

Management of CD is generally accomplished by medical rather than surgical means, although resection of affected bowel secondary to complications of disease occurs in about 40 percent of patients in their lifetime. Surgery is rarely curative as the disease often recurs after resection. In fact, endoscopic recurrence occurs in about 90 percent of patients after one year, usually at the site of anastamosis. In part, decisions regarding medical management depend on the location, severity of disease, and extraintestinal complications. Therapy is targeted to two goals: (1) to treat acute flare-ups and (2) to maintain remission. Immunomodulators such as azathioprine, 6-mercaptopurine, and methotrexate are targeted toward maintaining remission. In recent years, the discovery of drugs targeting TNF-α, an inflammatory cytokine, has resulted in significant improvement in morbidity in individuals with CD who are refractory to other medications. A better understanding of the immunopathogene-

sis of CD can help establish new and effective therapies. Emerging immunomodulatory therapies that are currently being tested include antibodies to IL-12 and the mucosal addressin, $\alpha 4\beta 7$.

ULCERATIVE COLITIS

In contrast to CD, histopathologic features and genetic factors are quite different in UC. Monozygotic twin studies in patients with UC only demonstrated a 6–14 percent concordance rate. Although this rate is much lower than that for CD, common genetic loci suggest there is some influence of genetic factors on UC disease susceptibility as well.

Development of UC has been associated with environmental factors. Appendectomy at a young age has been reported to have protective effects. The appendix is the site of abundant lymphoid tissue (PPs), and this may help generate protective mucosal immune responses. Surprisingly, cigarette smoking is associated with decreased risk. One possible, although not proven, reason for this association is the effect of nicotine on mucin production and possibly pro-inflammatory cytokine secretion.

UC is thought to be mediated by a mixed inflammatory immune response that is generally characterized by the secretion of cytokines IL-5, IL-13, and IFN-γ. Thus, it is neither T_H1 nor T_H2. Mouse models of colitis in which the haptenating agent, oxazolone, is introduced as well as the TCRα $-/-$ mouse demonstrate a similar cytokine profile.

UC only affects the colon and spreads proximally from the rectum in a continuous fashion. In cases in which it only affects the rectum, it is called *ulcerative proctitis*. It affects the superficial layers of the bowel wall with infiltration of lymphocytes, granulocytes, and mast cells. There are often ulcerations and crypt abscesses (collections of polymorphonuclear cells in the crypt). Clinically, patients often present with severe diarrhea, blood loss, and, with time and poor control, progressive loss of peristaltic function secondary to rigid "lead-pipe" colon. In severe cases, one can see the complications of this toxic megacolon and perforation. Of the IBDs, UC is strongly associated with an increased risk for colon cancer (occurs with long-standing – greater than ten years – disease) although this risk is present in CD as well (Figure 14.4).

Given that UC is generally confined to the colon, surgery is curative (total colectomy), in contrast to CD. Medical therapies include those that are used to treat CD – 5-ASA formulations, steroids, and immunomodulators. Surgery is reserved for those patients who are refractory to medications, develop intractable toxic megacolon, or show early or overt signs of colonic malignancy. The standard procedure up until fifteen years ago was a total proctocolectomy and end ileostomy. However, more recently, a procedure that spares the rectal musculature and

strips the rectal muscosa has been used, known as an *ileoanal pull-through* (restorative proctocolectomy with ileal pouch anal anastamosis). A total colectomy is performed, leaving the rectal musculature layer that is essentially stripped of its mucosa, as the disease is superficial, and an internal pouch is created from the distal ileum with outflow through the rectal muscular tube. A complication of this procedure is inflammation of the pouch, or pouchitis. Interestingly, this complication occurs in UC patients in up to 40 percent of the cases but does not occur in individuals in which this procedure is performed for noninflammatory disease (e.g., familial polyposis). These findings support an intrinsic defect in mucosal immunomoregulation in UC.

LIVER IMMUNOLOGY

The liver is essential in metabolism, the removal of pathogens and antigens from the blood, and the synthesis of proteins. As a result, it is exposed to numerous antigens and by-products of gastrointestinal metabolism on a daily basis. It is critical that the liver is able to mount active responses to eliminate microorganisms while avoiding unnecessary immune responses toward innocuous antigens, which could also result in injury to hepatocytes. Similar to the gut, the liver has a natural tendency toward immune tolerance rather than the induction of immunity.

Anatomically, the liver is divided into functional units termed *hepatic lobules* (Figure 14.5). These lobules are hexagonally shaped and consist of a central venule or vein and portal triads at its corners. Within the lobule, the hepatic sinusoids – the walls of which comprise liver sinusoidal

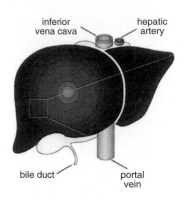

inferior vena cava

hepatic artery

bile duct

portal vein

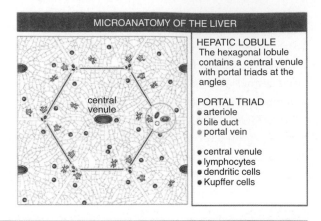

MICROANATOMY OF THE LIVER

HEPATIC LOBULE
The hexagonal lobule contains a central venule with portal triads at the angles

PORTAL TRIAD
- arteriole
- bile duct
- portal vein

- central venule
- lymphocytes
- dendritic cells
- Kupffer cells

central venule

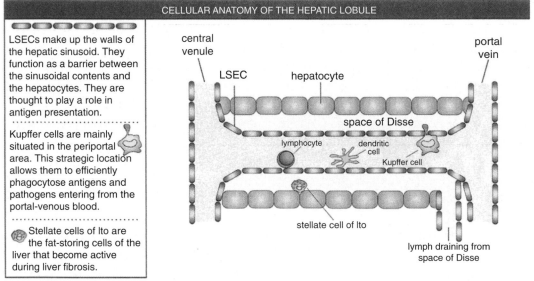

CELLULAR ANATOMY OF THE HEPATIC LOBULE

LSECs make up the walls of the hepatic sinusoid. They function as a barrier between the sinusoidal contents and the hepatocytes. They are thought to play a role in antigen presentation.

Kupffer cells are mainly situated in the periportal area. This strategic location allows them to efficiently phagocytose antigens and pathogens entering from the portal-venous blood.

Stellate cells of Ito are the fat-storing cells of the liver that become active during liver fibrosis.

central venule

LSEC   hepatocyte

portal vein

space of Disse

lymphocyte   dendritic cell

Kupffer cell

stellate cell of Ito

lymph draining from space of Disse

Figure 14.5 The hepatic microenvironment. Modified with permission from *Nature Reviews Immunology* (Crispe IN. Hepatic T cells and liver tolerance. *Nat Rev Immunol*, 2003;3(1):54.) © 2002 Macmillan Magazines Ltd.

endothelial cells (LSECs) – serve as a reservoir for the mixing of blood from both portal venous and arterial blood. Kupffer cells and lymphocytes are found in the sinusoidal lumen, adhering to the LSECs. Although the LSECs are fenestrated, it appears that they serve as a barrier to prevent leucocytes from reaching hepatocytes. The LSECs have a role in receptor-mediated endocytosis of macromolecules, which are believed to be subsequently transported to hepatocytes for metabolism. The LSECs are also believed to contribute to the activation of CD4+ and CD8+

cells as they constitutively express all molecules necessary for antigen presentation, and hence allow for immunity to harmful pathogens.

In vitro experiments have suggested that endothelial cells activate naïve T cells, but do not differentiate into effector T cells. Rather, these cells have been found to secrete cytokines and express a phenotype that is consistent with the induction of tolerance. Other cell populations such as dendritic cells and Kupffer cells may contribute to tolerance induction by deletion or apoptosis of T cells.

DISEASES OF THE LIVER

Hepatitis B

Hepatitis B virus (HBV) is thought to affect more than 400 million people worldwide. About 1.25 million Americans have chronic HBV. Chronic HBV infection contributes to 5,000 deaths annually from cirrhosis and hepatocellular carcinoma (HCC) in the United States. The rate of progression to chronic HBV infection is higher in individuals who are infected at a younger age (25–30 percent before five years of age; 3–5 percent after five years of age or as adults). HBV is especially prevalent in Southeast Asia, China, and Africa, where more than half the population is affected. It is passed on through vertical (mother to fetus) and horizontal (primarily child to child) transmission. In contrast, in the United States and Europe, infection occurs primarily by horizontal transmission among young adults.

HBV belongs to the family of hepadnaviruses. The virus is present in serum in large quantities (10^8 to 10^{10} virions) and can be transmitted not only through blood but also through bodily fluids such as semen, saliva, and cervical secretions. There is a 30 percent chance of transmission through needlestick. Acute infection is asymptomatic in 70 percent of adults and 90 percent of children younger than five years old. However, patients can present with nausea, anorexia, fatigue, fever, and right upper quadrant pain. Treatment for acute infection is generally supportive.

The HBV genome is composed of a partially double-stranded circular DNA that is enclosed within a nucleocapsid (or core antigen). This genome is surrounded by a spherical envelope or surface antigen. The genome encodes both core and surface proteins and a DNA polymerase, which also acts as a reverse transcriptase. The variable expression of core and surface antigens and antibodies to these proteins serve as useful markers of past, current, or chronic infection.

Four distinct stages of HBV infection have been described. The first stage is characterized by high levels of HBV DNA replication and normal serum transaminase levels. HBeAg, a marker of active viral replication, is positive. The second stage reflects the immune response in which inflammation results in destruction of HBV-infected cells and a subsequent elevation in transaminase levels. The highest risk of progression to cirrhosis and HCC occurs with chronic HBV infection when the patient stays in this stage beyond 6 months. The third stage is thought to indicate the end of viral replication although low levels of HBV DNA may still be present. HBeAg becomes negative, HBe antibody appears, and transaminase levels normalize. The final stage is defined by the clearance of hepatitis B surface antigen (HBsAg). Antibody to HBsAg confers protective immunity.

HBV replication is not directly cytotoxic. This is supported by the finding that despite ongoing viral replication within hepatocytes, many HBV carriers are asymptomatic and exhibit minimal liver injury. Rather, the liver injury that occurs with HBV infection is thought to be an unfortunate consequence of the immune response, which is directed at viral clearance. Clinical studies in patients with acute and self-limited hepatitis B infection have demonstrated strong T-cell responses involving both MHC class II restricted CD4$^+$ cells and MHC class I restricted CD8$^+$ cells to HBV antigens in contrast to the attenuated responses seen in chronic carriers of HBV. More specifically, cytotoxic T lymphocytes are targeted at epitopes in the HBV core, polymerase, and envelope proteins, suggesting the importance of cytotoxic T cells in the immune response.

To further characterize the role of cytotoxic T cells, transgenic mice that express HBV antigens or viral genomes in the liver have proven useful. These mice are tolerant to HBV proteins and therefore liver damage does not develop. However, when antiviral cytotoxic T cells from syngeneic mice are introduced to these mice, they develop acute liver injury similar to that seen in hepatitis B. Interestingly, the extent of hepatocyte injury cannot be entirely explained by the few interactions that occur between cytotoxic T cells and their targets. It is believed that the majority of the injury is the result of antigen nonspecific cytotoxic by-products such as TNF, free radicals, and proteases, which are released secondary to the effects of cytotoxic T lymphocytes.

Additional studies in mice suggest that the antiviral response does not necessarily involve killing the infected cells. When cytotoxic T cells are introduced in mice with active HBV replication, both DNA and RNA replication decreased even in hepatocytes that were uninjured and viable. Antibodies to TNF-α and IFN-γ inhibit this response, suggesting that these cytokines have antiviral effects.

Vaccination against HBV has been the cause of a tremendous decline of hepatitis B infection in the United States, from 300,000 cases per year to about 79,000 cases. A three-injection series with a recombinant vaccine has been found to induce protective antibody levels in 95 percent of children and 90 percent of adults.

Chronic HBV infection impairs the ability of the liver to respond to endogenous interferon. IFN-α-2b, a recombinant IFN, resembles naturally occurring antiviral cytokines. It is thought to up-regulate MHC class I molecules generally not expressed by hepatocytes, thereby increasing their susceptibility to recognition by CD8$^+$ T lymphocytes. In the first year after treatment, HBeAg seroconversion was seen in as many as 46 percent of patients treated with IFN-α-2b. The goal of immunomodulatory therapy using IFN is to accelerate the transition from stage II to stage III by eliminating the hepatocytes that house the replicating virus.

Lamivudine, a nucleoside analog first used to treat HIV infection, was approved for the treatment of HBV in 1999. It inhibits reverse transcriptase, thereby terminating viral DNA synthesis. Despite the advantages of lamivudine over IFN-α-2b in terms of its tolerability and safety in patients with decompensated cirrhosis, disadvantages include the uncertainty about the duration of therapy and the development of lamivudine-resistant strains of HBV. Recently, a nucleotide analog, adefovir dipivoxil has been approved for the treatment of HBV infection. One benefit of this drug over lamivudine is that no adefovir dipivoxil-resistant strains have been developed. It is speculated that because of its tolerability and oral route of administration, it may replace IFN-α-2b as first-line therapy in most patients.

Hepatitis C

Hepatitis C virus (HCV) affects 170 million people worldwide. Around 1.8 percent of the U.S. population is positive for HCV antibodies. Given that about 75 percent of these individuals demonstrate viral replication (viremia) in addition to seroconversion, about 2.7 million Americans have active HCV infection. For some time, blood transfusion was the primary cause of HCV infection in developed countries. With the introduction of blood-screening measures in the early 1990s, transmission by blood transfusion has decreased considerably. However, new cases continue to emerge, primarily as a result of intravenous drug use and percutaneous or mucous membrane exposure. Nosocomial infection is also a cause of HCV as the rate of transmission is estimated to be 3 percent in needle-stick injuries.

HCV belongs to the family of flaviviruses. The structural components include the core and two envelope proteins. One of the envelope proteins, E2, contains the binding site for CD81, which is present on hepatocytes and B lymphocytes and is thought to function as a cellular receptor for the virus. The regulatory proteins include helicase, protease, and polymerase. HCV replicates by means of an RNA-dependent RNA polymerase that lacks a "proofreading" function. This process can result in the evolution of genomic variations of the virus within an individual, making immune-mediated control of HCV difficult. In addition, six distinct genotypes and around 100 subtypes of HCV have been identified. Genotypes 1a and 1b are the most prevalent in the United States and western Europe, followed by genotypes 2 and 3. Genotype helps to predict effectiveness of antiviral therapy, with genotypes 2 and 3 demonstrating the best responses.

Study of acute HCV infection has been limited because these individuals are often asymptomatic. It is currently thought that the pathology, which results from HCV infection, is the result of both direct cytopathic effects of the virus and the immune response. The immune response to HCV, as with HBV, is still incompletely understood.

Due to the strict affinity of HCV for human cells, in the past only humans and higher primates such as monkeys could be infected with HCV. However, rodents make for a more appropriate and useful biological model in that their gestational periods are short, they are small, and cost less to maintain. Some models, which are currently being developed, include an immunotolerized rat and a Trimera mouse model. In the immunotolerized rat model, human hepatoma cells (Huh7) are introduced to fetal rats in utero and transplanted with the same cell line after birth. The rat is subsequently infected with HCV using HCV-positive human serum. In the Trimera model, mice are irradiated and reconstituted using SCID mouse bone marrow. HCV-infected liver fragments from patients with HCV or ex vivo infected HCV liver fragments are transplanted into the ear pinna or under the kidney capsule. More research is needed, but these particular models could be helpful in studying the effects of therapeutic regimens against HCV. In addition, several transgenic mouse models have been studied that have allowed for the analysis of the direct cytopathic effects of HCV protein and its correlation with the pathogenesis of chronic hepatitis C.

In the rare instances in which clinical acute hepatitis has been identified, symptoms have included jaundice, malaise, and nausea. Although infection becomes chronic in about 75–80 percent of affected individuals, it is often characterized by a prolonged asymptomatic period of anywhere from twenty to thirty years. Patients may present with nonspecific symptoms of fatigue (90 percent). Severe complications and death tend to occur primarily in individuals who progress to cirrhosis, which is around 15–20 percent of infected patients. Extrahepatic manifestations of HCV tend to be associated with autoimmune and lymphoproliferative states. These include cryoglobulinemia, vasculitis, and membranoproliferative glomerulonephritis. In addition, a correlation between HCV infection and lichen planus, sicca syndrome, and porphyria cutanea tarda has been noted. Co-infection with other viruses such as HIV-1 and HBV also tend to accelerate the disease process.

Liver biopsy is the gold standard for determining the activity of HCV-related disease as histologic staging is the only reliable predictor of prognosis. A biopsy can also help to rule out other causes of disease. Patients who demonstrate fibrosis or cirrhosis on liver biopsy, have genotypes 2 and 3, and present with symptoms such as fatigue and extrahepatic manifestations of disease should strongly be considered for medical therapy.

The mainstay of treatment for HCV includes the immunomodulatory drugs, pegylated (addition of polyethylene glycol prolongs the half-life and duration of activity) IFN-α-2a, -2b, and an antiviral agent, ribavirin. The HCV RNA level and HCV genotype must be obtained before starting medical therapy. Serum HCV RNA testing is the gold standard to determine effectiveness of medical therapy. Treatment is aimed at a sustained response – HCV RNA should be undetectable twenty-four weeks after discontinuation of medical therapy in individuals with either genotype 2 or 3 and for forty-eight weeks in individuals with genotypes 1a or 1b.

Patients with decompensated HCV-related cirrhosis and some patients with early stages of HCC require liver transplantation for survival. Complications include reinfection of the graft with HCV and recurrence of hepatitis and even cirrhosis. New therapies are necessary to improve long-term outcome of liver transplantation, either to prevent infection of the liver transplant or to treat HCV infection more effectively. With better characterization of the replicative cycle of HCV, it may be possible to develop virus-specific inhibitors. Potential targets include the HCV proteases, helicase, and polymerase as well as the cell surface receptor CD81.

Other Hepatitis Viruses

Hepatitis A virus (HAV) is a small RNA virus that belongs to the picornavirus family. Prevalence of the virus is generally correlated with areas of poor hygiene and sanitation. Even in countries such as the United States with relatively good sanitation, one-third of the population has evidence of previous infection from hepatitis A. Although infection is acute and resolves spontaneously in the majority of these individuals, a small number of cases result in fulminant hepatitis and death.

HAV replicates in the liver and is transported by bile into the stool. Transmission occurs through the fecal-oral route. Two formalin-inactivated hepatitis A vaccines are currently available in the United States. These vaccines cause formation of antibodies (seroconversion) to HAV in 94 percent of vaccine recipients after the first dose has been administered and in nearly all recipients after the second dose. In addition, immune globulin is available for individuals who require passive immunoprophylaxis. It is generally given within two weeks after exposure to HAV or two weeks before travel to areas where HAV is endemic.

Hepatitis D (delta hepatitis) is an RNA-containing "passenger" virus that requires co-infection with HBV. Hepatitis D needs the nucleocapsid assembly function of HBV in addition to the HBsAg-derived envelope. Without these, HDV replication cannot occur. The best prevention is vaccination against hepatitis B.

Hepatitis E virus (HEV), an RNA virus belonging to the family of caliciviruses, causes endemic and epidemic hepatitis mostly in Asia, the Middle East, North Africa, Mexico, and South America. Clinical illness generally occurs between the ages of 15 and 34, with a peak incidence from the age of 20 to 29. Most epidemics result from fecal contamination of water sources. Person-to-person transmission is uncommon and exposure to blood products and intravenous drug use do not seem to increase risk. The disease is acute and often resolves spontaneously. Fulminant hepatic failure is rare with mortality at 0.1 percent to 0.6 percent. However, infection in pregnancy has a mortality of 15 to 25 percent. Repeated episodes of infection are not uncommon as anti-HEV antibodies decline over time.

Primary Biliary Cirrhosis

Primary biliary cirrhosis (PBC) is an autoimmune disease of the liver that results in chronic injury to the intrahepatic bile duct epithelium. The gradual destruction of the bile ducts causes cholestasis with the subsequent retention of toxins, inciting further hepatic injury and resulting in fibrosis, cirrhosis, and eventual liver failure. Early detection is optimal, before significant liver injury has occurred.

PBC primarily affects middle-aged women. The ratio of affected women to men has been reported to be as high as 9:1.

The most common presenting symptoms include pruritis and fatigue. While pruritis can be severe, there is marked improvement by medications such as ursodiol. Fatigue on the other hand causes significant disability, as there are no medications that can provide relief. Other findings may include hyperlipidemia and osteoporosis. In addition, patients may have concurrent autoimmune diseases, which include but are not limited to Sjögren's syndrome and scleroderma. Patients with more advanced disease may present with symptoms commonly seen with other chronic liver diseases such as ascites, portal hypertension, and esophageal varices. An increased incidence of HCC in patients with longstanding advanced disease has been described.

The diagnostic criteria for PBC include an elevation in liver enzymes (most notably alkaline phosphatase) for a duration of six or more months, histologic findings, and the presence of antimitochondrial antibodies in the serum. The presence of two criteria is highly suggestive of the disease while a definite diagnosis requires all three.

Involvement of the liver is heterogeneous, so a biopsy may demonstrate different stages of disease. In such instances, the disease is assigned the most advanced stage. Stage I is characterized by portal inflammation comprised of predominantly lymphoplasmacytic infiltrates. The pathognomonic lesion of PBC, the florid duct lesion, represents focal duct obliteration by granuloma formation. In stage II there is extension of inflammation to the periportal areas. There is formation of fibrous septa that link adjacent portal triads and bile duct loss (ductopenia) in stage III. Finally, stage IV is defined by frank cirrhosis.

The targets of the antimitochondrial antibodies belong to the family of 2-oxo-acid dehydrogenase enzyme complexes located in the inner mitochondrial membrane. The major autoantigen is the E2 subunit of the pyruvate dehydrogenase complex (PDC-E2). Given that 90 to 95 percent of patients with PBC have anti-mitochondrial antibodies, some of which are asymptomatic, serologic detection has allowed for earlier diagnosis of disease and improvement in prognosis.

Molecular mimicry is the most widely proposed explanation as to the induction of autoimmunity in PBC. Briefly, a host is infected with a microorganism that contains antigens similar to antigens present in the host. These microbial antigens induce an immunologic response when presented to the immune system of the host. As a result, what began as a pathogen-specific response then cross-reacts with the host antigens and results in tissue injury and disease. This mechanism has also been associated with other autoimmune diseases of the liver such as primary sclerosing cholangitis (PSC) and autoimmune hepatitis (AIH).

Bacteria such as *Escherichia coli* have been implicated due to the reported high incidence of urinary tract infections in patients with PBC. Antibodies against human pyruvate dehydrogenase in PBC patients react well against the *E. coli* pyruvate dehydrogenase complex. More recently, a Gram-negative aerobe, *Novosphingobium aromaticivorans* has been demonstrated to have an even higher degree of homology with the immunodominant epitope on human PDC-E2 than *E. coli*. The titers of antibodies in PBC patients against pyruvate dehydrogenase in *N. aromaticivorans* are as much as 1,000 times higher than the titers of antibody against *E. coli*.

Other potential infectious triggers include *Chlamydia pneumoniae* and lactobacilli.

The exact mechanism of biliary destruction is not entirely clear, as it appears that the autoantibodies do not have a direct cytotoxic effect. This is supported by a lack of correlation between antibody titer and extent of hepatic involvement, the lack of immediate recurrence despite the persistence of antibodies status post-liver transplantation, and the absence of antibodies in about 5–10 percent of patients with histologically confirmed PBC.

The involvement of inflammatory cells in the pathogenesis of PBC is supported by several findings. The epitopes recognized by portal CD4$^+$ helper and CD8$^+$ cytotoxic T cells overlap on the lipoyl domain of PDC-E2. In patients with PBC, studies have demonstrated that the frequency of autoreactive CD4$^+$ T cells is higher in the hepatic lymph nodes than in the circulation. In addition, CD8$^+$ T cells and B cells that are reactive with PDC-E2 are higher in the liver than in the circulation. A decrease in CD4$^+$ CD25-high regulatory (Treg) cells may also contribute to an acceleration of autoimmunity in PBC. Bile duct destruction secondary to the accumulation of bile acids is thought to play a role in disease progression. Cholestasis increases the expression of HLA class I antigens in hepatocytes in PBC. The implication here is that there is increased presentation of antigens to cytotoxic cells.

Some puzzling observations are that the autoantibodies are specifically directed against the mitochondria in bile duct epithelial cells despite the fact that nucleated cells are ubiquitous in the body. One proposed theory is that the altered state of apoptotic biliary epithelial cells predisposes them to having antibodies developed against them. It is thought that the blockage of glutathione attachment to the lysine-lipoyl moiety of the E2 protein during biliary epithelial cell apoptosis renders the PDC-E2 susceptible to recognition by autoantibodies. When compared with PSC, the injury is limited to the intrahepatic ducts in PBC. The extrahepatic ducts often remain intact even at the cirrhotic stage. This selectivity for cholangiocytes may be attributed to inherent genetic differences (observed in mice) present in intra- and extrahepatic cholangiocytes.

Recently, studies have identified three murine models that spontaneously develop PBC. These models include the NOD.c3c4 mouse, a mouse with the dominant negative form of tTGF-β receptor II (dnTGFβ RII), and the IL-2Rα knockout mouse. In all three models, the target of the antimitochondrial antibodies is PDC-E2 and the immunodominant epitope is the lipoyl domain. In addition, they all demonstrate lymphocyte infiltration around the portal tracts accompanied by cholangiocyte injury. These animal models could help elucidate many unanswered questions.

Medical therapy is geared toward both symptomatic improvement and treatment of underlying disease. Cholestyramine and rifampin are common agents used to treat the pruritis. Ursodiol (ursodeoxycholic acid) is the only medical treatment for PBC that has received approval by the U.S. Food and Drug Administration. Ursodiol has been found to cause a normalization of enzymes and improve histologic findings in approximately 25 to 30 percent of patients with PBC. In addition, at least 20 percent of patients treated with ursodiol have no histologic progression over four years. Its effects are thought to be multifactorial. It promotes both endogenous bile acid secretion and membrane stabili-

zation. This compound is also associated with reduced aberrant HLA type 1 expression on hepatocytes and a fall in cytokine production. Colchicine and methotrexate are also commonly utilized if there is inadequate response to ursodeoxycholic acid. PBC still remains one of the top five indications for liver transplantation. The survival rates are 92 percent and 85 percent at one and five years, respectively. PBC recurs in 15 percent of patients at three years and 30 percent at ten years.

Primary Sclerosing Cholangitis

PSC is a chronic liver disease that is characterized by chronic inflammation and obliterative fibrosis of the intra- and extrahepatic bile ducts. Similar to PBC, the bile ducts are the initial target of injury with subsequent hepatic injury and progression to liver failure. Unlike PBC, there is a great deal more uncertainty as to the optimal means of diagnosis, monitoring, and therapy. Although the exact cause of PSC is unknown, it is considered autoimmune due to the presence of autoantibodies. However, therapy is limited because PSC does not respond as well to conventional immunosuppressive therapies as do other autoimmune diseases.

PSC typically presents in the fourth to fifth decades of life. Men are affected more often than women, which is in contrast to PBC. Patients often present with pruritis and fatigue. Essentially, the clinical course represents a progressive worsening of symptoms associated with bile stasis and eventual development of jaundice and end-stage liver disease. About a third of patients have bacterial cholangitis, especially following biliary intervention, during which time the disease can progress. In addition, PSC is closely related to IBD (typically UC) and 10 percent of patients develop cholangiocarcinoma, which can occur relatively early, before the onset of cirrhosis.

Similar to PBC, patients exhibit abnormalities in liver enzymes, characteristic histologic findings, and serum autoantibodies. However, the diagnosis of PSC requires demonstration of a "beaded" pattern by endoscopic retrograde cholangiopancreatography (ERCP) or magnetic resonance cholangiopancreatography, which represents alternating areas of stricture and dilatation of the bile ducts.

The primary injury is against medium- and large-sized bile ducts. The smaller ducts gradually disappear as a result of obstruction. The classic, nearly pathognomonic, lesion of PSC is concentric periductal fibrosis (onion-skinning) that causes narrowing and obliteration of the small bile ducts, ultimately leaving a scar. Other nonspecific changes commonly seen in chronic cholestasis include pseudoxanthomatous changes, Mallory bodies, and periportal copper accumulation. The staging and grading of PSC has not been tested for reliability. But similar to PBC, four stages have been described.

The autoimmune nature of PSC is supported by the presence of hypergammaglobulinemia, multiple autoantibodies, and specific MHC haplotypes commonly associated with autoimmune diseases. As mentioned earlier, it is also associated with other immune-mediated inflammatory disorders such as IBD. While many autoantibodies may be present in PSC, it is most closely linked to perinuclear antineutrophil cytoplasmic antibody (pANCA). Studies suggest that the antigen targeted by pANCA is either a nuclear envelope protein, myeloid-specific tubulin-beta isotype 5, or histone H1. These antibodies do not appear to be directly cytotoxic.

A recent study has suggested that the association between IBD and PSC is the result of inappropriate recruitment of mucosal lymphocytes to extraintestinal tissue. In PSC, the mucosal addressin, MAdCAM-1 and the gut-specific chemokine, CCL25, which are normally present in the intestine, are aberrantly expressed in the liver where they recruit mucosal lymphocytes. As a result, in PSC, the liver is infiltrated by activated mucosal T cells that secrete pro-inflammatory cytokines. The activated T cells bind to biliary epithelial cells. Whether this process represents a primary or a secondary change is not clear. In other studies, it has been suggested that toll-like receptors (TLRs), involved in the triggering of innate immune responses in IBD, may also play a role in the pathogenesis of PSC. TLRs are expressed in both gastrointestinal epithelial cells and cholangiocytes. It is possible that activation of TLRs can manipulate transepithelial resistance and decrease epithelial barrier function.

Unfortunately, no animal models are able to fully demonstrate the spectrum of clinical and pathological features of PSC. Although various toxins can induce cholangiocyte injury in rodents, the end result does not adequately mimic human disease. One model that shows promise is that of the $Mdr2$ knockout mouse. Normal bile secretion depends on the presence of bile acid and lipid transporters. In humans, $MDR3/ABCB4$ (the murine analog is $Mdr2$) encodes a canalicular flipase that is responsible for transporting phospholipids into bile. Humans with $MDR3$ mutations have been found to develop progressive familial intrahepatic cholestasis. Mice that have $Mdr2$ knocked out have spontaneous sclerosing cholangitis with serum as well as histologic features resembling human PSC. These mice also develop autoantibodies to pANCA. These mice have been utilized as models for therapy in PSC. In this model, nor-ursodeoxycholic acid improved histologic findings and liver enzymes.

The improvement in PSC using ursodeoxycholic acid is controversial. While there may be an improvement in liver enzymes, there is no actual improvement in liver histology or liver transplant-free survival. Between 10 and 15 percent of patients with PSC will experience high-grade obstruction from a discrete area of narrowing within the extrahepatic tree. In the past, these were managed surgically. Since then, improvements in endoscopic techniques have allowed for management by ERCP with balloon or coaxial dilatation or stenting. Clinical response can be achieved in 80 percent of patients without cirrhosis. Liver transplant survival is excellent with 90 percent at one year and 84 percent at two years. Retransplantation rates are higher for PSC patients than those with other diagnoses (9.6 percent versus 4.6 percent within two years) potentially due to the persistence of underlying immunologic defects.

Autoimmune Hepatitis

AIH is a chronic hepatitis of unknown cause that affects children and adults of all ages. It tends to present with a waxing and waning course. As with PBC and PSC, diagnosis is based on an elevation of liver enzymes (transaminase levels tend to be affected the most), histology, and the presence of antibodies in serum. In addition, variant, overlapping, or mixed forms of AIH have been described that share features with PBC and PSC. It is important to distinguish AIH from PBC and PSC, as a high percentage of patients with AIH respond to anti-inflammatory and immunosuppressive therapy.

Although the exact mechanisms underlying AIH are not known, environmental triggers such as infection with hepatitis, measles, cytomegalovirus, and Epstein-Barr virus are thought to be involved in molecular mimicry. Certain drugs such as oxyphenisatin, methyldopa, nitrofurantoin, diclofenac, IFN, pemoline, minocycline, and atorvastatin can also cause hepatocellular injury, which resembles AIH.

Histologically, AIH can be indistinguishable from a chronic hepatitis. Virology panels and cholangiography are especially helpful in narrowing the differential diagnosis. AIH is characterized by a mononuclear infiltrate that permeates the limiting plate (the row of hepatocytes lining the portal triad), in what is referred to as *piecemeal necrosis* or *interface hepatitis*, which progresses to hepatocyte inflammation (lobular hepatitis). Plasma cells and eosinophils are frequently present and fibrosis is often present in all but the mildest of cases.

Classification of AIH is based on autoantibody patterns. Type 1 AIH is characterized by antinuclear (ANA) and anti-smooth muscle antibodies. Anti-actin is more specific. Atypical pANCA and autoantibodies against soluble liver antigen and liver pancreas antigen (SLA/LP) may also be present. Type 1 is also associated with HLA-DR3 and HLA-DR4. Type 2 AIH, which is rare, is characterized by antibodies to liver kidney microsome (LKM-1) and liver cytosol (ALC-1).

The autoantigens responsible for AIH are still being explored. One popular contender is the liver-specific membrane protein, asialoglycoprotein receptor. It is expressed in high levels in periportal hepatocytes and shares some common amino acid sequences with SLA/LP antigen. Even more compelling is the discovery that LKM-1 antibodies in type

2 AIH react with epitopes on the 2D6 isoform of cytochrome P450 (CYP2D6). One study found that the sera of 38 percent of chronic hepatitis C patients reacted specifically with CYP2D6, whereas the sera of hepatitis B patients did not show CYP2D5 reactivity. This lends credence to the role of HCV in molecular mimicry.

CD4$^+$ regulatory T cells (Treg) that express the IL-2 receptor α chain (CD25) are known to suppress the proliferation and effector function of autoreactive CD4$^+$ and CD8$^+$ cells. Absence of these T cells has been shown to result in spontaneous autoimmune disease such as autoimmune thyroiditis, gastritis, and insulin-dependent diabetes in animal models. A study in humans demonstrated that Treg cells were decreased in patients with AIH as compared with normal controls. In addition, the percentage of Treg cells was significantly decreased at diagnosis rather than remission and was inversely proportional to the titers of anti-LKM and soluble liver antigen antibodies. The suppressor activity of the Treg cells, however, was maintained. This suggests that therapeutic measures in the treatment of AIH may include increasing Treg cells.

Several animal models of AIH have been described. The major limitations to most models are that they require complicated induction protocols and the hepatitis observed is generally transient. One of the more recently proposed models is based on CYP2D6 and its involvement in molecular mimicry. In this model, mice express human CYP2D6 under their own promoter in the liver. To break tolerance, these CYP2D6 mice were infected with adenovirus-CYP2D6 vector, which resulted in long-lasting hepatic damage, infiltration with B cells, CD4 and CD8 T cells, and a transient elevation in serum aminotransferases. These CYP2D6 mice also had high titers of anti-CYP2D6 antibodies, which were found to react with the same immunodominant epitope in AIH patients.

Early diagnosis is essential as medical treatment is successful at improving long-term outcomes for patients. Prednisolone alone or in combination with azathioprine is the mainstay of treatment. Most patients require lifelong immunosuppression as maintenance therapy. Liver transplantation is required in patients who are refractory to or intolerant of immunosuppressive therapy and in whom end-stage liver disease develops. The survival rate among patients and grafts five years after liver transplantation is approximately 80 to 90 percent, the ten-year survival rate is approximately 75 percent, and the recurrence rate has been reported to be as high as 42 percent.

REFERENCES

MUCOSAL IMMUNOLOGY

Mayer L. Mucosal immunity and gastrointestinal antigen processing. *J Pediatr Gastroenterol Nutr* 2000;30(suppl):S4–S12.

Mayer L. Mucosal immunity. *Pediatrics* 2003;111(6):1595–1600.

PERNICIOUS ANEMIA

Alderuccio F, Sentry JW, Marshall ACJ, Biondo M, Toh BH. Animal models of human disease: experimental autoimmune gastritis—a model for autoimmune gastritis and pernicious anemia. *Clin Immunol* 2002;102(1):48–58.

Oh R, Brown DL. Vitamin B12 deficiency. *Am Fam Physician* 2003;67(5):979–986.

Toh BH, van Driel IR, Gleeson PA. Pernicious anemia. *N Engl J Med* 1997;337(20):1441–1448.

Waters HM, Dawson DW, Howarth JE, Geary CG. High incidence of type II autoantibodies in pernicious anaemia. *J Clin Pathol* 1993;46:45–47.

GLUTEN-SENSITIVE ENTEROPATHY

Green PH, Jabri B. Coeliac disease. *Lancet* 2003;362(9381):383–391.

Mention JJ, Ben Ahmed M, Begue B, et al. Interleukin-15: a key to disrupted intraepithelial lymphocyte homeostasis and lymphomagenesis in celiac disease. *Gastroenterology* 2003;125(3): 730–745.

Sollid LM. Coeliac disease: dissecting a complex inflammatory disorder. *Nat Rev Immunol* 2002;2(9):647–655.

INFLAMMATORY BOWEL DISEASE

Bach SP, Mortensen NJ. Ileal pouch surgery for ulcerative colitis. *World J Gastroenterol 2007*;13(24):3288–3300.

Bouma G, Stober W. Immunological and genetic basis of inflammatory bowel disease. *Nat Rev Immunol* 2003;3(7): 521–533.

Knutson D, Greenberg G, Cronau H. Management of Crohn's disease – a practical approach. *Am Fam Physician* 2003;68(4):707–714.

Podolsky DK. Inflammatory bowel disease. *N Engl J Med* 2002;347(6):417–429.

LIVER IMMUNOLOGY

Crispe, IN. Hepatic T cells and liver tolerance. *Nat Rev Immunol* 2003;3(1):51–62.

Knolle PA, Gerken G. Local control of the immune response in the liver. *Immunol Rev* 2000;174(1):21–34.

VIRAL HEPATITIS

Craig AS, Shaffner W. Prevention of hepatitis A with the hepatitis A vaccine. *N Engl J Med* 2004;350(5):476–481.

Flamm SI. Chronic hepatitis C virus infection. *JAMA* 2003;289(18):2413–2417.

Ganem D, Prince AM. Hepatitis B virus infection – natural history and clinical consequences. *N Engl J Med* 2004;350(11):1118–1129.

Kremsdorf S, Brezillon N. New animal models for hepatitis C viral infection and pathogenesis studies. *World J Gastroenterol* 2007;13(17):2427–2435.

Lauer GM, Walker BD. Hepatitis C virus infection. *N Engl J Med* 2001;345(1): 41–52.

Lin KW, Kirchner JT. Hepatitis B. *Am Fam Phys* 2004;69(1):75–82.

Marsano LS. Hepatitis. *Prim Care* 2003; 30(1):81–107.

PRIMARY BILIARY CIRRHOSIS

Kaplan MM. Primary biliary cirrhosis. *N Engl J Med* 2005;353(12):1261–1273.

Talwalkar JA, Lindor KD. Primary biliary cirrhosis. *Lancet* 2003;362(9377): 53–61.

Ueno Y, Moritoki Y, Shimosegawa T, Gershwin ME. Primary biliary cirrhosis: what we know and what we want to know about human PBC and spontaneous PBC mouse models. *J Gastroenterol* 2007 42(3):189–195.

PRIMARY SCLEROSING CHOLANGITIS

LaRusso NF, Shneider BL, Black D, et al. Primary sclerosing cholangitis: summary of a workshop. *Hepatology* 2006;44(3):746–764.

AUTOIMMUNE HEPATITIS

Christen U, Holdener M, Hintermann E. Animal models for autoimmune hepatitis. *Autoimmun Rev.* 2007;6(5): 306–311.

Krawitt EL. Autoimmune hepatitis. *N Engl J Med.* 2006;354(1):54–66.

15. Immunological Aspects of Endocrine Disease

Jean-François Bach, M.D.

INTRODUCTION

Endocrine cells may be localized in a defined glandular organ such as the pancreas (islet cells) or in the adrenal gland. Others may be distributed throughout a nonendocrine gland such as the stomach. Functional disorders of the endocrine gland may result from overactivity of the glands or atrophy. The former results in overproduction of a given hormone, while the latter is a failure to produce the hormone.

Although a number of endocrine glands are involved in this process and other organs such as the thyroid and adrenal gland will be discussed in other chapters (see "Autoimmunity," Chapter 6), we will concentrate our discussion on a single organ, the pancreas, and the disease insulin-dependent diabetes mellitus (IDDM).

INSULIN-DEPENDENT DIABETES MELLITUS

IDDM is a T-cell-mediated autoimmune disease. Its etiology is multifactorial, involving several predisposing genes and complex environmental factors. The analysis of disease pathogenesis and the search for new treatments have benefited enormously from the availability of two spontaneous animal models of the disease: (1) the nonobese diabetic (NOD) mouse and (2) the bio-breeding (BB) rat.

CLINICAL PRESENTATION

Most commonly, IDDM starts suddenly in a previously healthy individual, usually a child. The initial clinical symptoms include polyuria and polydipsia as a consequence of osmotic diuresis induced by glycosuria. If the disease is not diagnosed early, weight loss is observed, and in some cases ketoacidosis, leading to coma. The biological hallmarks of the disease are hyperglycemia and glycosuria. The treatment is based on the regular administration of exogenous insulin in doses and with a timing adapted to each individual patient. Once it has appeared, insulin dependency is definitive, as explained by the complete destruction of β cells, the insulin-producing cells in the islets of Langerhans of the pancreas in patients with longstanding disease. In some patients, however, the disease may regress for a few months after initiation of intensive insulin therapy (the so-called honeymoon). This remission is linked to the relief of B cells from glucotoxicity.

An important and yet unsettled question is the percentage of β cells that are still alive at the time of diagnosis. This is a crucial question for immunotherapy strategies. Only limited data are available in human IDDM, since pancreas biopsies have only

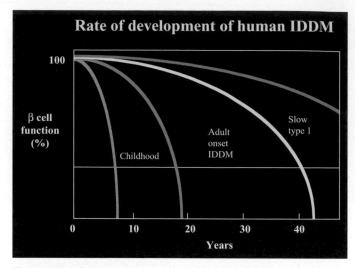

Figure 15.1 Rate of development of human IDDM.

occasionally been performed because of the risk of biopsy-induced pancreatitis. Data obtained in the NOD mouse indicate, however, that before being destroyed, β cells show reversible signs of inflammation.

IDDM usually starts abruptly in most patients. However, IDDM may be preceded by a long phase of non-insulin-dependent diabetes (latent autoimmune diabetes of the adult, or LADA). It is generally assumed that LADA represents a slowly progressing form of autoimmune diabetes (see Figure 15.1).

ANIMAL MODELS

Five main animal models of IDDM have been described.

The NOD Mouse

This mouse strain is characterized by the onset of IDDM at three or four months of age. Disease incidence and age of onset vary according to gender (with a marked female predominance) and to the sanitary conditions in which the mice are bred (the cleaner the facilities, the higher the disease incidence).

Diabetes onset is preceded for several weeks by insulitis (cellular infiltration of the pancreas, including T cells and macrophages), starting at three weeks of age. At six to eight weeks of age, islet-specific autoantibodies and T cells are detected (see Figures 15.2 and 15.3). NOD mice, particularly females, do not develop only IDDM. They also often show thyroiditis and sialitis as well as various extrapancreatic autoantibodies (essentially antierythrocytic and antinuclear antibodies).

The relevance of the NOD mouse model to human IDDM is a matter of debate. Some minor differences are seen with the human disease: the female predominance is not observed in humans, except in the less common form of IDDM associated with extrapancreatic autoantibodies. Islet-specific antibodies are less prevalent in NOD mice than in human diabetes. In fact, with these two reservations, all other clinical, biological, and immunological characteristics of NOD mouse and human IDDM are remarkably similar. The only troublesome point is the unexpected sensitivity of NOD

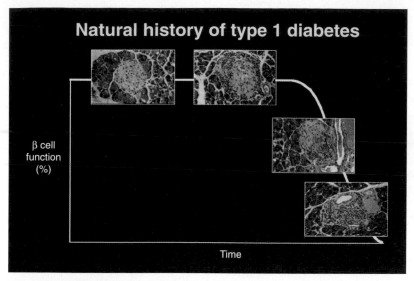

Figure 15.2 Natural history of type I diabetes.

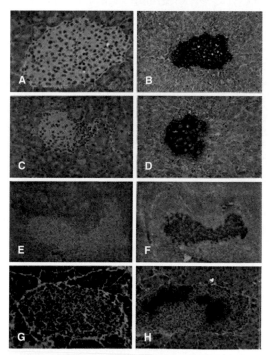

Figure 15.3 Progression of insulitis and of decrease of insulin-secreting β cells in the course of the natural history of diabetes in nonobese diabetic (NOD) mice. Left column (a, c, e, g) T-cell infiltration. Right column (b, d, i, h) β-cell number (as assessed by insulin staining).

mice to immunointervention. More than 150 therapeutic maneuvers have been shown to prevent diabetes onset when they are applied to young NOD mice. It appears difficult to some diabetologists to believe that human diabetic patients would be as sensitive as NOD mice to immuno-intervention, considering the severity of disease progression in the human species. Immunotherapy has not been applied in humans as early as it is usually performed in NOD mice. Additionally, when NOD mice are treated at diabetes onset or just before it, most of the methods that were successful in the young mice fail, with the exception of a few robust therapies that are described later.

Collectively, these data validate the NOD mouse as a good model for human IDDM.

The Bio-breeding Rat

The bio-breeding (BB) rat is historically the first known spontaneous model of IDDM. It also resembles human IDDM with, however, a major difference, which consists of a major state of lymphocytopenia selectively involving the T-cell subset of Rt6⁺ cells. Most immunodiabetology laboratories now use the NOD mouse rather than the BB rat because it is easier to handle, it breeds very well, and there are many more genetic and immunological markers available in the mouse than in the rat. However, remarkable studies have been performed in the BB rat, notably the Rossini groups, including the demonstration of IDDM prevention by administration of antilymphocyte serum and neonatal thymectomy that played a considerable role in drawing attention to the autoimmune origin of the disease.

T-Cell Receptor Transgenic Mice

Several islet-specific CD4$^+$ and CD8$^+$ diabetogenic T-cell clones have been derived from diabetic NOD mice. When the T-cell receptor (TCR) genes of such clones were used to generate transgenic NOD mice, IDDM developed in an accelerated fashion. The most popular mice produced with this strategy were the BDC2.5 mouse (for CD4 T-cell clones) and the 8.1 mouse (for a CD8$^+$ T-cell clone). A large proportion of T cells (but not all) in such mice express the transgenic TCR. This is usually sufficient for transgenic mice to develop rapid diabetes. This is not, however, an absolute rule, since in some genetic backgrounds the disease develops slowly or does not even appear. In all cases, the disease is remarkably accelerated after backcrossing to severe combined immunodeficiency (SCID) or Rag knock out −/− mice that lack both B and T cells, an observation explained by the lack in such backcrossed mice of T cells having undergone endogenous TCR rearrangements (which probably include regulatory T cells) that normally delay diabetes onset. In fact, T cells from these backcrossed mice are monoclonal, all expressing the diabetogenic TCR.

RIP Mice

When transgenes are coupled to the rat insulin promoter (RIP), they are selectively expressed in the β cells. This observation has allowed the generation of a wide variety of transgenic models of IDDM. The T antigen of the Simian virus (SV) virus was expressed in β cells of non-autoimmune-prone mice. Depending on individual mice, animals developed insulinoma or major insulitis (not sufficiently severe, however, to induce IDDM).

Later on, other antigens were used, including influenza virus hemagglutinin (HA) and lymphochoriomeningitis virus (LCMV) glycoprotein. The expression of high amounts of these antigens did not induce diabetes by themselves because the mice were tolerant to the antigens, which, in that context, behaved as bona fide autoantigens. Diabetes could be induced, however, when mice were infected by LCMV (in the case of the RIP-LCMV mice) or when they were crossed to other transgenic mice expressing an HA-specific TCR (in the case of RIP-HA mice). Double transgenic mice were also produced with RIP-LCMV mice, but they did not become diabetic unless they were infected by LCMV.

The Low-Dose Streptozotocin Model

Streptozotocin (STZ) is a selective β-cell toxic agent. Administered at high doses, it induces the quasi-immediate apoptosis of all β cells with subsequent IDDM. When administered at low doses in a repeated fashion, toxic IDDM does not appear. Diabetes is, however, observed after a few days because of autoimmune aggression of the pancreas. Neonatal thymectomy and anti-T-cell antibody treatment prevent low-dose STZ-induced IDDM. This IDDM model has the great advantage of being rapidly induced and obtained in a large variety of mouse strains. Not all strains are equally sensitive to STZ in a genetically controlled fashion. STZ doses must be selected with caution because only a small difference between toxic and immune-triggering doses is apparent. The mechanisms leading to STZ-induced diabetes are ill defined but probably involve T-cell triggering by β-cell autoantigens released by apoptotic β cells.

THE β-CELL LESION: NATURE OF EFFECTOR CELLS

IDDM is characterized by the selective destruction of β cells (other islet cells, notably glucagon-producing cells remain intact). The β-cell destruction is due to apoptosis. It is preceded by a long phase of prediabetes that has been well characterized in animal models. Initial insulitis is essentially of peripheral nature (perinsulitis) without β-cell aggression. It becomes progressively more active, resulting in "malignant" insulitis. Even at a late stage (diabetes onset), much of this aggression is reversible because of T-cell-mediated inflammation. One can thus explain that hyperglycemia in recently diagnosed diabetic mice is corrected within twenty-four to forty-eight hours by treatment with an anti-T-cell antibody (anti-TCR or anti-CD3) and that islets derived from recently diagnosed diabetic NOD mice recover the capacity to produce insulin after in vitro culture in the absence of T cells or autoantibodies.

The nature of the cellular and molecular events at the origin of β-cell inflammation

and destruction is still a matter of debate. The role of T cells is unquestionable. Diabetes can be transferred to NOD-SCID mice (which do not spontaneously develop diabetes because they lack T cells) after infusion of purified T cells or T-cell clones. Both CD4 and CD8 T cells are necessary to obtain diabetes transfer when using polyclonal T cells, even though transfer can be obtained with CD4$^+$ or CD8$^+$ T-cell clones injected alone. Emphasis has recently been put on the role of CD8$^+$ T cells, but there has not yet been a clear demonstration of islet-specific cytotoxic T lymphocytes capable of destroying β cells in a FAS or a perforin-dependent manner (probably because of the difficulties met in using 51Cr release assay with β cells). Using major histocompatibility complex (MHC) class I tetramers with islet antigen mimetopes, it was shown that diabetes progression in the NOD mouse is associated with increasing numbers of high-avidity islet-specific CD8 T cells. CD4$^+$ T cells are also important. They may have direct diabetogenic action through cytokine release. They may also intervene as helper T cells for CD8 T cells. A number of studies have attempted to dissect the molecular events leading to β-cell apoptosis. The role of free radicals and various cytokines, notably IL-1, has been the matter of particular attention.

No role for islet-specific autoantibodies has been demonstrated so far. Transfer of sera from diabetic mice does not induce diabetes onset. Pure T-cell populations derived from diabetic mice injected into syngeneic recipients still induce diabetes when the recipients have previously been rendered agammaglobulinemic by postnatal anti-IgM antibody treatment. These observations do not preclude the possibility that B cells may play a role in the pathogenesis of IDDM since B-cell-less

NOD mice ($Ig^{-/-}$) do not develop diabetes. One may assume that in this context, B cells act as antigen-presenting cells, rather than as producers of diabetogenic autoantibodies. The only evidence in favor of the pathogenic role of autoantibodies is the observation that newborns from diabetic autoantibody-positive NOD mouse mothers develop diabetes more rapidly than newborns from antibody-negative mothers. This intriguing observation does not fit with clinical studies showing the higher IDDM incidence in descendants of diabetic fathers than of diabetic mothers and with the absence of difference in the incidence of diabetes in children from antibody-positive or antibody-negative mothers.

THE RUPTURE OF TOLERANCE TO β-CELL ANTIGENS

β-Cell-Specific T Cells Are Present in Healthy Individuals but Do Not Attack β Cells

It is possible to derive T-cell lines and to produce T-cell clones specific to various β-cell autoantigens (insulin, glutamic acid decarboxylase, or GAD) in healthy individuals. Diabetes does not develop, though such β-cell-specific T cells are likely to have access to β cells. Similarly, double-RIP LCMV transgenic mice (in which large amounts of LCMV glycoprotein are expressed in β cells and a large proportion of CD8 T cells expressed an LCMV glycoprotein-specific TCR) do not become diabetic unless they are infected with LCMV. This state of ignorance implies that development of diabetes requires that autoreactive T cells be activated to become pathogenic.

Is IDDM Associated with a Defect in Intrathymic Negative Selection?

T cells differentiate in the thymus where they undergo two successive stages of selection: the first positive, giving rise to the emergence of the TCR repertoire, and the second negative, eliminating high-affinity self-reactive TCR-carrying T cells. In any event, negative selection is not absolute, because autoreactive T cells are found in the periphery. They can then be stimulated by the corresponding autoantigen when it is adequately presented to them in the context of MHC molecules. The hypothesis has recently been put forward that IDDM could result, at least in part, from defective intrathymic negative selection due to either underexpression of intrathymic β-cell autoantigens (perhaps under the control of the *AIRE* gene) or to partial expression of these autoantigens in the thymus due to alternative splicing. Also, NOD mouse thymocytes show a defect in thymocyte apoptosis, which could reduce the efficacy of negative selection.

Driving of the Islet-Specific Response by β-Cell Antigens Search for IDDM Autoantigen(s)

There is strong evidence that the diabetogenic autoimmune response is driven by β-cell autoantigens. (Diabetogenic T cells are rapidly exhausted in the absence of β cells.) The nature of the IDDM target autoantigens remains elusive. Several candidates have been proposed, namely, insulin (or proinsulin), GAD, IA.2, a tyrosine phosphatase, and IGRP. All four molecules have an exclusive or a preferential β-cell distribution. They induce the production of T cells or autoantibodies in NOD mice or diabetic patients. Insulin was recently proposed as the primary autoantigen.

The Role of Regulatory T Cells

Strong experimental evidence in the NOD mouse indicates that regulatory T cells slow down disease progression. Diabetes onset is accelerated by thymectomy performed at weaning (three weeks of age) or by high doses of cyclophosphamide, which selectively destroys regulatory T cells. Disease transfer by diabetogenic T cells derived from overtly diabetic mice into prediabetic syngeneic recipients only operates when the recipient is immunoincompetent (neonate, NOD-SCID). The protective role of such regulatory T cells is demonstrated by the capacity of purified CD4$^+$ T cells to inhibit diabetes transfer when they are co-injected with T cells from diabetic mice into NOD-SCID or irradiated NOD recipients. This model has allowed the phenotyping of the regulatory T cells, which are either CD4$^+$, CD25$^+$, or CD4$^+$, CD25$^-$, CD62L$^+$ (CD62L is l-selectin). It has also allowed the demonstration of their dependency on TGF-β (but not on IL-4 or IL-10).

The question remains to determine whether regulatory T-cell function declines at the time of diabetes onset or whether it is overridden by a burst of effector cells. Another possibility is that effector cells resist regulation. There is experimental evidence in favor of each of these three hypotheses, which are not mutually exclusive.

Conclusion

Collectively, these data suggest that the triggering of diabetogenic T cells leading to diabetes onset is a multifactorial event.

Autoreactive β-cell-specific T cells are initially present in the periphery, perhaps in higher number than in non-diabetes-prone individuals. These β-cell-specific T cells are activated by ill-defined mechanisms. The local inflammation of the pancreas, perhaps of viral origin, enhances the expression of the molecules contributing to antigen recognition (MHC, co-stimulation adhesion molecules). The differentiation and the activation of effector cells are initially controlled by regulatory T cells, but the efficacy of the control progressively declines and clinical diabetes appears (Figure 15.4).

ETIOLOGY OF IDDM

Like most other autoimmune diseases, IDDM is multifactorial, resulting from the unfavorable interaction of genetic and environmental factors.

Genetic Factors

IDDM has a strong hereditary component, as assessed by the high disease

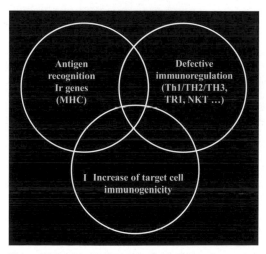

Figure 15.4 Multifactorial origin of insulin-dependent diabetes mellitus.

concordance rate in monozygotic twins (30 to 40 percent). Approximately half of this heredity is due to MHC genes (the IDDM concordance rate in HLA identical siblings is on the order of 15 percent).

HLA-predisposing genes are essentially HLA DR3 and DR4 or their DQ counterparts. In fact, there are two predisposing haplotypes: DQA1*0501 DQB1*0201 and DQA1*0301 DQB1*0302. The relative risk associated with these genes (or set of genes, the haplotype) remains relatively small (less than five), except when considering DR3/DR4 heterozygotes, which is surprising considering the major influence of HLA on IDDM heredity. It has thus been assumed that other genes within the MHC could be in operation, in particular a gene located between HLA-B and TNF.

Non-MHC genes are also important. A large number of them (approximately twenty) have been recognized in the NOD mouse and in human IDDM thanks to systematic genome scanning rather than by the study of candidate genes, which has proven rather disappointing, with the exception of the insulin and CTLA-4 genes. Much more work remains to be done to identify the precise genes in question. One may hope that the complete knowledge of the sequence of the human genome will help in achieving this major goal. One should add that in addition to predisposition genes, there are a number of HLA (DR2) and non-HLA-protective genes that oppose the effect of predisposition genes.

Environmental Factors

The 60 to 70 percent discordance rate observed in monozygotic twins, despite sharing many environmental factors, indicates the importance of the environment in IDDM predisposition. The two categories of environmental factors are triggering and protective. Triggering factors have proven to be elusive. Pancreatotropic viruses are the best candidates. There is some epidemiological evidence for a role for enteroviruses, notably Coxsackie B4, but the data have never been fully convincing, even though there is a renewed interest in their validity. The lack of clear epidemiological or serological evidence could be due to the long lapse in time between the initial infection and its clinically detectable consequence (diabetes). In fact, the virus could be cleared long before its pathogenic effect is visible (hit-and-run hypothesis). Viruses could act in two ways. Viral proteins could resemble certain β-cell autoantigens (antigen mimicry). More likely, the local inflammation induced by the virus enhances the immunogenicity of β-cell autoantigens.

No clear evidence has been collected for other triggering environmental factors. Cow's milk proteins have been incriminated through antigen mimicry between a lactalbumin peptide and a β-cell autoantigen (p69) but the hypothesis remains to be confirmed. However, the environment may have a protective effect. This hypothesis was initially suggested by the previously mentioned observation that the incidence of IDDM in NOD mice tightly depends on the sanitary conditions of the facilities where they are bred (the cleaner, the higher the disease incidence). A large number of pathogens (bacteria, viruses, or parasites) prevent diabetes onset in NOD mice infected at an early age. These observations fit with considerable epidemiological evidence, indicating that human IDDM occurs frequently in countries or people with high socioeconomic levels who are protected from infections (better quality of water and food, better conditions of lodging, more common usage of vaccinations and antibiotics; see Figures 15.5, 15.6, 15.7). Mechanisms underlying the protective effect of infections on IDDM, which are reminiscent of those observed in other autoimmune diseases and allergic disorders are multifactorial: homeostatic competition, bystander suppression through the effect on regulatory cytokines, and toll-like receptor stimulation.

Viral Considerations

Viruses have been considered major potential candidates in the etiology of IDDM for several decades. The viral hypothesis was initially based on the temporal relationship between defined virus infections and onset of overt diabetes. This sequence was notably evoked for Coxsackie B4 virus. The argument is not very robust if one considers that T-cell-mediated islet aggression probably begins many years before clinical onset in most patients and thus the incriminated infection. The infection could at most exacerbate the anti-islet response and accelerate disease onset. One should add that serological evidence (detection of antiviral antibodies in type I diabetes patients) has always been elusive have the episodic claims of virus isolation from pancreatic tissue. The interest in enteroviruses has recently been renewed by a set of observations. It has thus been reported that the frequency of enterovirus infections studied using both serology and testing for the presence of enterovirus RNA was correlated with islet-specific autoantibodies in subjects at risk of developing type I diabetes. An increased T-cell response to Coxsackie B4 antigens was also observed in a recently onset diabetic patient. All these data show significant differences, but their contribution to the

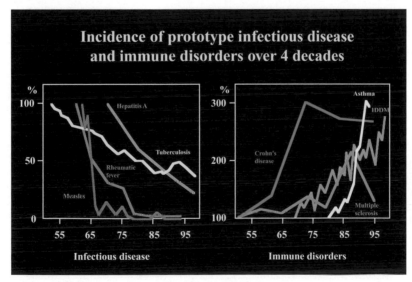

Figure 15.5 Incidence of prototype infectious diseases and immune disorders over four decades. Reprinted by permission: Bach JF. The effect of infections on susceptibility to autoimmune and allergic diseases. *N Engl J Med*. 2002;347:912, Figure 1.

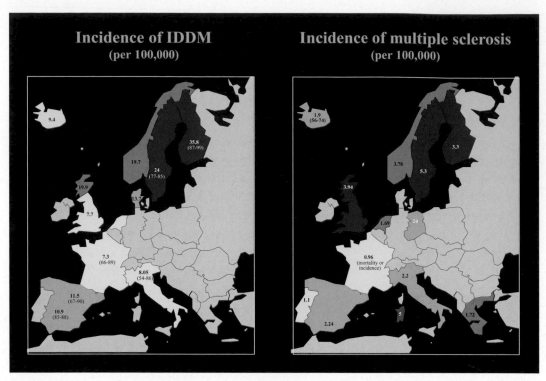

Figure 15.6 North-South gradient of frequency of insulin-dependent diabetes mellitus (IDDM) and multiple sclerosis in Europe. Reprinted by permission: Bach JF. The effect of infections on susceptibility to autoimmune and allergic diseases. *N Engl J Med*. 2002;347:913, Figure 2.

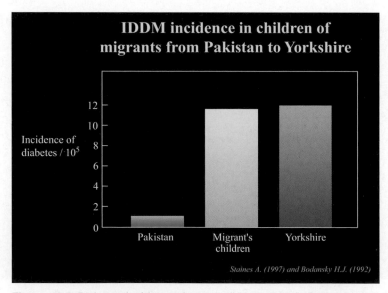

Figure 15.7 Diabetes incidence dramatically increases in Pakistani immigrants to England in children of the first generation, reaching the incidence observed in the English children. This data shows that geographical differences in diabetes incidence involve major environmental factors.

Immunological Aspects of Endocrine Disease

etiologic role of enteroviruses remains indirect since positive results are also observed in a large percentage of the normal population.

At the experimental level, there are rather limited data also. Encephalomyocarditis virus has been reported to induce IDDM in mice, but IDDM is of the cytopathic type in that case without much immunological involvement. The Coxsackie B4 virus can induce diabetes in mice with some features of autoimmune type I diabetes, but it is not clear whether disease pathogenesis involves a direct cytopathic effect or an immune β-cell attack secondary to virus-induced inflammation. This interpretation is compatible with data showing that Coxsackie B4 infection of BDC 2.5 mice, which have a limited nontransgenic TCR repertoire, show accelerated diabetes.

Other interesting data have been derived from the RIP-LCMV transgenic mice. These mice develop IDDM after LCMV infection, according to a hit-and-run mechanism. The virus infection stimulates the induction of LCMVgp-specific CD8 cytotoxic T lymphocytes, which cause the disease even though the virus is rapidly cleared through the action of such cytotoxic T cells.

Collectively, these data are compatible with a viral etiology of type I diabetes even though the diabetogenic virus is still unidentified. The etiological infection may take place many years before clinical onset, questioning the role of preclinical infections and the disease's seasonal nature. This lag time would explain the difficulty in identifying the diabetogenic viruses, which in addition might not be unique. Several pancreatotropic viruses could operate through nonspecific inflammatory mechanisms. Antigen mimicry is possible, but there is no good evidence for this hypothesis in humans (except a questionable homology between a Coxsackie B4 virus protein and GAD) and very little evidence in the mouse. IDDM is accelerated in BB rats infected with Kilham virus.

CLINICAL CONSIDERATIONS

Diagnosis

IMMUNOASSAYS

Several assays have been proposed to detect and quantitate islet-specific autoimmunity. Because IDDM is T-cell mediated, one would certainly prefer to use T-cell-based rather than humoral assays. Unfortunately, this has proven difficult. No fully reliable T-cell assay has so far been described that is sufficiently sensitive (positive in a significant proportion of patients) and disease-specific (negative in most controls). Some hope relies in more recent studies using peptides eluted from IDDM-predisposing HLA molecules, but the results obtained must be confirmed and rendered applicable to their routine usage. One may also hope that other new T-cell targets will become available, such as IGRP, which stimulates CD8 T cells. The emergence of the tetramer technology could prove useful, particularly for CD8+ T cells.

At variance with T-cell-based assays, autoantibody detection has been extremely informative. Islet cell-specific autoantibodies (ICA) were first detected by indirect immunofluorescence using sections of human pancreas (ICA). These tests proved extremely useful for several decades. It is not fully quantitative and has now been replaced by assays using chemically defined β-cell antigens. There is not a single IDDM target autoantigen, but rather autoantibodies are found against a variety of islet autoantigens using highly reliable assays. Anti-insulin autoantibodies are measured using a radioimmunoassay rather than ELISA, whose interpretation is hampered by low-avidity autoantibodies. Anti-GAD and anti-IA-2 autoantibodies are measured by radioligand assays in which the autoantigen is synthesized de novo in vitro as a radiolabeled (35S) recombinant protein in cell-free translation systems.

HELP FOR DIAGNOSIS

The diagnosis of IDDM is essentially made on a metabolic basis (hyperglycemia and glycosuria). There are certain settings, however, where confirmation of the presence of islet-specific autoimmunity may be useful.

At the onset of clinical diabetes, there may be some hesitation about the autoimmune origin of the disease even in relatively young subjects (young adults) particularly in non-HLA DR3 non-DR4 subjects. It may be important to confirm the presence of islet-specific autoimmunity, which will become critical when more patients are enrolled in immunotherapy trials in which nonautoimmune patients are excluded.

Another important setting in this context is that of LADA. These patients appear to be conventional type II diabetes patients (with the exception of an unusual absence of excess weight). Orientation toward LADA (slowly progressing IDDM) is done in the presence of β-cell-specific autoantibodies. Recognition of LADA is important clinically because the knowledge of a likely short- or medium-term evolution toward insulin dependency will prompt clinicians to accelerate the onset of insulin therapy, protecting patients from exposure to the risk of degenerative complications associated with unsatisfactory metabolic control (usually observed when insulin dependency is progressively recognized).

PREDIABETES

A large (and yet ill-defined) proportion of β cells are destroyed at the clinical onset of IDDM, even though there is still a significant number of living β cells that are rescuable by anti-CD3 antibodies. In any event, reserving immunotherapy for subjects with high β-cell mass would be highly desirable. This can be achieved by identifying subjects progressing toward IDDM but still capable of maintaining normal glycemia despite some reduction of the β-cell mass. These subjects can be recognized by the early presence of islet-specific autoantibodies using the reliable assays described earlier. These prediabetic subjects can be identified with a high degree of precision. Subjects with the three autoantibodies (insulin, GAD, and IA-2) will become diabetic within five years in more than 90 percent of cases. However, the situation is less clear for subjects with only one or two antibodies. Furthermore, diabetes prediction in the general population (in the absence of an IDDM heredity) is much less efficacious than in relatives of diabetic patients in whom it is essentially performed today both because of the higher risk (7 percent versus 0.2 percent) and the higher prediction value of the autoantibody assays.

One may complement autoantibody detection by genetic testing, which is today essentially limited to HLA, DR3, and DR4 (or their DQ equivalents). This approach has been used for systematic DR3/DR4 screening of young children born of diabetic parents, starting antibody monitoring at birth.

IMMUNOTHERAPY

Insulin is not a fully satisfactory treatment for IDDM. It is associated with major constraints (monitoring) and hazards (hypoglycemia) and above all does not completely prevent the onset of degenerative complications; hence, the interest given over the past two decades to the immunotherapeutic approach.

On the basis of results obtained in animal models, treatment was first attempted with recently diagnosed IDDM patients with nonspecific immunosuppressants, namely, cyclosporin A and azathioprin. A significant retardation of disease progression was obtained with observation of complete disease remission in a statistically significant percentage of cases. Drug-specific side effects were observed and the disease relapsed when treatment was stopped. Inasmuch as chronic immunosuppression is hardly possible in young subjects like IDDM patients, it was considered that the immunotherapy research should be oriented toward induction of long-term restoration of islet-specific tolerance after a short course of induction treatment, considering the side effects of long-term immunosuppression. Two approaches were undertaken. The first one was inspired by the remarkable ability of some β-cell autoantigens to induce long-term tolerance and diabetes prevention in NOD mice when administered at an early age either parenterally or orally. It was rapidly realized that oral insulin did not slow IDDM progression in recently diagnosed subjects. Similar negative results were observed when administering parenteral insulin in prediabetic subjects, even though the trial was performed in a

large number of patients. More recently, a new approach was developed based on the demonstration that administration of nonmitogenic anti-CD3 antibodies could induce long-term remission of recently diagnosed diabetes, an effect associated with the parallel elimination of effector cells and resetting of immunoregulatory TGF β-dependent regulatory T cells. An open phase I/II trial provided promising results that have now been confirmed in a phase II randomized placebo-controlled study. Importantly, in the latter trial, there was not only maintenance of β-cell function but also real rescue in a large proportion of patients, confirming that at the time of diabetes onset, there is a significant role for reversible islet inflammation in addition to β-cell destruction.

Other trials are now in progress using β-cell-antigen peptides or altered peptides. It will be important to determine whether the antigen-specific approach is operational in advanced disease. Perhaps the solution will be the combined usage of tolerance-inducing regimens of the CD3 antibody type complemented in a second phase by antigen-specific therapy.

One should also follow with interest the prolific research of new immunotherapeutic methods tested in the NOD mouse, with the caveat of not overinterpreting data obtained in early treatments that may act in a nonspecific fashion or at least in conditions that do not correspond to the clinical setting.

GENERAL CONCLUSION

Insulin-dependent diabetes mellitus is an autoimmune disease essentially due to β-cell aggression (inflammation and killing) by CD4[+] and CD8[+] T cells. The autoimmune nature of the disease and the complex underlying mechanisms (triggering of β-cell-specific responses by local inflammation overriding regulatory T cells) should not mask the importance of etiologic initial events, which probably involve an as-yet-unraveled pancreatotropic virus. The major present issue and logical corollary of the multitude of clinical and experimental studies performed over the past three decades is to establish a safe and efficacious immunotherapy active before disease onset, which means that major efforts should be developed to detect prediabetic subjects with high reliability. When this goal is achieved, one may envision, thanks to the use of tolerance-inducing regimens, the progressive eradication of the disease using vaccination strategies to achieve these goals.

BIBLIOGRAPHY

REVIEWS

Bach J-F. The effect of infections on susceptibility to autoimmune and allergic diseases. *N Engl J Med*. 2002;347: 911–920.

Bach J-F. Insulin-dependent diabetes mellitus as an autoimmune disease. *Endocr Rev*. 1994;15:516–542.

Bach J-F. Immunotherapy of insulin-dependent diabetes mellitus. *Curr Opin Immunol*. 2001;13:601–605.

Bach J-F, Chatenoud L. Tolerance to islet autoantigens in type 1 diabetes. *Annu Rev Immunol*. 2001;19:131–161.

SUGGESTED READING

Christen U, Juedes A, Homann D, Von Herrath MG. Virally induced inflammation and therapeutic avenues in type 1 diabetes. *Endocrinol Metab Clin North Am*. 2004;33:45–58.

Greenbaum CJ. Type 1 diabetes intervention trials: what have we learned? A critical review of selected intervention trials. *Clin Immunol*. 2002;104: 97–104.

Hanninen A, Hamilton-Williams E, Kurts C. Development of new strategies to prevent type 1 diabetes: the role of animal models. *Ann Med*. 2003;35:546–563.

Hirschhorn JN. Genetic epidemiology of type 1 diabetes. *Pediatr Diabetes*. 2003;4:87–100.

Ide A, Eisenbarth GS. Genetic susceptibility in type 1 diabetes and its associated autoimmune disorders. *Rev Endocr Metab Disord*. 2003;4:243–253.

Jun HS, Yoon JW. 2003. A new look at viruses in type 1 diabetes. *Diabetes Metab Res Rev*. 2003;19:8–31.

Karvonen M, Sekikawa A, La Porte R, Tuomilehto J, Tuomilehto-Wolf E. Type 1 diabetes: global epidemiology. In: Ekoe JM, Zimmet P, Williams R. eds. *The Epidemiology of Diabetes Mellitus: An International Perspective*. Chichester: Wiley; 2001:71–102.

Knip M. Natural course of preclinical type 1 diabetes. *Horm Res*. 2002;57(suppl 1):6–11.

Knip M. Environmental triggers and determinants of beta-cell autoimmunity and type 1 diabetes. *Rev Endocr Metab Disord*. 2003;4:213–223.

McDevitt H. The role of MHC class II molecules in the pathogenesis and prevention of type I diabetes. *Adv Exp Med Biol*. 2001;490:59–66.

Pociot F, McDermott MF. Genetics of type 1 diabetes mellitus. *Genes Immun*. 2002;3:235–249.

Roep BO. The role of T-cells in the pathogenesis of type 1 diabetes: from cause to cure. *Diabetologia*. 2003;46:305–321.

Varela Calvino R, Peakman M. Enteroviruses and type 1 diabetes. *Diabetes Metab Res Rev*. 2003;19:431–441.

Yang Y, Santamaria P. Dissecting autoimmune diabetes through genetic manipulation of non-obese diabetic mice. *Diabetologia*. 2003;46:1447–1464.

16. Immune-Mediated Neurological Syndromes

Jacqueline Friedman, M.D.

This chapter will discuss the clinical phenomena and underlying theories of autoimmune diseases affecting the human nervous system. Examples will be drawn from diseases affecting (1) the central nervous system (CNS): brain and spinal cord, multiple sclerosis (MS); (2) a disease of the peripheral nerves, Guillain-Barré syndrome (GBS); and (3) an autoimmune disease affecting the endplate between nerve and muscle: myasthenia gravis (MG). In these diseases, the nervous system or motor endplate is the unique target of autoimmunity. Systemic lupus erythematosus (SLE), an example of a systemic autoimmune disease with nervous system involvement, will also be discussed.

Animal models for the study of pathogenesis and treatment have played a large role in the study of immunologically mediated neurological diseases. The success has been variable and not always well correlated with the human condition. Animal models will be mentioned within the context of each disease addressed, and a general discussion of this topic is included at the end of the chapter.

MULTIPLE SCLEROSIS

MS is the most prevalenat inflammatory disease of the CNS in humans, affecting 1 person per 1,000 adults. This disease affects women in a 2:1 ratio to men, and,

for the most part, respects the latitudinal geographic presentation; that is, it occurs mostly in the northern European population or those of northern European descent. The incidence of MS gradually decreases as one approaches the equator. MS increases in incidence as one moves south, away from the equator. Epidemiological studies have also determined that the risk rate is fixed at the age of puberty; that is, if a person moves from an area of high risk to low risk before the age of fifteen that person takes on the risk rate of the new location. If a person moves after the age of 15, that person maintains the risk rate from the area he or she migrated from. The reverse is true in going from low-risk areas to high-risk areas. Epidemiologists have interpreted this to mean that the inciting event or exposure that will ultimately lead to the clinical picture of MS occurs decades before the disease is manifested in the mid-twenties and thirties.

Some epidemiologists point to the geographical parameters of the disease as evidence of a genetic predisposition. In fact, even within the northern latitudes, the Laplanders and Inuits are not susceptible to MS. Specific human leucocyte antigens (HLA) types, such as DR2, occur more frequently in MS patients than in the general population. Twin studies also support this hypothesis, with identical twins experiencing concordance for the disease at a rate twenty to fifty times higher than expected from the population as a whole.

Newer studies are focusing on the role of 25-hydroxy vitamin D, an immuno-modulating factor, in the pathogenesis of MS vis-à-vis the latitudinal gradient. High levels of vitamin 25-hydroxy vitamin D in the serum significantly lower the odds ratio of MS risk in large population studies. Possibly, the higher exposure to sunlight in the equatorial latitudes enhances natural absorption of vitamin D from the skin, resulting in higher serum levels, which may protect against MS.

By definition, the disease must affect two parts of the CNS at two discrete periods. Historically, the neurological examination and patient's clinical history were used to fulfill these criteria. More recently, the MRI scanner has become a powerful adjunct to the history and examination in these patients. Multiple areas of the CNS can now be imaged to confirm the presence of more than one lesion. Serial MRI scans can now confirm multiple episodes in time, even when the patient is asymptomatic. A scan may be performed at three-month intervals from the first symptom to determine whether new lesions present themselves. New evidence of inflammation fits the criterion for separate episodes in time and thus the definition of MS. This is called the McDonald criterion for MS and has strengthened the practice of treating patients earlier in the disease course before significant disability sets in.

Cerebrospinal fluid (CSF) analysis has also proven helpful in diagnosing MS. The CSF is usually normal in terms of protein and cells but may have a slight protein elevation or increase in lymphocytes, rarely more than 50 cells/ml. Spinal fluid analysis, which directs one to the diagnosis of MS, includes evidence of intrathecal synthesis of immunoglobulins and the presence of oligoclonal bands. These antibody bands, primarily IgG, are found in approximately 90 percent of patients at some point in their disease course. These antibodies are detected on an agarose gel in the presence of an electric field and isoelectric focusing. The bands present in the basic area of the gel were initially felt to show a specific immune response to an autoantigen or infectious agent in MS patients. However, years of investigation have detected no consistent antibody response in MS patients. In fact, the pattern differs from patient to patient. Newer interpretation for the presence of oligoclonal antibodies is that they represent polyclonal dysregulation, rather than B-cell populations with specific immune responses induced. Nonetheless, the oligoclonal bands are a useful adjunctive test in the diagnosis of MS. Other diseases, which can produce bands, can be readily ruled out by other means, such as syphilis with a rapid plasma reagin (RPR) test or Lyme disease with enzyme-linked immunosorbent assay (ELISA) and Western blotting against *Borrelia* antigens.

The symptoms of MS depend on their localization in the nervous system. If the optic nerves are affected, the patient can present with decreased vision, ranging from color blindness to total loss of vision, which is accompanied by pain due to eye movement. Lesions of the brain stem can present with double vision, trigeminal neuralgia, severe pain on the face, or speech or swallowing difficulties. Lesions in the spinal cord can present with numbness, tingling, or weakness of the upper or lower extremities, as well as bladder/bowel and sexual dysfunction. Symptoms are often accompanied by severe fatigue, possibly caused by release of cytokines in the CNS. The symptoms are manifest because nerve conduction is significantly slowed in demyelinated fibers. Saltatory conduction between the nodes of Ranvier is disorganized, and the slowed conduction results in neurological symptoms of nerve dysfunction.

In addition, local edema in the area of the plaque may interrupt function temporarily. Some patients develop symptoms that last a few hours or less. It is believed that low-affinity antibodies present in MS directly interact with antigens composing the sodium channels on neurons directly. The attachment and subsequent freeing of the antibodies from these channels may be responsible for a rapid change in symptoms not involving an entire autoimmune/inflammatory cascade.

This finding points to the premise that MS is not solely a disease of white matter and demyelinating pathology but may also be a neuronal disease as well. MRI scanning using the neuronal marker NAA (N-acetyl-aspartate) has demonstrated that neuronal dysfunction occurs earlier in MS patients than would be expected from destruction of neurons based only on demyelination secondarily. This may open up new avenues of therapy in the future, directed not only toward remyelination but also in the area of nerve growth factors as well.

The overall pathological lesion has been categorized as a demyelinated area within the CNS white matter, with the presence of inflammation, gliosis remyelination, or axonal pathology. More recently, the pathology of MS has been categorized into four distinct patterns. Two patterns show lesions induced by autoreactive T cells (type I), or T cells plus antibodies and complement (type II). These are similar to the pathology induced by animal models discussed later. Patterns III and IV appear to be caused more by a dystrophy of the oligodendrocyte, and apoptosis, rather than an autoimmune reaction. The pathologies are homogeneous within the demyelinated lesions in each patient but differ from patient to patient. This may suggest that different disease pathologies may be linked to one clinical state, MS, or that there are clinical subcategories of MS presentations that may be clinically tied to the pathology, which is yet to be determined. This will ultimately reflect different treatment modalities for the different presentations of MS.

Experimental allergic encephalomyelitis (EAE) in rodents, which has been the hallmark animal model of MS, is induced following immunization with whole myelin or antigens related to myelin (i.e., myelin oligodendrocyte glycoprotein, or MOG, or myelin basic protein, or MBP with complete Freund's adjuvant). These myelin antigens are also cross-reactive with T cells and antibodies directed against the Semliki Forest virus, used to promote an immune-mediated demyelinating viral encephalitis model. Antibodies to MOG induce demyelination in EAE and exacerbate the clinical disease, while antibodies to MBP reduce disease severity. A polymer of a peptide sequence of MBP is an approved immuno-modulating drug for MS in humans, which is believed to stabilize disease by changing the T-cell repertoire from T_H1 to T_H2 in the CNS.

The pathogenesis of the EAE model involves immune cells migrating from the peripheral lymphoid system, where activation takes place, to the CNS. These cells then mediate tissue damage in the CNS. In addition, epitope spreading occurs where autoreactive T cells and antibodies become more diverse.

This model also allows for the concept of microbial-induced autoimmune reactions in genetically susceptible mice strains with

Theiler's murine virus or Semliki Forest virus. Blood-brain barrier passage by CD4$^+$ cells, CNS immigration, demyelination lesion induction, and clinical neurological deficit in the rodent have all been achieved in this model. However, the cause of permanent neurological deficit in MS and EAE is still not entirely understood. CNS and inflammation and demyelination do not account for irreversible neurological symptoms. Recently, axonal pathology has been also implicated not only in MS but also in EAE as well and may lead to future therapies. In terms of therapies for MS, many biologic agents are species specific, and nonhuman primates such as marmosets and rhesus monkeys are the more appropriate model to use. For studying MS, nonhuman primates have proved the most useful model thus far, despite the history of EAE in rodents. They also provide species-specific therapeutic options to be investigated, as well as an easier ability to do longitudinal sampling of body fluids.

Treatment of the disease is aimed at three levels. The first level, the use of intravenous corticosteroids, is the treatment and shortening of acute attacks, such as visual loss with optic neuritis, a spinal cord syndrome, or hemiparesis. Patients are also treated with oral steroids for less severe attacks, with the exception of optic neuritis. In addition to its anti-inflammatory properties, steroids may strengthen the blood-brain barrier and decrease edema in a lesion, causing a rapid reversal of symptoms.

The next level of therapy for patients is the daily management of ongoing symptoms. This might include muscle relaxants for spasticity, amantadine, or modafinil for fatigue, antidepressants or anticonvulsants for pain and mood changes, and anticholinergic medication for bladder spasticity and incontinence. Fortunately, most MS patients have a limited constellation of symptoms, but some require significant polypharmacy.

Ongoing physical therapy and a course of psychotherapy are often prescribed for patients. Physical therapy optimizes the muscle capabilities of the patient and has an effect on psychological well-being as well. Depression plays a major role in MS, but it is unclear whether it is a reactive or endogenous mood disorder. Nonetheless, suicide attempts are a considerable risk with MS patients and psychological counseling is often suggested.

Interferons and immunomodulating agents have become the mainstay of treatment of the long clinical course of MS. Specifically, IFN-β, given subcutaneously or intramuscularly has become recommended lifelong for patients at this time. Statistical significance was achieved in these patients, both in terms of MRI effects and the frequency and severity of attacks. The clinical relapse rate diminished by one-third, and MRI data suggest an even more dramatic drop in lesion volume (−17.3 percent) and number (−83 percent) compared with placebo. The literature is somewhat contradictory about the goal of slowing the gradual progression or worsening of the disease overall, but some studies are able to confirm this finding. While interferons have several immunomodulating effects and may also be antiviral, the main function of these medications in this setting may be to block adhesion of lymphocytes and macrophages to the blood-brain barrier and thus limit trafficking into the CNS. Natalizumab, a newly approved immunomodulator in MS also inhibits the attachment of lymphocytes to the endothelial cells and limits trafficking of the cells across. It is an antibody directed against the integrin-4α adhesion molecule on lymphocytes and monocytes.

Glatiramer acetate (Copaxone) has a similar effect profile in MS patients in terms of reduction of MRI lesions and clinical attack rate. The drug is a polypeptide polymer of myelin, eight amino acids long, and is believe to function by a different mechanism from the interferons. The drug appears to act directly within the CNS by altering the immune profile from a helper to suppressor predominance. It is hoped that these immunomodulating agents will change the course of disease in the long term, especially if they are started early after diagnosis or presumptive diagnosis.

GUILLAIN-BARRÉ SYNDROME

GBS is a hallmark disease of molecular mimicry, resulting in several different clinical manifestations. It was initially characterized as a disease of the peripheral nervous system because of the earliest detection of cases of flaccid paralysis in 1859 by Landry. By 1916, Guillain, Barré, and Strohl had characterized the disease as having a rapidly developing symmetrical flaccid paralysis, loss of reflexes, and autonomic dysfunction, followed by a spontaneous remission. There is a pathognomonic dissociation in the spinal fluid of the presence of high protein, without a concomitant significantly elevated cell count. The category of pathology is primarily a cellular immune system–mediated demyelinating disease with infiltration of nerves by macrophages and lymphocytes (see Figure 16.1).

The humoral and cellular target is myelin directly or the Schwann cells that produce myelin in the peripheral nervous system (see Figure 16.2). The other name for this phenomenon is acute inflammatory demyelinating polyneuropathy (AIDP). Similar in pathology, but manifesting differently clinically is the Miller-Fisher variant of GBS, described as the triad opthalmoparesis, ataxia, and absent reflexes, which may then encompass the clinical AIDP form. Another variant of the disease includes the finding of cranial nerve abnormalities, which can also evolve into AIDP. These variants have variations in their immunopathology as well.

Most patients present with neurological complaints two to four weeks after a mild gastrointestinal or upper respiratory illness. The first symptoms may be tingling in the extremities, followed by weakness in the legs and loss of reflexes, all of which may develop rapidly and ascend into the arms, cranial nerves, and respiratory muscles. The respiratory decline can occur rapidly in some patients and may be life threatening. Twenty to 30 percent require respiratory ventilators. In addition, patients can develop life-threatening autonomic changes, including cardiac arrhythmias and hypotension. Most patients are at their worst clinical state within two to four weeks and start to recover within weeks to months. A chronic, or relapsing, form of inflammatory demyelinating neuropathy also exists and is considered a different disease (chronic inflammatory demyelinating polyneuropathy).

Similar to MS, a demyelinating inflammatory disease of the CNS, an animal model exists for this peripheral demyelinating disease entity, EAN. This is produced by inoculation with whole myelin or specific proteins of peripheral nervous system myelin in complete Freund's adjuvant. This produces a cell-mediated immune attack on native myelin proteins.

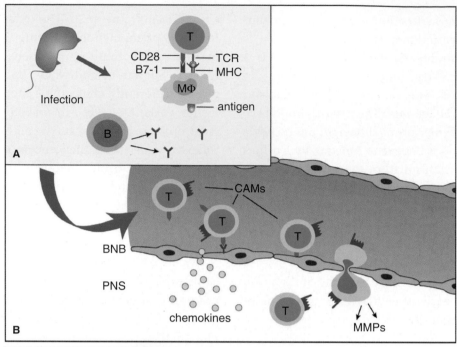

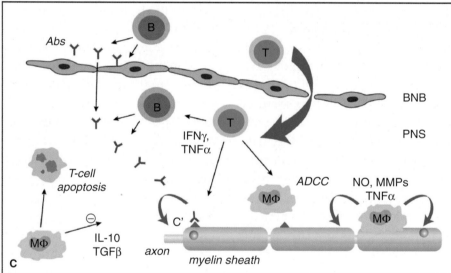

Figure 16.1 Immune response in immune-mediated demyelination of the peripheral nervous system. Depicted are the basic principles of the cellular and humoral immune responses: The initiating event may be infection triggering molecular mimicry. *A*, Autoreactive T cells (T) recognize a specific autoantigen presented by major histocompatibility complex (MHC) class II molecules and the simultaneous delivery of co-stimulatory signals on the cell surface of antigen-presenting cells, such as macrophages (M[PHI]), in the systemic immune compartment. *B*, Activated T lymphocytes cross the blood-nerve barrier (BNB) to enter the peripheral nervous system (PNS), a process partly mediated by chemokines, cellular adhesion molecules (CAMs), and matrix metalloproteinases (MMPs). *C*, Within the PNS, T cells activate macrophages that enhance phagocytic activity, the production of cytokines, and the release of toxic mediators, such as nitric oxide (NO), MMPs, and pro-inflammatory cytokines, such as TNF-α or IFN-γ. In the humoral arm autoantibodies (Abs), crossing the BNB or locally produced by B

However, more recently, basic premises of this disease have been redefined. It is now recognized that there may be a distinct axonal form of GBS. Electromyography has been able to distinguish these two forms. An attack against myelin and axons may be found concurrently in the same patient, with both demyelination and periaxonal macrophages.

Molecular mimicry has been found to be the major pathogenic force and the basis for autoimmunity. Various preceding infections can initiate the immune response that causes the clinical state of GBS. The two major agents are *Campylobacter* and *Cytomegalovirus*, with Epstein-Barr virus considered an inciting agent as well. Specific features of the inciting organism may play a major role in the development of GBS. For instance, although *Campylobacter jejuni* often may cause diarrhea, the strains that have been linked to GBS (O-serotypes) are different from those strains causing diarrhea only but are genetically similar to each other. Only 70 percent of those infected with *Campylobacter* in the presence of GBS give a previous history of gastrointestinal complaints in the three months before the neurological onset, but the risk of developing GBS within two months of a symptomatic *Campylobacter* infection is 100-fold higher than the general population. GBS following *C. jejuni* and intestinal symptoms are felt to have a more dire clinical course, involving axonal destruction in addition to demyelination.

The Miller-Fisher variant, which involves primarily the cranial nerves, demonstrates the close association between antiganglioside antibodies and a specific syndrome. Anti-GQ1b has a high specificity and sensitivity for this symptom complex. GQ1b is a ganglioside that is a component of cranial nerve myelin. Similarly, anti-GM1 (anti-GD1a) antibodies have been linked specifically to the axonal form of the disease, acute motor axonal neuropathy. Although GM1 antigens can be found on motor and sensory nerves, there are variable reports in the literature about whether these antigens are on the axon or in the myelin sheath. However, antibodies to GM1 can bind to the nodes of Ranvier and activate complement. Other factors may be necessary for the disease to occur, as many patients with *Campylobacter* infections produce antibodies to GM1 ganglioside but do not develop neurological symptoms. Because the disease can improve rapidly, an association between sodium channels and the antibody has been studied, but there has been no consistent association with sodium channels.

Influenza vaccine has been implicated as a causative agent for GBS as well. However, careful epidemiological studies have not borne this out. Combining the 1992–1993

Figure 16.1 (*Caption continued*)

lymphocytes (B), contribute to the process of demyelination and axonal damage. Abs can mediate demyelination by antibody-dependent cell-mediated cytotoxicity (ADCC), can block functionally relevant epitopes for nerve conduction, and can activate the complement system (C′) by the classic pathway, yielding pro-inflammatory mediators and the lytic C5b-9 terminal complex. The termination of the inflammatory response is partly mediated by macrophages, inducing T-cell apoptosis and the release of anti-inflammatory cytokines, such as IL-10 and transforming growth factor-β (TGF-β). Modified from Hartung, H. et al., Acute immunoinflammatory neuropathy: update on Guillain-Barre′ syndrome: *Curr Opin Neurol.* 2002;15(5):571–577.

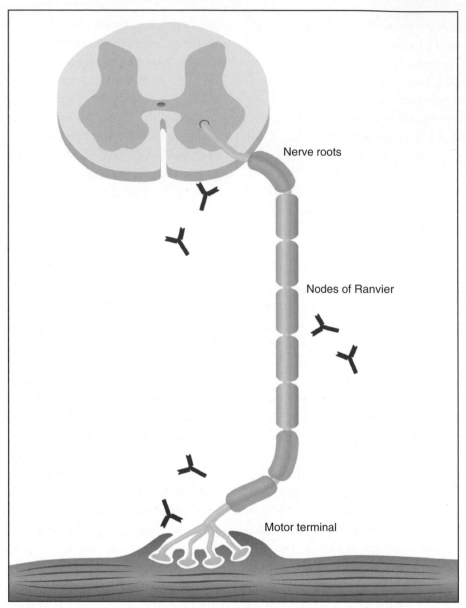

Figure 16.2 Sites of action for autoantibodies in inflammatory demyelination disorders. There are various sites of vulnerability in the peripheral nervous system to autoimmune attack. The blood-nerve barrier, separating the systemic immune compartment (blood) from the nerve tissue, is absent or relatively deficient at the roots and at the motor terminal. These anatomic areas can thus become targets for autoantibodies. Also, the nodes of Ranvier, where receptors required for nerve conduction are exposed, represent locations for antibody binding. Besides provoking an immune response, antibodies exhibit neurochemical effects, such as the blockade of neuromuscular transmission. Modified from Hartung, H. et al., Acute immunoinflammatory neuropathy: update on Guillain-Barre´ syndrome: *Curr Opin Neurol.* 2002;15(5):571–577.

and 1993–1994 seasons, only one additional case of GBS occurred than expected in 1 million vaccinated patients. Nonetheless, the

American Academy of Neurology suggests that patients at low risk for severe influenza but who have a history of GBS developing within six weeks of a previous flu vaccine should not be vaccinated.

The host may play a significant role in this disease as well. GBS has been associated with certain major histocompatibility complex (MHC) class II genes and may determine a heightened immune response to C. jejuni, resulting in GBS in these patients compared with controls who do not go on to develop the neurological disease after exposure to Campylobacter. GBS patients may be high producers of tumor necrosis factor alpha 2 compared with controls.

In the Fisher variant, anti-GQ1b antibodies affect acetylcholine release at the nerve terminals. In one mouse model of disease, applying serum from patients on a mouse model is similar to that of the black widow spider venom – the inception of a large release of acetylcholine, which is calcium dependent. Complement is required for this reaction, either by the classical or alternative pathway. Presumably, humoral immunity is the inciting factor.

For the classic AIDP form of the disease, the target antigen is still unknown. Two candidate antigens are the myelin protein PMP22 and the heparin sulfate glycosoaminoglycans. The virulence of some C. jejuni strains may be due to several factors. First, specific cross-reactive antigens may be more common in these strains. These strains may also have higher immunogenicity or may have greater invasiveness. The O-19 strains (overly presented in GBS) do have GM1-like epitopes composed of lipopolysaccharides. However, other organisms do as well, including those causing enteritis only, and humans are frequently exposed to C. jejuni with GM1 cross-reactivity. Therefore, these epitopes do not alone explain GBS.

Therapy for GBS has been directed at the immune mechanisms, but interestingly, corticosteroids have been shown to have no clinical effect, as has been established in many other neurological manifestations of autoimmune mechanisms. Instead, the two mainstays of therapy have been plasma exchange and intravenous immunoglobulins (IVIG). These treatments are suggested for those with illness severe enough to limit walking ability. Plasma exchange using fresh frozen plasma or albumin has been shown to increase muscle strength and decrease the time needed for a respirator to assist ventilation. Intravenous immune globulin has similar efficacy, but there is no additive effect of combining the two therapies. In animal models, IVIG has been shown to neutralize neuromuscular blocking antibodies and inhibit binding of anti-GQ1b antibodies to GQ1b. These prevent initiation of the destructive complement cascade. Overall, 80 percent of patients recover fully or are left with only minor deficits. Up to 10 percent are left with weakness, imbalance, or loss of sensation and 3 to 8 percent die from sepsis, pulmonary emboli, cardiac arrest, or acute respiratory distress syndrome even despite care in an intensive care unit. These patients are usually older, have preexisting pulmonary disease, or were on prolonged respirator assistance.

MYASTHENIA GRAVIS

MG is an autoimmune disease that causes muscle weakness believed to be primarily mediated by antibodies to the acetylcholine receptor (AChR) on the motor endplate of muscles (Figure 16.3). There are four criteria that meet the definition of an antibody-mediated autoimmune disease and MG meets all of them. First, the presumed antibody is present in 80 to

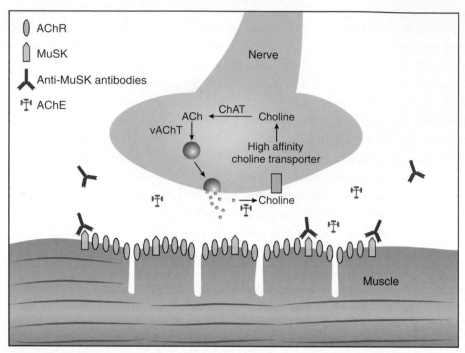

Figure 16.3 Nicotinic cholinergic neuromuscular junction. Various sites of autoimmune attack of the nicotinic cholinergic neuromuscular junction. In addition to the more prevalent acetylcholine receptor blockade, the presence of anti-MuSK antibodies is demonstrated, often detected in "seronegative" myasthenia and by mutations underlying congenital myasthenic syndromes: muscle-specific tyrosine kinase (MuSK), acetylcholine receptor (AChR), choline, acetyltransferase (ChAT), asymmetric acetylcholinesterase (AChE), and vesicular acetylcholine transporter (vAChT). Modified from Palace J, Vincent A, Beeson D. Myasthenia gravis: diagnostic and management dilemmas. *Curr Opin Neurol*. 2001;14(5):583–589.

90 percent of patients. Second, the clinical syndrome can be passively transferred to an animal model. Third, injection of the human antigen, in this case the AChR into an animal can produce a model of the disease. Fourth, an improvement in the clinical disease state is associated with a decrease in antibody levels.

In the case of MG, a major diagnostic test after physical exam would be to assay for the AChR antibody. The more severe the clinical manifestation, the more likely the antibody will be detected and is diagnostic of the illness. However, absence of the antibody does not exclude MG (see discussion about seronegative MG). Clinically, these patients present with a muscle weakness only, associated with demonstrable fatigability of the muscles on exam. For instance, if the extraocular muscles are involved, weakness can be detected by the development of lid ptosis or drooping when having the patient sustain an upward gaze. Patients usually report a decrease in strength later in the day, a hallmark symptom of this disease, rather than uniform weakness throughout the day. Weakness often begins in the ocular muscles producing double vision or a drooping lid but can go on to cause weakness of the muscles of speech and swallowing (bulbar MG) as well as the extremities. The respiratory muscles can be affected later on, in the setting of

Immune-Mediated Neurological Syndromes

a "myasthenic crisis," which can be life threatening.

In infants, congenital myasthenia occurs from transplacental passage of antibodies from a woman with MG or may be caused by a mutation of the neuromuscular junction itself. It is accepted as conventional wisdom in the medical community that MG is antibody mediated because an autoantibody specifically reactive to the acetylcholine receptor in the neuromuscular junction is present in 80–90 percent of patients. Reduction of this antibody is associated with improvement in clinical symptoms. A decrease in the number of acetylcholine receptors has been shown to occur directly because of binding of antibody to the receptors, possibly by clustering these receptors. These receptors may be destroyed ultimately via the activation of the complement system.

The Lambert-Eaton syndrome is an immunological and clinical variation of MG and is a paraneoplastic syndrome in the setting of small cell lung cancer (70 percent of patients). More than 90 percent of patients with this syndrome have autoantibodies to P/Q-type calcium channels.

Patients usually present with hip girdle weakness, which is more notable in the morning and improves with exercise and over the course of the day. Autonomic dysfunction is also found in addition to muscle weakness.

Animal models for myasthenia gravis can be produced by injecting the human antigen or by passively transferring the disease to an animal by injection of the antibodies. However, the antibodies are far from homogeneous. The subtypes of antibodies may vary among patients and even among muscles within the same patient. The antibody may also have variations in light chain type and subclass within one patient. Most likely these variations are due to the receptor on the muscle, which consists of five subunits. These subunits associate to form a transmembrane ion channel. It is likely that the populations of B lymphocytes, producing the receptor antibodies, are also heterogeneous.

T lymphocytes are also felt to play an important role in MG, although they are not found in biopsy specimens. Their main function in this setting might be to stimulate the B cells. It has been demonstrated that anti-T-cell antibodies may be used for immunoregulation in this disease. The naturally occurring anti-T-cell receptor (anti-V beta 5.1) IgG antibody is found to occur in those patients with milder disease and less so in more severe MG. Although this antibody occurs in higher titers in MG patients than in controls, the higher the antibody titer, the less severe are the clinical symptoms, suggesting that therapy targeting pathogenic T-cell receptors (TCRs) may be a useful avenue of exploration.

The thymus gland has been considered to be the source of the autoimmune state of patients with MG. Most patients with MG have thymic hyperplasia and 10 to 12 percent have a thymoma. The thymus gland contains myoid-type cells, which have striations and acetylcholine receptors. The thymic cells may act as antigen-presenting cells with MHC class II molecules. Cathepsin V, an enzyme responsible for cleaving the invariant chain in the antigen-presenting cleft of the MCH II molecule is overexpressed in MG patients in the thymic tissue and in the thymoma when present. However, mRNA and cathepsin V protein are not expressed in patients who have a thymoma but do not have MG. Patients who have thymoma also may have antibodies directed against muscle antigens as titin or the ryanodine receptor in addition to the acetylcholine receptor.

The thymus gland may also play a role because of the presence of acetylcholine receptor on the myoid cells. Theories include the possibility that a virus might alter the myoid cells, and the proximity to the antigen presenting cells and helper T cells in the gland increases the possibility of an autoimmune response. Molecular mimicry may play a role as well.

Herpes viruses and bacteria have been shown to share cross-reactivity with the acetylcholine receptor. A genetic predisposition is most likely a requisite of acquiring the disease. HLA types have been associated with MG such as HLA-B8, DRw3, and DQw2. Other autoimmune diseases are found to occur concomitantly in these patients or in their families such as lupus, rheumatoid arthritis, and Graves' disease.

There is also a subset of patients (10–20 percent) with clinical MG, who do not produce antibodies to the acetylcholine receptor. They are designated as "antibody-negative myasthenia." This may be a misnomer. Some patients (40–70 percent) with this disorder produce antibodies to another antigen, the MuSK. The antibodies are of the subclass IgG4 and strongly activate complement cascade. In contrast, the ACh-R-Abs are primarily of the IgG1 and IgG3 subclasses, which can also fix complement. The MuSK antibody is also found in 10 percent of patients with antibody-positive MG, or alone without the AChR-Ab.

Of interest, although no animal studies have shown that this particular antibody can cause muscle weakness, a myasthenic syndrome can be passively transferred with plasma from these patients into an animal model. In addition, seronegative patients respond to plasmapheresis and immunosuppressive therapy, similar to seropositive MG.

The experimental animal model of MG, experimental autoimmune MG (EAMG) requires CD4$^+$ helper T cells needed for the antibody-mediated autoimmune response. In mice, the T-cell response to the AchR is predominantly to a single peptide in about 50 percent of the cells. These T cells use a restricted set of TCR genes and have a conserved CDR3 region. This is in contrast to the human manifestation of the disease, where AChR-specific T cells are very low in frequency. The specific T cells, when they have been cloned from patients are heterogeneous in MHC restriction, and recognize various epitopes of the AChR.

There are three levels to treatment of myasthenic patients, cholinesterase inhibitors, thymectomy, and immunosuppression. The mainstay of medications that treat the symptoms, but not the course of the disease, are the cholinesterase inhibitors. These medications increase the availability of acetylcholine in the neuromuscular junction and thereby help to overcome the effect of decreased acetylcholine receptors due to the autoantibodies, AChR-Ab.

However, while this medication may maintain patients on a stable course for some time, they will not induce remission of the disease. The two approaches to this goal are thymectomy and immunosuppressants. The reason for thymectomy is that most MG patients have thymic abnormalities, either hyperplasia (60–70 percent) or a thymoma (10–12 percent). Computerized tomography or MRI scanning of the mediastinum should be routine in all patients suspected of MG. Although the clinical response is very variable

Immune-Mediated Neurological Syndromes

according to the literature, thymectomy is the most frequently used treatment for myasthenia and is generally suggested to be performed very early. The rationale is that the thymus gland serves as a source for the antigens involved in the autoimmune response detected in patients, even without the presence of thymoma.

The third arm of treatment is immunosuppression. Steroids improve 45 percent of patients and cause remission in 30 percent. Steroids can initially cause a worsening of the clinical symptoms in the first few weeks, which is unique to this disease, and patients are often initiated on them in a hospital setting. Plasmaphoresis may be performed preventively before steroids are initiated. Patients are often on steroids for one or two years before tapering is begun. Immunosuppressive agents, such as azathioprine or cyclosporine, are also administered in some cases because they act as T-cell suppressors. The antibody production in this disease is T-cell dependent, as demonstrated in the animal model.

Plasmapheresis or intravenous immunoglobulin is sometimes used in the setting of a clinical crisis. The plasmaphoresis removes the AChR-antibody from the circulation and the clinical response correlates with the decrease in antibody titer. Sometimes the plasma is processed through a staph-protein A immunoabsorbant column to more effectively remove the IgG. Clinical trials are also under way using an AChR-Ab specific immunoabsorbant column. Intravenous immunoglobulin also has been demonstrated to reverse an acute exacerbation for reasons unknown. For both treatments, while the response time is rapid, a matter of days, the result is short lived, lasting only a few months. It is hoped that within that time other modalities of treatment have begun to be effective.

CENTRAL NERVOUS SYSTEM SYSTEMIC LUPUS ERYTHEMATOSUS

CNS SLE is an example of an autoimmune pathology with abnormalities also detected in other organs outside the central or peripheral nervous system. Over ten years' follow-up, approximately 25 percent of SLE patients will develop CNS manifestations.

One hypothesis is that the neuropsychiatric symptoms of SLE may result from secondary causes. Infarctions may be experienced by patients, felt to be related to antibodies found in SLE, which affect the clotting system, such as circulating lupus anticoagulant or antiphospholipid antibodies (APLAs). Another mechanism may be symptoms secondary to CNS infections such as meningitis or encephalitis. Treatments of SLE require immunosuppressive medications or steroids, which may predispose patients to these etiologies. Metabolic issues may also present as neuropsychiatric symptoms, such as in the case of uremia secondary to renal involvement of SLE.

Lupus cerebritis is the term used to convey that the CNS symptomatology is due to the SLE immune process. This broad etiology of neuropsychiatric symptoms may result from a demyelinating pathology. The symptoms associated with CNS SLE may be diffuse in nature, rather than a focal symptom suggestive of a vascular territory and therefore stroke. These symptoms may include aseptic meningitis, headache, chorea, myelopathy, cranial neuropathy, seizures, confusion, and cognitive dysfunction. Also felt to be due to diffuse etiology are psychiatric symptoms, such as mood disorders and psychosis. Other neurological symptoms outside the CNS include peripheral neuropathy or mononeuritis multiplex.

The combination of pathological studies and positron emission tomography scanning form a hypothesis: hypoperfusion causes a breakdown of the blood-brain barrier. The loss of integrity allows antineuronal antibodies to cross over and ultimately lead to demyelination, similar to theories in MS. The inciting factors that would cause hypoperfusion are unknown. Evidence of a vasculopathy is present in pathological specimens, which demonstrate a perivascular accumulation of mononuclear cells, without destruction of the blood vessels. There may also be small infarctions secondary to occlusion of the vessel lumen. APLAs are associated with stroke syndromes and may play a role in the vasculopathy of CNS SLE.

The effects of these APLAs may include a prothrombotic state with coagulation pathway abnormalities and cause thromboembolism, stroke, focal seizures, migraines, and multi-infarct dementia. In this setting, the treatment of the disease would be directed more at the antithrombotic state, with aspirin and consideration of anticoagulation, rather than with steroids or immunosuppressants.

Steroids are used only if there is coexisting serological evidence of active SLE. Steroids may be detrimental in a pure stroke setting, without evidence of active immune disease. Clinically, CNS diffuse vasculitis presents as fever, severe headaches, and confusion, with symptoms that progress rapidly to psychosis, seizures, or coma. Serologically active SLE is detected with elevated anti-dsDNA (double-stranded DNA) and hypocomplementemia.

MRI scanning is the clinical tool of choice in investigating the diagnosis of CNS SLE. Infarctions can be identified, as well as diffuse demyelinating disease. Some lesions may resolve on subsequent MRI testing and therefore point away from infarction as the etiology of the clinical manifestation. Infarctions are permanent, whereas demyelination may be reversible. In fact, clinical improvement has been correlated with resolving lesions, following immunosuppressive therapy on MRI scanning, and resolving lesions may actually predict an improved clinical course.

Diffuse CNS SLE is difficult to diagnose and manage. CSF studies, anti-DNA antibody titers, complement levels, and even imaging may be nonspecific or insensitive. For instance, if a psychosis develops in the SLE patient, it may be due to the SLE, or the use of steroids, a mainstay of the pharmacopoeia in this disease. Depression may also be a manifestation of lupus cerebritis or may be a reactive depression to having the disease. However, missing the diagnosis of lupus cerebritis or mistreating it carries high mortality and morbidity.

In 1986, the first reports of an antibody population to ribosomal P proteins and association to lupus cerebritis came to the literature. This work was based on earlier findings that patients produced antibodies that bound to ribosomes. The antigens were found to be phosphoproteins or "P proteins" located on the 60S subunit of ribosomes. These three proteins were labeled P0 (35 kD molecular weight), P1 (19 kD), and P2 (17 kD). These proteins are felt to be involved in protein synthesis; monoclonal antibodies to these proteins inhibit the elongation factors EF-1 and EF-2 to ribosomes and inhibit protein synthesis. In addition to being on ribosomes, the P proteins are also on the cell surfaces of

Immune-Mediated Neurological Syndromes

neuronal, hepatoma, and activated T cells. ELISA testing is the assay of choice against purified human ribosomal P proteins.

This antibody is specific to SLE when tested against other autoimmune diseases, such as rheumatoid arthritis, scleroderma, and myositis, but the incidence rate is variable among different studies of SLE patients. The antibody is especially linked to patients with lupus-related psychosis (18/20 patients) and severe depression (88 percent). Others in the literature have not been able to confirm these results. Small patient numbers confound the conclusions of many of these studies.

Ribosomal P protein–targeted antibodies do not appear to be synthesized in the CNS and are much more prevalent in the serum of SLE patients. One possible explanation is that the antibodies are cell bound in the CNS, as normal neuronal tissue may also express the ribosomal P proteins. Overall, these antibodies might be considered specific for CNS SLE, although not very sensitive. They are present independently of other SLE-associated antibodies such as to dsDNA and may be helpful in diagnosis if the other marker antibodies have returned to normal.

Other antibodies are being investigated for specificity for CNS SLE. An antineuronal antibody was produced against human neuroblastoma cell lines. These were detected in 45 percent of patients with CNS SLE, but on 5 percent of those with SLE but without CNS involvement. Lymphocytotoxic antibodies have been associated with decreased cognitive function. Cross-reactive antibodies have been found in the sera and CSF of SLE patients that bind to double stranded DNA and excitatory N-methyl-D-aspartate (NMDA) receptors on neurons. Still it is not known if all of these antibody populations are causative

Table 16.1 Possible Relationships of Pathogenetic Mechanisms to Type of CNS SLE

Mechanism	Presentation
Phospholipid antibodies	Focal Neurologic
Neuronal antibodies	Diffuse neurologic or psychiatric; emotional distress
Lymphocytotoxic antibodies	Visuospatial cognitive disturbances
Ribosomal P antibodies	Depression; psychosis
IL-2	Organic brain syndrome
IL-6	Aseptic meningitis; Neurobehavioral dysfunction

of CNS symptoms or produced in reaction to the tissue.

Neurological manifestations can be divided into diffuse symptoms and focal symptoms, which may be correlated with different immune event (Table 16.1). It is generally believed that diffuse symptoms, such as seizures, psychosis, or mental status changes may be associated with anti-lymphocyte antibodies cross-reactive with neuronal antigens. Autoimmune antibodies can be directed against neurofilaments, phospholipids, glycolipids, glycoproteins, and neuronal cell surface antigens. Widely studied autoantigens are the 32-kD cell surface antigen, the 50–52-kD cell surface antigen, and the 97–98 kD antigen. Patients with lymphocytotoxic antibodies have been shown to have visuospatial abnormalities and verbal deficits on neuropsychological testing, not detected in those without these antigens. In this setting, the treatment would aim for anti-inflammatory and immunosuppressive mechanisms, using steroids and possibly cyclophosphamide and plasmapheresis. Meningitis may present as well and may be secondary to bacterial infections due to immunosuppression. In addition, aseptic meningitis may be caused by medications, such as ibuprofen and immunosuppressive medication.

Partial or generalized seizures may also occur in the setting of SLE and generally portend a poor prognosis. Patients are generally treated with anticonvulsants, and steroids are only added if it is felt that the patient is in an active flare, to prevent potential permanent scarring and a seizure focus.

Although migraine headaches occur frequently in the setting of SLE, a causative effect has not been determined. More seriously, patients may have other types of headache, such as pseudotumor cerebri, cerebral venous, or sagittal sinus thrombosis. This is usually due to a secondary cause of SLE, such as renal dysfunction and a hypercoagulable state. The sudden development of headaches in a previously headache-free patient or neurological symptoms or signs requires rapid work-up and imaging.

More uncommon CNS syndromes occur and may be varied. Movement disorders such as chorea or ataxia point to disease in the basal ganglia or cerebellum. These disorders are usually self-limited to two to six weeks and may not require therapy. If they are associated with APLA, anticoagulation may be considered.

Patients may have cranial neuropathies causing symptoms such as double vision or hearing loss, trigeminal neuralgia, or dysarthria. Steroids are generally used in these conditions, and if refractory, cyclophosphamide, an immunosuppressant medication, is used. When patients present with these symptoms, the question of MS should be ruled out. Both diseases may have optic neuritis, transverse myelitis,

or inflammation of the spinal cord (which must be treated aggressively with, at the very least, steroids, and possibly plasmapheresis and cyclophosphamide for recovery), or internuclear ophthalmoplegia, and may have similar MRI scans. Patients who do have similar scans and who have lupus are referred to as having "lupus sclerosis." APLA in this setting often help with differentiation of the syndromes. MS should have no peripheral manifestations outside of the CNS.

Cytokine release may play a role in these pathologies. IL-1, IL-2, IL-6, TNF-α, IFN-α, and IFN-γ have all been demonstrated to be released by CNS microglial cells and astrocytes by LPS stimulation. In the CNS, a cascade of pro-inflammatory cytokines causes events of inflammation similar to peripheral macrophages and monocytes. These cytokines not only mediate inflammation but also may directly affect brain function, as there are cytokine receptors on the hypothalamus. Antibodies can cause functional dysregulation by blocking the release of neurotransmitters and neuropeptides, resulting in abnormal electrophysiological testing, such as the electroencephalogram.

Animal models have been used to investigate the human disease with mixed success. The MRL/P mice have neurobehavioral abnormalities such as timidity, phobic behavior, and anxiety. This manifests at age 7 to 8 weeks, when autoantibodies to brain tissue also present. The pathology demonstrates B lymphocytes around the choroid plexus with MHC class II antigen presentation. This differs from the vasculitis that is more typical of the human SLE syndrome. However, like humans with an exacerbation of SLE, IL-6 is elevated in the CSF and the animal behavior can be significantly improved by treating with immunosuppression and steroids. The clinical improvement is correlated with a decrease in IL-6 levels in the CSF.

The SLE syndrome of focal events secondary to APLA can also be demonstrated in a mouse model by injecting MRL/pr mice with APLA and anti-neuronal antibodies. Antigen derived from limbic brain structures, which also react to human sera, the B2 glycoprotein, causes production of APLA and ischemic events/stokes.

The future of CNS SLE may lie in stem cell transplant. One study of seven patients using chemotherapy followed by autologous stem cell transplantation yielded excellent clinical results at a median follow-up of twenty-five months. The patients had initially suffered from cerebritis, myelitis, vasculitis, or glomerulonephritis and were unresponsive to multiple courses of cyclophosphamide. At follow-up, all patients were free of signs of active lupus and serological markers had improved. The theory of the treatment is that when memory T cells are removed from influence, maturation of new lymphocyte progenitor cells occurs without recruiting autoimmune activity.

ANIMAL MODELS

A unique difficulty in developing treatment strategies and pathogenic theories of neurological immune diseases is that often the human end organ is unavailable for study. The morbidity of taking CNS tissue purely for research places that option beyond ethical boundaries in most cases. Therefore, reliance is mainly on autopsy material, when usually only end-stage disease pathology is available, keeping the natural history of the disease unknown. Therefore, reliance on animal models in these diseases

is paramount in testing treatment strategies and theories of etiology. Controversy arises when one considers how closely the animal model follows the human disease state under study. The animal model should reflect the susceptibility of the host, and the clinical findings of the disease, and should be similar to the histopathological findings in the human.

MS and EAE provide good examples of strengths and difficulties of animal models based on differences between human and murine immunology. For example, in EAE IFN-γ was demonstrated in several studies to be a protective cytokine. Antibodies to the cytokine exacerbated EAE, possibly by blocking induction and activation of suppressor activity. However, when this principle was applied to patients, the study was discontinued because of exacerbation of MS by administration of IFN-γ in a clinical trial.

IFN-α is another example of differing cytokine responses. In humans, this cytokine is secreted by several types of cells, inclining macrophages in response to exposure to viral antigens. The cytokine induces T cells to T_H1 development, a process that depends on signal transducer and transcription-4 (STAT-4) activation. In mice, however, INF-α dose not activate STAT-4, therefore; T_H1 is not induced by IFN-α. Multiple other differences abound in the immune systems between mice and humans; therefore, responses to treatment protocols in models compared with human disease may vary greatly.

Differences in the immunology of mice and human are numerous (see Table 16.2). For example, in delayed-type hypersensitivity (DTH) in humans, neutrophils are the first responders, followed by a mix of mononuclear cells composed of T cells and macrophages. In mice, there are relatively

Table 16.2 Some Immunological Differences Between Mouse and Human Immune Function

	Mouse	Human
IFN-γ effects in demyelinating disease	Protective in EAE	Worsens MS
IFN-α promotes T$_H$1 differentiation	No	Yes
Delayed-type hypersensitivity (primary cell type)	Neutrophils	Lymphocytes
Epithelial cell presents AG to CD4$^+$ T cells	No	Yes
CD4 on macrophages	Absent	Present
CD38 on B cells/plasma cells	Low/Off	High/High
Hematopoiesis in spleen	Into adulthood	Prenatal
Lymphocytes in peripheral blood	75–90%	30–50%
Neutrophils in peripheral blood	10–25%	50–70%
Vascularized grafts tolerogenic	Yes	No
Microchimerism induces graft tolerance	High success	Low success
Caspace-8 deficiency	Lethal	Viable
Caspace-10	Absent	Present

far fewer neutrophils in the peripheral blood system than in humans. However, the murine response to antigens in DTH is richer in neutrophils compared with humans and a far greater amount of antigen is needed to elicit a response.

Human endothelial cells are now believed to be antigen-presenting cells to memory CD4$^+$ and CD8$^+$ T lymphocytes. This is not the case for CD8$^+$ cells in mice. Therefore, in humans, antigen transport to lymphoid tissue by Langerhans cells may not be required for DTH, and the endothelial cells may locally trigger a response to antigen. The peripheral lymphoid system would be required in mice for DTH, compared with local presentation in humans.

Human and mouse endothelial cells both express MHC class I molecules, but only humans express class II, as well as CD40, ICOS ligand 50, and CD58. This has practical interactions in terms of the response to transplantation, where mice

may readily adapt to vascularized graphs, whereas humans rapidly reject them. This is also felt to be secondary to the ability of human endothelial cells to present antigen compared with mice.

The mouse and human immune systems are felt to have diverged 65 million years ago, although thus far, only 300 genes are felt to be unique to each species. The adaptations were in response to various pathological challenges based on ecological niche. For example, that mice are closer to the ground would change the exposure and response to microorganisms encountered. Even the difference in life spans would account for the difference in the immune response. For example, transit times of immune cells are different between mice and humans and a larger T-cell and B-cell repertoire must be continued for many years in humans. Humans would encounter more somatic mutations over time, and greater control of the immune system must be generated to control for autoimmunity and to control larger, widely varied antigen-specific clones.

Thus, one can see multiple reasons for often wide discrepancies between animal models and the human condition, particularly in the response to potential therapeutic treatments. Perhaps the focus of effort and funding should be placed on direct human studies, whether on the molecular, tissue, or organism level, to unravel the designs of these diseases.

BIBLIOGRAPHY

REVIEW ARTICLES

Chitnis T, Khoury SJ. Immunologic neuromuscular disorders. *J Allergy Clin Immunol*. 2003;111(2 suppl):S659–S668.

Denburg J, Denburg S, Carbotte R, and Szechtman H. Nervous system lupus: pathogenesis and rationale for therapy. *Scand J Rheum*. 1995;12:263–273.

Ho T, Grifin J. Guilain-Barré syndrome. *Curr Opin Neurol*. 1999;12(4):389–394.

Huizinga T, Steens S, van Buchem M. Imaging modalities in central nervous system systemic lupus erythematosis. *Curr Opin Rheum*. 2001;13:383–388.

Lucchinetti C, Bruck W, Parisi J, et al. Heterogeneity of multiple sclerosis lesions: implications for the pathogenesis of demyelination. *Ann Neurol*. 2000;47:707–717.

McDonald W, Compston A, Edan G, et al. Recommended diagnostic criteria for multiple sclerosis: guidelines from the International Panel on the Diagnosis of Multiple Sclerosis. *Ann Neurol*. 2001;50:121–127.

Newswanger D, Warren C. Practical therapeutics: Guillain-Barré syndrome. *Am Fam Phys*. 2004;69(10):2405–2410.

Palace J, Vincent A, Beeson D. Myasthenia gravis: diagnostic and management dilemmas. *Curr Opin Neurol*. 2001;14(5):583–589.

Schur P, Khoshbin S Neurologic manifestations of systemic lupus erythematosis. Online: http:/uptodateonline.com/application/topicText.asp?file = rheumatic/1974&type=A&selecte...; 2004.

SUGGESTED READING

Mestas J, Hughes C. Of mice and not men: differences between mouse and human immunology. *J Immunol*. 2004;172:2731–2738.

't Hart B, Amor S. The use of animal models to investigate pathogenesis of neuroinflammatory disorders of the central nervous system. *Curr Opin Neurol*. 2003;16(3):375–383.

't Hart B, Laman J, Bauer J, Blezer E, van Kooyk Y, Hintzen R. Modelling of multiple sclerosis: lessons learned in a non-human primate. *Lancet Neurol*. 2004;3:588–597.

Infante AJ, Kraig E. Myasthenia gravis and its animal model: T cell receptor expression in antibody mediated autoimmune disease. *Int Rev Immunol*. 1999;18(1–2):83–109.

17. Immunological Aspects of Renal Disease

Gil Cu, M.D., and John B. Zabriskie, M.D.

INTRODUCTION

Human kidneys play an integral role in the development of primary or secondary immunologic diseases. As a major filtering organ, the kidneys, which represent about 0.5 percent of the human body mass, receive 20 percent of the total cardiac output. The enormous blood flow (1 L/min) to the renal microcirculation exceeds that observed in other major vascular organs (heart, liver, and brain). Urine is produced after a complex process of glomerular filtration, tubular transport, and reabsorption at a rate of 1 ml/min. Cellular elements involved in immunity thereby have a high probability of interacting with glomerular and tubular cells that may or may not cause renal disease.

Sufficient knowledge of the anatomy and histology of the kidney is vital in understanding the pathogenesis of renal diseases. The renal corpuscle, or glomerulus (Figure 17.1), is composed of capillary tuft lined by a thin layer of endothelial cells; central region of mesangial cells and its surrounding matrix; and visceral and parietal epithelial cells with their respective basement membranes. The glomerulus is primarily responsible for production of ultrafilrate from the circulating plasma. The filtration barrier between the bloodstream and urinary space is made up by the fenestrated endothelium, the glomerular basement membrane (GBM), and the slit pores seen between the foot processes of the visceral epithelium (Figure 17.2).

The endothelial cells form as initial barriers to cellular elements of the blood (red blood cells, leucocytes, and platelets) in reaching the subendothelial space. The endothelial cells produce nitric oxide (a vasodilator) and endothelin-1 (a potent vasoconstrictor), chemical substances implicated in inflammatory processes. The surface of the endothelial cells is negatively charged, which may contribute to the charge-selective properties of the glomerular capillary wall.

The GBM is composed of a central dense layer called the *lamina densa* and two thin layers called the *lamina rara externa* and *lamina rara interna*. The GBM is formed by the fusion of the endothelial and epithelial basement membrane during development. Biochemical analyses of the GBM have identified the presence of glycoproteins (type IV collagen, laminin, fibronectin, and endotactin/nidogen) and heparan sulfate proteoglycans (perlecan and agrin). Type IV collagen is the major constituent of the GBM. Gene mutations involving those encoding $\alpha3$, $\alpha4$, and $\alpha5$ isomeric chains of the type IV collagen can cause Alport's syndrome. This is a progressive form of glomerulopathy associated with ocular abnormalities, hearing loss, and microscopic hematuria. Electron microscopic examination shows thinning of the GBM in early stages of the disease. With

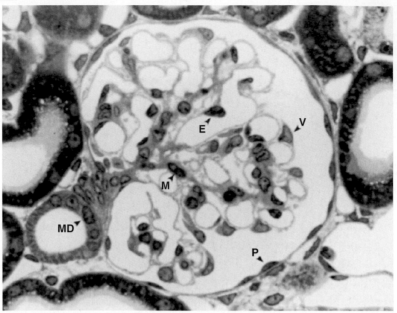

Figure 17.1 Light micrograph of a normal glomerulus from a rat, demonstrating the four major cellular components: mesangial cell (M), endothelial cell (E), visceral epithelial cell (V), and parietal epithelial cell (P). MD, macula densa. Reproduced with permission from: Brenner BM, ed. *Brenner and Rector's The Kidney.* 7th ed. Philadelphia, PA: W. B. Saunders; 2004.

progression of the renal disease, there is a longitudinal splitting of the GBM, producing a laminated appearance.

The presence of glycosaminoglycans rich in heparin sulfate renders the GBM to have an anionic charge. Combined with the negatively charged endothelial cell lining and the epithelial slit diaphragm, the GBM becomes a formidable sieve that is both size and charge selective. Although it restricts passage of large molecules like albumin, it allows small molecules and large cationic molecules like ferritin to pass through. Enzymatic digestion of the glycosaminoglycans increases permeability to large molecules like bovine serum albumin. This strongly suggests that glycosaminoglycans play a significant role in the permeability properties of the GBM.

The visceral epithelial cells, or podocytes, wrap around individual capillary loops to form pedicels, or foot processes, that come in direct contact with the lamina rara externa of the GBM. The gaps between the podocytes become the slit pore, which is bridged by a thin membrane called *filtration slit membrane*, or *slit diaphragm* (Figure 17.2). It appears that two membrane proteins, nephrin and CD2-associated protein (CD2AP), are involved in maintaining the integrity of the filtration slit membrane. The CD2AP has been identified as an adapter molecule that binds nephrin to the cytoskeleton of the GBM. Deletion of the CD2AP is known to cause congenital nephrotic syndrome with morphologic evidence of effacement or fusion of foot processes. Other membrane proteins like the human glomerular

Immunological Aspects of Renal Disease

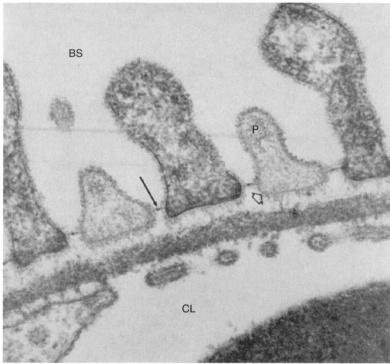

Figure 17.2 Electron micrograph of a normal rat glomerulus. Note the relationship among the three layers of the glomerular basement membrane and the presence of pedicels (P) embedded in the lamina rara externa (thick arrow). The filtration slit diaphragm with the central dense spot (thin arrow) is especially evident between the individual pedicels. The fenestrated endothelial lining of the capillary loop is shown below the basement membrane. A portion of an erythrocyte is located in the extreme right lower corner. BS, Bowman's space; CL, capillary lumen. Reproduced with permission from: Brenner BM, ed. *Brenner and Rector's The Kidney*. 7th ed. Philadelphia, PA: W. B. Saunders; 2004.

C3b receptor, Heymann nephritis antigen (gp330 or megalin) and podoplanin have been associated with the visceral epithelial cells. Animal experiments that cause efface-ment or fusion of foot processes (such as injection of antipodoplanin IgG antibod-ies in rats) or disruption of the negatively charged GBM causes proteinuria. In addi-tion, visceral epithelial cells are capable of endocytosis, can synthesize and maintain the GBM, and produce prostaglandins.

Mesangial cells are specialized peri-cytes with functional properties similar to that of smooth muscle cells. In addition to providing structural support for the glo-merular capillary loop, its contractile prop-erties help regulate glomerular filtration. The presence of actin and myosin allows the mesangial cells to contract in the pres-ence of vasoactive agents like angiotensin II, vasopressin, norepinephrine, leukotri-enes, thromboxanes, and platelet-activat-ing factors. However, prostaglandins, atrial peptides, and dopamine cause mesangial relaxation. The surrounding mesangial matrix consists of glycosaminoglycans, fibronectins, laminin, and other collagens. The presence of cell surface receptors in the matrix (e.g., β-integrin receptor) are implicated in signal transduction mechanisms that promote synthesis of various inflammatory cytokines, vasoactive substances, and growth factors. Finally, mesangial cells have phagocytic properties. During endocytosis of immune complexes, intracellular production of prostaglandins and reactive oxygen species cause injury to the glomerulus.

Parietal cells are squamous cells that make up the epithelium that forms the outer wall of the Bowman's capsule. At the vascular pole, the parietal epithelium is continuous with the visceral epithelium. At the urinary pole, there is a transition to the cuboidal cells of the proximal tubule. The exact role of parietal cells is not well defined. However, as pointed out by Brenner (2004), these cells can proliferate and become crescents like in rapidly progressive glomerulonephritis (RPGN).

MECHANISMS OF IMMUNE INJURY TO THE KIDNEYS

Cells of both innate and adaptive immunity mediate human defense against microbes. The principal components of innate immunity are composed of physical and chemical barriers (e.g., epithelial cells and antimicrobial substances produced by the cells), phagocytic cells (neutrophils and macrophages), natural killer cells, complement systems, and cytokines. These represent the first line of defense against microbial agents. In contrast, adaptive immunity is represented by B and T lymphocytes. These cells are initially stimulated by exposure to offending agents. Subsequent exposure to similar agents cause specific cells to mount a defense in increasing magnitude.

Adaptive immunity is distinguished as having the ability to "remember" specific molecules and therefore provide specific immunity. Both types of immunity work in tandem to provide comprehensive defense against offending microbes.

Diseases caused by immune responses are often called *hypersensitivity diseases*. These are classified according to the type of immune responses and the effector mechanisms that are responsible for cell and tissue injury. In this chapter, we will attempt to elucidate the nature of renal diseases in relation to the immune system.

Immediate hypersensitivity or type I disease is mediated by immunoglobulin E (IgE), which is produced in response to an allergen. After exposure to a specific allergen, T_H2 cells specific for the allergen are activated. IgE antibodies are then produced, which subsequently bind to the Fc receptor of mast cells and basophils. This binding releases biogenic amines (histamine), neutral serine proteases, lipid mediators, and cytokines. Biogenic amines and lipid mediators cause vascular leakage, vasodilation, and airway bronchoconstriction. Serine proteases cause tissue damage. Cytokines are implicated in late phase reaction. Certain drugs, especially methicillin, nonsteroidal agents, rifampin, sulfa, cimetidine, cephalosporins, and 5-aminosalicylates, can cause allergic interstitial nephritis. Affected patients present with acute renal failure three to five days after intake of the offending drug. Fever, rash, hematuria, proteinuria, and eosinophiluria are typical findings. On kidney biopsy, tubulointerstitial inflammation is prominent with occasional demonstration of eosinophils. The glomeruli appear spared of any inflammatory effects. Treatment consists of withholding the offending drug and use of steroids.

Antibody-mediated or type II disease is caused by antibodies against fixed cell and tissue antigens. Although most cases demonstrate the presence of autoantibodies, some antibodies can be produced by a foreign antigen that is immunologically cross-reactive to human tissue. Three mechanisms have been described to explain this phenomenon. First, antibodies may opsonize cells or activate the complement system that eventually produces complement proteins that assist in opsonization of cells. Macrophages bind to Fc receptors of antibodies or complement protein receptors to cause endocytosis and destruction of the offending antigen. This appears to be the main mechanism in hemolytic anemia and autoimmune thrombocytopenic purpura. Second, antibodies bound in target tissues recruit neutrophils and macrophages by binding to Fc receptors or by activating complement. Activated neutrophils and macrophages release intracellular enzymes and reactive oxygen radicals that cause tissue injury. Examples of glomerular disease that can be explained by this pathway include Goodpasture's syndrome and anti-neutrophil cytoplasmic antibody (ANCA) mediated disease. Third, antibodies may bind to normal cellular receptors and interfere with their function to cause disease. However, no actual tissue injury is demonstrated. Graves' disease represents this mechanism where the TSH receptor is targeted by the anti-TSH-receptor antibody. This mechanism causes hyperthyroidism. No glomerular disease has been associated with this mechanism (see Table 17.1).

Immune-complex-mediated, or type III, disease is caused by deposition of antibodies bound to self- or foreign antigens into target tissues. Although the glomerulus is a common target for immune complexes, other organ systems are involved, which suggests the systemic nature of this disease. A classic example is the serum disease or serum sickness, which was originally described by Clemens von Pirquet in 1911. During his time, diphtheria infections were treated with passive immunization using serum from horses immunized with diphtheria toxin. He noted that joint inflammation (arthritis), rash, and fever occurred in patients injected with the antitoxin-containing horse serum. On further investigation, similar symptoms were seen in patients injected with horse serum without the antitoxin. The symptoms usually occurred at least one week after the first injection and more rapidly on subsequent injections. He concluded that the host had developed antibodies to the horse serum, and deposition of antibody–serum protein complexes (immune complexes) to different tissues of the host caused the symptoms described earlier. In experimental animals like the rabbit, injection of a large dose of a foreign protein antigen leads to the formation of antibodies against the antigen (see Figure 17.3). Subsequent formation of antibody–antigen complexes leads to enhanced phagocytosis and clearance of the antigen by the macrophages in the liver and the kidney. With subsequent injection of the antigen, more of the immune complexes are formed and may be deposited in the vascular bed, renal glomeruli, and synovia. These activate the complement, which leads to recruitment of inflammatory cells (predominantly neutrophils) to cause injury to the affected tissues. Clinical and pathological manifestations are vasculitis, glomerulonephritis, and arthritis. Clinical symptoms are

Table 17.1 Examples of Diseases Caused by Cell- or Tissue-Specific Antibodies

Disease	Target Antigen	Mechanism of Disease	Clinicopathologic Manifestations
Autoimmune hemolytic anemia	Erythrocyte membrane proteins (Rh blood group antigens, I antigen)	Opsonization and phagocytosis of erythrocytes	Hemolysis, anemia
Autoimmune thrombocytopenic purpura	Platelet membrane proteins (gpIIIb: IIIa integrin)	Opsonization and phagocytosis of platelets	Bleeding
Pemphigus vulgaris	Proteins in intercellular junctions of epidermal cells (epidermal cadherin)	Antibody-mediated activation of proteases, disruption of intercellular adhesions	Skin vesicles (bullae)
Vasculitis caused by ANCA	Neutrophil granule proteins, presumably released from activated neutrophils	Neutrophil degranulation and inflammation	Vasculitis
Goodpasture's syndrome	Noncollagenous protein in basement membranes of kidney glomeruli and lung alveoli	Complement- and Fc receptor-mediated inflammation	Nephritis, lung hemorrhage
Acute rheumatic fever	Streptococcal wall antigen; antibody cross-reacts with myocardial antigen	Inflammation, macrophage activation	Myocarditis, arthritis
Myasthenia gravis	Acetylcholine receptor	Antibody inhibits acetylcholine binding, down-modulates receptors	Muscle weakness, paralysis
Graves' disease (hyperthyroidism)	TSH receptor	Antibody-mediated stimulation of TSH receptors	Hyperthyroidism
Insulin-resistant diabetes	Insulin receptor	Antibodies inhibit binding of insulin	Hyperglycemia, ketoacidosis
Pernicious anemia	Intrinsic factor of gastric parietal cells	Neutralization of intrinsic factor, decreased absorption of vitamin B12	Abnormal erythropoiesis

Abbreviations: ANCA, anti-neutrophil cytoplasmic antibodies; TSH, thyroid-stimulating hormone

short-lived and resolve with discontinuation of the injection. As will be noted in later discussion, the majority of immune-related disease falls into this category.

T-cell-mediated, or type IV, hypersensitivity diseases involve activation of CD4$^+$ T cells of the T$_H$1 subset and CD8$^+$ T cells. Both types of T cells release interferon-γ and activate macrophages, which can release tumor necrosis factor (TNF), interleukin-I (IL-1), and other chemokines that are involved the inflammatory processes. In delayed-type hypersensitivity (DTH), tissue injury is mediated by hydrolytic enzymes, reactive oxygen intermediates, and nitric oxide.

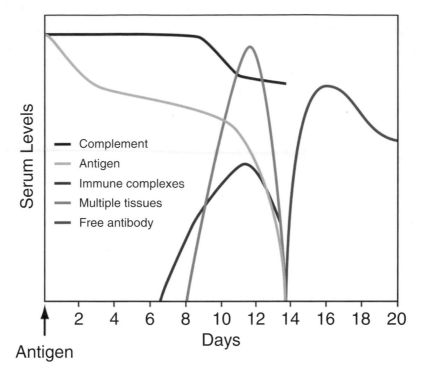

Figure 17.3 Sequence of immunologic responses in experimental acute serum sickness. Injection of bovine serum albumin into a rabbit leads to the production of specific antibody (blue) and the formation of immune complexes (red). These complexes are deposited in multiple tissues (green), activate complement (black), leading to a fall in serum complement levels, and cause inflammatory lesions, which resolve as the complexes and the remaining antigen (yellow color) are removed.

There is also up-regulation of adhesion molecules and class II molecules in vascular endothelial cells. Chronic DTH processes cause fibrosis because of continuous secretion of cytokines and growth factors. In some instances, CD8[+] cytolytic T cells (CTL) directly kill target cells bearing class I MHC cells.

T-cell-mediated renal diseases are best exemplified in kidney allograft rejection. In acute allograft rejection, T cells react to alloantigens, including MHC molecules, which reside on the vascular endothelial and renal parenchymal cells. Microvascular endothelitis is an early finding in acute rejection. Later involvement of the medium-sized arteries signifies severe rejection. Experimental evidence that points to the involvement of CD8[+] CTL in allograft rejection include the presence of RNAs encoding CTL-specific genes (e.g., perforin and granzyme B), presence of cellular infiltrates enriched with CTL population, and ability to adoptively transfer alloreactive CD8[+] CTL cells. CD4[+] T cells mediate rejection by secreting cytokines and inducing DTH-like reactions in the allograft. Adoptive transfer of alloreactive CD4[+] T cells in experimental animals has been known to cause rejection of the allograft as well. In chronic allograft rejection, histopathological findings are compatible with by-products of a chronic inflammatory state (interstitial fibrosis, vascular occlusion, and glomerulosclerosis) (Abbas and Lichtman 2005).

SPECIFIC IMMUNE-RELATED RENAL DISEASES

IgA Nephropathy

IgA nephropathy or Berger's disease is the most common cause of glomerulonephritis in the world. Rarely seen in blacks, this disease afflicts mainly Asians and Caucasians. Clinical features include gross hematuria (40–50 percent), microscopic hematuria (30–40 percent), and rarely, renal insufficiency with edema and hypertension (less than 10 percent). These usually occur after a respiratory infection. Minimal proteinuria is noted. IgA nephropathy is made by kidney biopsy only. The hallmark of this disease is mesangial deposition of IgA, which is prominently noted on immunofluorescence. This deposition is associated with focal mesangial expansion, which can be seen on light microscopy. Electron microscopy confirms the presence of electron-dense deposits in the mesangium, which correspond to the immune complex deposits. An abnormality in the regulation of IgA may exist because of an environmental stimuli. This is supported by higher circulating levels of IgA in about 50 percent of cases, circulating immune complexes that parallel the duration of the disease, and increased number of IgA-specific B and T lymphocytes. Its strong association with respiratory infection has led authorities to believe that mucosal immunity plays a role in this disease. Exaggerated mucosal IgA response or decreased clearance may explain the elevated levels of plasma IgA in this disease. In the glomeruli, IgA-containing immune complexes activate the alternative complement pathway but do not bind C1, which may slow the removal of circulating complexes and thereby promote deposition in the glomeruli.

The role of fibronectin and uteroglobin (an anti-inflammatory protein) in IgA nephropathy remains unclear. Most of the IgA-containing complexes are bound to fibronectin. In experimental animals, uteroglobin–fibronectin heteromerization prevented formation of fibronectin–IgA complexes and binding to glomeruli. Deletion of the uteroglobin gene in mice by gene knockout or suppression of the uteroglobin gene by antisense technology has histological features similar to IgA nephropathy. Interestingly, polymeric but not monomeric IgA binds only to mesangial cells, which stimulate release of IL-6, further leading to mesangial expansion.

IgA nephropathy usually follows a benign course, although about 15 percent of cases may reach end-stage renal disease at ten years and 20 percent at twenty years. Clinical and histopathological predictors of progression of renal disease include worsening proteinuria (>1 g/day of proteinuria) and biopsy findings of glomerular sclerosis, tubular atrophy, interstitial fibrosis, and crescent formation. Treatment of IgA nephropathy has radically changed over the past decade. Aggressive use of angiotensin-converting enzyme (ACE) with and without angiotensin-receptor blocker (ARB) is recommended to decrease the proteinuria and for their renoprotective properties. Cytotoxic agents and steroids are reserved for aggressive renal disease.

MINIMAL CHANGE DISEASE

Minimal change disease (MCD), or nil disease, is the most common cause of nephrotic syndrome in children under age 10. It accounts for about 90 percent of cases in children and about 10–15 percent in adult cases. Patients usually present with heavy proteinuria (>3 g/day), hypoalbuminemia, dyslipidemia, and anasarca. Urine sediment is benign. Diagnosis rests on kidney biopsy. Under light microscopy, the glomeruli appear normal. There is absence of immune deposits by immunofluorescence. Electron microscopic findings show effacement of the epithelial foot processes. Investigators believe that MCD is a T-lymphocyte disease because of its sensitive response to steroids and cyclosporine. It is strongly associated with Hodgkin's lymphoma, a hematologic malignancy. Proteinuria appears to disappear when the malignancy goes into remission. A glomerular permeability factor (GPF) derived from a T-cell hybridoma has been identified to cause fusion of the foot processes and proteinuria, when injected into experimental rats. The T-cell hybridoma was made from T cells harvested from a patient with minimal change disease. It is thought that this GPF has TNF-like activity. In addition, epithelial damage causes loss of polyanions like heparin sulfate. This loss of charge selectivity allows macromolecules like albumin to pass through the filtration barrier and leak into the urine.

In children with idiopathic nephrotic syndrome, treatment with steroids produces immediate results with about 50 percent of cases going into remission in two weeks, and almost all within eight weeks of treatment. Clinical response in adults tends to be slower, but the majority will achieve remission after twelve to sixteen weeks of treatment. Cytotoxic agents, which include cyclophosphamide, chlorambucil, azathioprine, mycophenolate mofetil, and cyclosporine are reserved for relapsers and steroid-resistant cases.

FOCAL SCLEROSING GLOMERULOSCLEROSIS

Focal glomerulosclerosis or focal segmental glomerulosclerosis (FSGS) is a common cause of idiopathic nephrotic syndrome in adults, accounting for about 35 percent of all cases. About 50 percent of all FSGS cases appear to afflict black people, suggesting possible involvement of their genetic background and socioeconomic status. FSGS is classified as primary or secondary. Primary or idiopathic FSGS usually presents with overt nephrotic syndrome. Secondary FSGS presents with nonnephrotic-range proteinuria (<3.5 g/day) and renal dysfunction. The latter form has been considered to be a physiologic response to hyperfiltration or glomerular hypertrophy as a result of nephron loss. This loss can be seen in unilateral nephrectomy, unilateral agenesis of one kidney, reflux nephropathy, renal vasodilation, obesity, and preeclampsia. Secondary FSGS may be seen as a response to a prior injury of any cause (e.g., acute glomerulonephritis, or vasculitis). The transforming growth factor–beta (TGF-β), which is released from affected glomerular cells and platelets, appears to contribute to the development of glomerulosclerosis. TGF-β promotes extracellular matrix production, prevents matrix degradation, and facilitates migration and adhesion of inflammatory cells to the matrix. In experimental animals, inhibition of TGF-β with use of antibodies or inhibitors appears to decrease or abrogate glomerular scarring.

FSGS is diagnosed with a kidney biopsy. On light microscopy, some of the glomeruli show segmental areas of mesangial collapse and sclerosis. There is minimal mesangial hypercellularity. No immune deposits can be found except for nonspecific binding of IgM and complements in sclerotic lesions. Like MCD, there is diffuse fusion of the epithelial foot processes. The histologic similarities between FSGS and MCD have led many investigators to believe that the former may be a more severe form of the latter. Like MCD, a circulating toxin has been identified from the serum of FSGS patients that can increase permeability of isolated glomeruli to albumin. This toxin (or cytokine) appears to cause injury to the podocytes similar to the GPF found in MCD. This finding is also supported by rapid recurrence of FSGS in kidney transplant patients.

Primary FSGS can cause progressive renal disease if not treated aggressively. Like MCD, primary FSGS will respond to steroids and immunosuppressive agents, albeit it entails a more prolonged therapy. The degree of proteinuria is an important prognostic factor. Patients with nonnephrotic proteinuria have better survival rates that those with nephrotic-range proteinuria. Poor prognostic factors include advanced renal insufficiency at the outset of treatment and presence of interstitial fibrosis on the biopsy. Treatment of secondary FSGS is directed to modifying the underlying primary disease (e.g., antiviral therapy for HIV-associated nephropathy). In both types of FSGS, use of ACE inhibitors and ARBs are used for their antiproteinuric properties and renoprotective potentials.

MEMBRANOUS NEPHROPATHY

Membranous nephropathy is the most common cause of nephrotic syndrome in adults in developed countries. This renal disease affects males more than females.

The term *membranous* refers to the thickening of the capillary walls of the glomeruli as seen on light microscopy. The thickening appears to be seen on the epithelial side of the basement membrane where electron-dense deposits can be found. These deposits appear to represent in situ formation or deposition of immune complexes. Immunofluorescence studies show granular deposits of IgG and C3 (including the membrane attack complex) along the capillary walls. There is minimal mesangial involvement. In about 75–80 percent of cases, the disease is idiopathic. Secondary causes are associated with systemic lupus erythematosus (SLE), malignancy, infections (hepatitis B and C viruses and syphilis), and drugs (gold, penicillamine, mercury compounds, tiopronin, captopril, diclofenac, and other nonsteroidal agents).

The presence of subepithelial deposits suggests that the offending antigen may be cationic in its charge to be able to cross the anionic GBM. Antibodies to endogenous antigens (e.g., megalin or gp 330) have been implicated in the Heymann nephritis model of membranous nephropathy. Megalin appears to function as a receptor for aminoglycosides, advanced glycation products, and vitamin D.

The benign course of idiopathic membranous nephropathy has led clinicians to withhold treatment. About 5 to 20 percent of cases go into spontaneous remission without treatment. Partial remissions (<2 g/day proteinuria) can be seen in another 25 to 40 percent of cases. However, if progressive renal disease is noted, use of steroids and cytotoxic agents are recommended. Treatment of secondary membranous nephropathy involves treatment of the underlying disease (e.g., treatment of malignancy) or withholding offending drugs.

MEMBRANOPROLIFERATIVE GLOMERULONEPHRITIS

Membranoproliferative glomerulonephritis (MPGN) or mesangiocapillary glomerulonephritis is a severe type of glomerulonephritis that is often idiopathic in nature. It affects patients from age 8 to 30. Patients usually present with a nephritic picture (hematuria with red cell casts, nonnephrotic-range proteinuria, hypertension, and renal insufficiency). Characteristic histologic changes seen on light microscopy include thickening of the GBM, hypercellularity as a result of mesangial cell proliferation and influx of monocytes, and narrowing of the capillary lumens. Immunofluorescence shows extensive complement deposition along the capillary wall. MPGN is classified into three types, depending on the location of dense deposits seen on electron microscopy. In type I MPGN, immune deposits are found in the mesangium and subendothelial space. This type is a rare finding but appears to be the most benign lesion. Systemic diseases associated with type I MPGN include hepatitis C infection with and without mixed cryoglobulinemia, SLE, hepatitis B infection, subacute bacterial infection (SBE), and infected ventriculo-peritoneal shunt (VP shunt). Type II MPGN is also called dense-deposit disease due to the presence of continuous dense, ribbonlike material in the subendothelial area, tubules, and Bowman's capsule. Although C3 has been detected on immunofluorescence, no immune complexes have been demonstrated. Its high recurrence after kidney transplantation suggests that a circulating factor is present. This factor was previously identified as a circulating C3 nephritic factor (C3NeF), an IgG autoantibody against the alternative complement pathway C3

convertase that normally cleaves C3 into C3a and C3b. This binding to the enzyme creates a stable C3bBb complex that is resistant to enzymatic inactivation but allows consumption of C3. The exact role of C3NeF remains to be defined because it does not correlate with the activity of the disease. It is proposed that persistent hypocomplementemia and accumulation of terminal C5b-9 complement complex deposits in the glomeruli will eventually cause tissue damage. Type III MPGN is characterized by marked thickening of and disruption of the GBM. Subepithelial deposits are found that are suggestive of immune complexes. Causes of type III MPGN are unknown. A report links a gene that causes familial MPGN type III in an Irish family to chromosome 1.

The clinical course of MPGN varies according to the type and etiology. Type I MPGN has the best prognosis and appears to respond to steroids. Treatment of the underlying disease with antiviral agents (for hepatitis B and C) and antibacterial agents (for SBE and infected VP shunt) is effective in stabilizing renal function. Use of antiplatelet agents has limited use.

RAPIDLY PROGRESSIVE GLOMERULONEPHRITIS

RPGN, or crescentic glomerulonephritis, is a severe form of glomerulonephritis that leads to end-stage renal disease invariably in a matter of weeks. Patients present with acute nephritis picture associated with progressive loss of renal function. The histology on kidney biopsy shows extensive presence of circumferential crescents that tends to compress the glomerular tuft and occlusion of capillary lumens. Rents along the glomerular capillary wall allow inflammatory cells such as macrophages that release cytokines such as IL-1 and TNF. Also, movement of plasma products into the Bowman's space induces fibrin formation. This process is usually followed by formation of fibrocellular crescents, which are not amenable to therapy. Prognosis is worse when about 80 percent of glomeruli are affected.

There are three types of RPGN, depending on the mechanism of injury. RPGN type I or anti-GBM disease (Goodpasture's syndrome) refers to the presence of circulating antibodies to an antigen in the GBM. The antigen has been identified to be the NC1 domain of the alpha-3 chain of type IV collagen. In addition to the role of B cells in producing this antibody, T cells isolated from affected patients also reacted to the same antigen. An anti-CD8 monoclonal antibody appears to prevent anti-GBM disease in a rodent model (Reynolds et al. 2002). This finding suggests that T cells may enhance production of the antibody to the alpha-3 chain of the GBM. In addition to renal failure, pulmonary hemorrhage and hemoptysis can be seen in affected patients. The circulating antibody binds to the alveolar basement membrane, which contains the same alpha-3 chain and causes lung injury. Chest radiograph will show bilateral infiltrates because of pulmonary hemorrhage. The presence of pulmonary involvement is variable, which appears to reflect access of the circulating antibody to the alveolar basement membrane. Recent reports have indicated genetic susceptibility to this disease, which is supported by a murine model. In mice immunized with the alpha-3(IV) NC1, development of crescentic glomerulonephritis and lung hemorrhage appears in mice with MHC haplotypes H-2s, b and d. Laboratory diagnosis can be made by measurement of anti-GBM antibody titer. Indirect immunofluorescence is done by incubating the patient's serum with normal renal tissue. Fluorescein-labeled anti-human IgG is then added and checked if linear deposition of IgG can be seen. An ELISA test has been developed using native and recombinant alpha-3(IV) NC1. This test appears to be more accurate. If the tests described are negative, a kidney biopsy is performed. Immunofluorescence will show the characteristic linear deposition of IgG along the glomerular capillaries and tubules. The main treatment for anti-GBM disease includes a combination of plasmapheresis, steroids, and cyclophosphamide. Plasmapheresis is designed to remove circulating antibodies. Steroids and cyclophosphamide will prevent further antibody production. About 40 percent of cases respond to this regimen. Early diagnosis is crucial because a serum creatinine of 5 mg/dl or greater suggests irreversible damage.

Type II RPGN is often considered an immune-complex RPGN. Immune complex deposits in the glomeruli suggest the presence of a systemic disease. Diseases associated with this type include PSGN, post-infectious glomerulonephritis, IgA nephropathy, lupus nephritis, and mixed cryoglobulinemia. Treatment of the underlying disease may or may not improve the clinical picture, especially in advanced renal failure.

Type III RPGN, or pauci-immune glomerulonephritis, is a form of necrotizing glomerulonephritis characterized by minimal or absence of immune deposits on immunofluorescence or electron microscopy. In addition to renal failure, affected patients will exhibit systemic symptoms related to the respiratory tract, skin, nervous system, and musculoskeletal system. Most patients will have ANCA, an antibody that is invariably present in other form of vasculitides (Wegener's granulomatosis, polyarteritis nodosa, Churg-Strauss syndrome, microscopic polyangiitis, and drug-induced vasculitis). Two target antigens have been identified by ANCA – proteinase 3 (PR-3) and myeloperoxidase. Both can be found in the azurophilic granules of neutrophils and lysosomes of monocytes. When ethanol-fixed neutrophils are incubated with serum from affected patients, two distinct immunofluorescent patterns can be identified. The first is C-ANCA, which pertains to the diffuse staining of the cytoplasm, in contrast to clear nuclear staining. Antibodies against PR-3 antigen appear to exhibit this pattern. The majority of active Wegener's granulomatosis will exhibit the C ANCA pattern. P-ANCA refers to the perinuclear staining around the nucleus, which appears to be an artifact of ethanol fixation. Antibodies to the myeloperoxidase antigen are associated with this pattern. About 75–80 percent of pauci-immune glomerulonephritis cases exhibit the P-ANCA pattern. ANCA patterns for the other vasculitides are variable, making it a difficult marker for diagnostic use. Like anti-GBM disease, use of steroids, plasmapheresis, and cytotoxic agents can be attempted to treat this disease.

LUPUS NEPHRITIS

SLE is an autoimmune disease characterized by overproduction of antibodies to self-antigens, which are mostly derived from cell components like the nucleus, cytoplasm, ribosomes, and cell membranes. Most affected patients are women of childbearing age. In the United States,

SLE is more common in black people. Clinical symptoms include polyarthralgias, malar rash, photosensitivity, alopecia, serositis, myocarditis and endocarditis, anemia, and thrombocytopenia. Although about 50–70 percent of SLE cases will have renal involvement (abnormal urinalysis, hematuria, proteinuria, or pyuria), the incidence may actually reach 100 percent because kidney biopsies on patients without clinical evidence of lupus nephritis often show mesangial and even proliferative glomerulonephritis. Hypertension and renal insufficiency occur in later stage of the disease. The degree of proteinuria correlates with the severity of the renal disease. Nephrotic-range proteinuria is more common in membranous and diffuse proliferative forms.

Immune complex deposits in the glomeruli are primarily responsible for the inflammatory process that causes glomerular damage. If deposited into the mesangium and subendothelial space, immune complexes will activate the complement (cause hypocomplementemia) and generate chemoattractants (C3a and C5a). The result is an influx of neutrophils and mononuclear cells that secrete proteases, reactive oxygen species, and cytokines, causing glomerular injury. Histologically, these can be seen in mesangial, focal, or diffuse proliferative lesions. However, subepithelial deposits do not cause influx of inflammatory cells because of the restriction of the chemoattractants from reaching the subepithelial space. The urine sediment is benign. Proteinuria is often in the nephrotic range and is mainly seen in membranous type (Roseet al. 2007). Immune complexes identified in lupus nephritis include DNA-anti-DNA, nucleosomes, chromatin, C1q, laminin, Sm, La (SS-B), Ro (SS-A), ubiquitin, and ribosomes. On electron microscopy, tubuloreticular structures can be identified in lupus nephritis. These inclusions are made of ribonucleoproteins and membranes and appear to be synthesized in response to interferon-alpha. Similar structures can be seen in HIV-nephropathy, a renal disease that has high levels of circulating interferon-alpha.

Lupus nephritis is currently classified into six types based on kidney biopsy findings. Class I refers to presence of mesangial deposits without mesangial hypercellularity. Class II refers to presence of mesangial deposits with mesangial hypercellularity. Class III refers to focal glomerulonephritis (involving <50 percent of the total number of glomeruli). Class IV refers to diffuse glomerulonephritis (involving >50 percent of the total number of glomeruli) with either segmental class (Class IV-S) or global (Class IV-G). Class V refers to membranous nephropathy. Class VI refers to advanced sclerosing lesions. The latter may have features similar to that of end-stage renal disease.

The clinical course and treatment of lupus nephritis depends on the kidney biopsy findings and presence of systemic symptoms. Class I and II lesions have good prognosis and do not require treatment. In class V disease, steroids and cytotoxic agents can be used to induce and maintain remission. Likewise, class III and IV require more aggressive treatment with pulse steroids and cyclophosphamide, followed by oral steroids and mycophenolate mofetil or azathioprine. Concurrent treatment of hypertension, dyslipidemia, and proteinuria (with low-protein diet and ACE inhibitors, or ARBs) is also indicated. If treated early, renal function may stabilize and prevents patients from reaching end-stage renal disease.

ACUTE POSTSTREPTOCOCCAL GLOMERULONEPHRITIS

APSGN is an immune complex disease that follows pharyngitis and skin infections from nephritogenic strains of group A streptococci. Most affected patients are children in developing countries. About ten days after streptococcal pharyngitis or twenty-one days after streptococcal skin infection (impetigo), susceptible individuals may develop microscopic hematuria or full-blown acute nephritis (red cell casts, proteinuria, edema, hypertension, and acute renal failure). Diagnosis is made by history of throat or skin infection. In addition to throat or wound culture, serology for ASO, anti-DNAase B and antihyaluronidase may be obtained to confirm the infection. Circulating immune complexes appear early in the course of the disease and are associated with hypocomplementemia. The majority of affected children recover and kidney biopsy is not always indicated. When kidney biopsy is obtained, prominent findings are compatible with a diffuse proliferative nephritis picture (hypercellularity and marked neutrophilic infiltration). On immunofluorescence, there is granular deposition of complements and IgG in the glomerular tuft. On electron microscopy, subepithelial dense deposits, or "humps," are considered hallmarks of PSGN. Damage to the epithelial cells appears to be responsible for the proteinuria noted in this renal disease. Subendothelial deposits are also seen, which are primarily responsible for complement activation and influx of inflammatory cells.

Over the past two decades, many attempts to identify the nature of the streptococcal antigen in the immune complex have been made by several investigators.

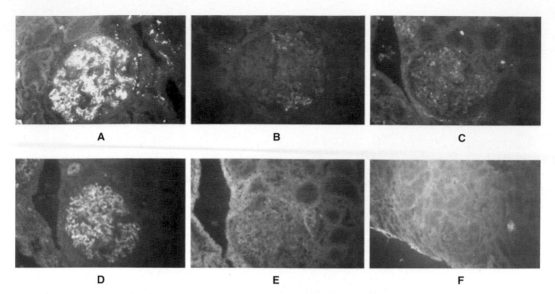

Figure 17.4 Immunofluorescent staining of kidney biopsy section of one case of APSGN using different antibodies (×40). *A*, Extensive deposition of C3 in mesangium and glomerular capillary walls. *B, C*, Minimal staining for IgG and IgM. *D*, Extensive deposition of streptococcal pyrogenic exotoxin B (SPEB) in mesangium and glomerular capillary wall. *E*, Staining for SPEB can be abolished by preabsorbing the rabbit sera against purified SPEB. *F*, Absence of SPEB in a non-APSGN kidney biopsy section (case of IgA nephropathy). Reproduced with permission from: Cu GA, Mezzano S, Bannan JD, Zabriskie JB. Immunohistochemical and serological evidence for the role of streptococcal proteinase in acute post-streptococcal glomerulonephritis. *Kidney Int.* 1998;54:824, Figure. 4.

Two prominent proteins have been implicated in the pathogenesis of APSGN: streptokinase (Ska) and SPEB. Ska is produced by all strains of group A streptococci, but SPEB appears to be secreted in abundance in nephritogenic strains causing APSGN. Ska cleaves cell-surface-bound plasminogen to active plasmin. Plasmin then cleaves fibrin into degradation products, which are also seen in inflammatory processes. Bound plasmin apparently cannot be inhibited by endogenous antiproteases, thereby causing unopposed formation of fibrin degradation products. The role of streptokinase, however, was in doubt when immunostaining studies on kidney biopsy specimens using rabbit anti-Ska antibody failed to detect this protein.

SPEB, or streptococcal proteinase, however, behaves as a cysteine protease, which can activate endothelial metalloprotease and cause tissue destruction. Although structurally unrelated to streptokinase, SPEB can also bind plasmin to form a complex that can activate the complement cascade system. SPEB and other streptococcal pyrogenic exotoxins (SPEA and SPEC) are considered superantigens, which can stimulate T-cell proliferation. The result is excessive production of cytokines, which mediate inflammation and tissue injury. As demonstrated by Cu and coworkers, immunohistochemical and serologic studies (see Figures 17.4 and 17.5) on kidney biopsy specimens and sera from affected patients have shown strong and specific reactivity to SPEB in the biopsies and in the sera of these patients. This suggests a significant role of this protein in the pathogenesis of APSGN. This observation was recently

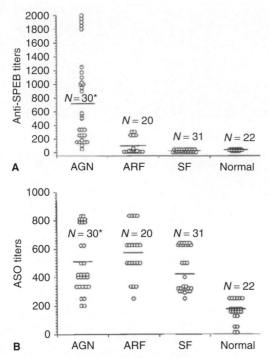

Figure 17.5 *A*, Anti-SPEB (streptococcal pyrogenic exotoxin B) titers in sera from patients with acute post-streptococcal glomerulonephritis (APSGN), acute rheumatic fever (ARF), scarlet fever (SF), and normal children.*P < 0.001 when AGN sera are compared with the other groups. *B*, ASO titers from the same group of patients, indicating a definite serological response to a streptococcal extracellular product in the streptococcal infections groups. *P < 0.001 for AGN, ARF, and SF vs. normals. P = NS vs. AGN, ARF, and SF. Reproduced with permission from: Cu GA, Mezzano S, Bannan JD, Zabriskie JB. Immunohistochemical and serological evidence for the role of streptococcal proteinase in acute post-streptococcal glomerulonephritis. *Kidney Int*. 1998;54:822, Figure. 17.3.

confirmed in a much larger study by Batsford and coworkers with essentially the same results.

APSGN follows a relatively benign course. The majority of cases will recover spontaneously with only less than 1 percent of children and slightly higher percentages of adults needing long-term dialysis treatment. Hematuria may resolve in three to six months. Proteinuria may persist for years, which may be later associated with hypertension and renal insufficiency.

MIXED CRYOGLOBULINEMIA

Circulating cryoglobulins are immunoglobulins that precipitate at cold temperatures and dissolve on rewarming. Three types of cryoglobulins have been described. Type I refers to monoclonal immunoglobulin that is associated with multiple myeloma or Waldenstrom's macroglobulinemia. Type II, or essential mixed cryoglobulinemia, refers to cryoglobulin, which contains both polyclonal IgG (as an antigen or formed against another circulating antigen) and monoclonal IgM rheumatoid factor against the IgG. Most cases have been associated with chronic hepatitis C virus infection. Type III is also a mixed cryoglobulin, but both the IgG and rheumatoid IGM are polyclonal. This latter type is associated with hepatitis C infection, autoimmune disorders (e.g., lupus), and lymphoproliferative disorders. Although hepatitis C antibodies were found in the precipitates in both type II and III, antibodies to HIV-1 can be found as well.

Clinical symptoms of mixed cryoglobulinemia are related to the deposition of the cryoglobulins in medium-sized arteries. Palpable purpura is a major skin finding. Other symptoms include polyarthralgias, hepatosplenomegaly, lymphadenopathy, peripheral neuropathy, and hypocomplementemia. About 20 percent of cases will have renal involvement. MPGN is commonly seen, including the presence of precipitated cryoglobulins that may occlude the capillary loops. Immunofluorescence will show diffuse deposition of IgM in capillary loops. Electron microscopy will show subendothelial deposits, which may have a "fingerprint" appearance.

Until the discovery of hepatitis C and HIV-1 in cryglobulin precipitates, steroids and cytotoxic drugs (cyclophosphamide or chlorambucil) were mainstays of treatment. These drugs are now reserved for severe cases of progressive renal failure, necrotic extremities that may require amputation, and severe neuropathy. Plasmapheresis is initially done to remove circulating cryoglobulins. Pulse steroids and cytotoxic agents are used to prevent new antibody formation. Antiviral therapy is directed to hepatitis C and HIV disease to prevent further cryoglobulin formation.

BIBLIOGRAPHY

REVIEWS

Abbas AK, Lichtman AH, Pober JS, eds. *Cellular and Molecular Immunology.* . Philadelphia, PA: W. B. Saunders; 2005.

Brenner BM, ed. *Brenner and Rector's The Kidney.* 7th ed. Philadelphia, PA: W. B. Saunders; 2004.

Lewis EJ, Schwartz MM, Korbet SM, eds. *Lupus Nephritis.* Oxford, UK: Oxford University Press; 1999.

Pereira BJG, Sayegh MH, Blake P, eds. *Chronic Kidney Disease, Dialysis & Transplantation.* 2nd ed. Elsevier Health Sciences; 2004.

Rose BD, ed. UpToDate Online 15.3. Waltham, MA; 2007.

SUGGESTED READINGS

Batsford SR, Mezzano S, Mihatsch M, Schiltz E, Rodríguez-Iturbe B. Is the nephritogenic antigen in post-streptococcal glomerulonephritis pyrogenic exotoxin B (SPE B) or GAPDH? *Kidney Int.* 2005;68:1120–1129.

Cu GA, Mezzano S, Bannan JD, Zabriskie JB. Immunohistochemical and serological evidence for the role of streptococcal proteinase in acute post-streptococcal glomerulonephritis. *Kidney Int.* 1998;54: 819–826.

Farquhar MG, Saito A, Kerjaschki D, Orlando RA. The Heymann nephritis antigenic complex: megalin (gp330) and RAP. *J Am Soc Nephrol.* 1995; 6:35–47.

Reynolds J, Norgan VA, Bhambra U, Smith J, Cook HT, Pusey CD. Anti-CD8 monoclonal antibody therapy is effective in the prevention and treatment of experimental autoimmune glomerulonephritis. *J Am Soc Nephrol.* 2002;13(2): 359–369.

Johnson RJ, Feehally J, eds. *Comprehensive Clinical Nephrology,* 2nd ed. Elsevier Health Sciences; 2003.

Rose BD, Appel GB, Schur PH. Types of renal disease in systemic lupus erythematosus. In: Rose BD, ed. *UpToDate.* Waltham, MA; 2007.

18. Immunological Aspects of Transplantation

Jeffrey M. Venstrom, M.D., and James W. Young, M.D.

INTRODUCTION

More than fifty years have passed since the first identical twin transplant was performed, and we can now look on organ transplantation as an extremely successful treatment for hundreds of thousands of patients who would otherwise have been doomed to organ failure or to death. This successful kidney transplant between identical twins in 1954, performed at the Peter Bent Brigham Hospital by Dr. Joseph Murray and his colleagues, helped to usher in the field of solid organ transplantation. Within the ensuing decade, this transplant was followed by the first successful transplants from a non-twin living donor and later on from a cadaveric donor. The shortage of donor organs is now the chief stumbling block to further development.

The first twin transplant confirmed that a young, healthy donor could survive with one kidney with no disability, as long as the single remaining kidney was not damaged. Indeed, the donor of the first twin transplant is still alive more than fifty years later. This achievement, which was quickly repeated in a number of other twin transplants, confirmed the surgical aspects of this operation. Two other important observations were made. First, if the patient suffered from an autoimmune nephritis, this could recur in the transplanted kidney. The same disease could also develop in the donor's remaining kidney because of the genetic susceptibility of identical twins to similar diseases.

The immunological obstacles, however, proved to be stubborn. Medawar and colleagues had shown that skin grafts were destroyed by a mechanism that had immune characteristics. Having reacted against one skin graft, the recipient of a second skin graft from the same donor would react more violently, demonstrating an acquired immunity and a memory for the first tissue. A few years later, Medawar and colleagues demonstrated a natural way of overcoming graft rejection, which occurs in fraternal animal twins. The definitive experiment, injecting cells from an inbred strain of mice into the fetus of another strain, resulted in graft acceptance in survivors of this procedure and established the concept of immunological plasticity in the embryo before the immune system fully develops. Although this had no obvious clinical application, it raised the question about whether this state of immunological plasticity could be temporarily induced in a potential organ graft recipient so that the graft would be accepted even though the immune defenses would be rapidly restored.

The ensuing story of immunosuppression still has this aim of "tolerance" in view. Clinical immunological tolerance occurs when the recipient's immune system is ablated and replaced by hematopoietic stem cells from a donor matched according to expression of human leucocyte antigens

(HLAs). Refinements in immunosuppression include more precisely dosed irradiation as well as drug and antibody treatment to support engraftment. Clinicians tend to add more potent immunosuppressive agents to the patient's therapy. More recent attempts to achieve graft acceptance with minimal immunosuppression are beginning to meet with some success. One example is the use of the lympholytic monoclonal antibody, alemtuzumal (Campath-1H), as an inducing agent, followed by maintenance therapy with reduced-dose calcineurin inhibitor monotherapy.

The interest in organ transplantation greatly stimulated the science of immunology. Mechanisms of graft rejection are now well understood, and the fate of a graft depends not only on surgical technique but also on the degree of HLA matching between donor and recipient. The specific transplanted organ also has relevance, such as the liver, which is more tolerogenic than others. The HLA system of antigenic determinants arises from genes on human chromosome 6. The ABO antigen system is also important in solid organ graft outcome but does not directly affect hematopoietic stem cell transplantation (HSCT).

Of the drugs used to suppress the immune system, each has some side effects specific to the agent in question and others common to all immunosuppressive agents, namely, increased susceptibility to infections and tumors, especially lymphoproliferative disorders. A strategy of using different agents together to maximize immunosuppression and minimize side effects has been partially successful, and the new approach of minimal immunosuppression should be of additional benefit. Active agents vary from small molecules (azathioprine and corticosteroids) to complicated peptides and macrolides (cyclosporine, tacrolimus, and sirolimus) and onto large polyclonal and monoclonal antibodies.

Much interest has recently focused on blocking the secondary and tertiary signals of antigen recognition. In animal models, such blockade can result in long-term graft acceptance without other potentially toxic immunosuppressive agents. These and other immunosuppressive agents are in the process of early clinical trials and no doubt will have an effect on immunosuppression in the future.

IMMUNOLOGICAL CONSIDERATIONS OF TRANSPLANTATION

The human major histocompatibility complex (MHC) comprises a set of genes on the short arm of chromosome 6. These genes are highly polymorphic and are codominantly expressed, each individual having inherited one set of MHC genes from each parent. MHC molecules present foreign antigens, as well as self-peptides, to T cells for recognition and response. In general, class I MHC molecules present peptides to $CD8^+$ T cells, while class II MHC molecules present peptides to $CD4^+$ T cells. In the context of transplantation, this process can determine acceptance or rejection of the donor graft.

Class I and II MHC loci carry the greatest significance for transplantation compared with other loci within the complex. While their polymorphisms are inherently critical to the species' ability to resist various pathogens, these polymorphisms also pose one of the major obstacles to transplantation tolerance. Every individual expresses three different pairs of class I molecules (designated as HLA-A, HLA-B, and HLA-C) and three different pairs of class II molecules (designated as HLA-DP, HLA-DQ, and HLA-DR). In addition, the MHC contains other genes that encode complement proteins, cytokines, and other proteins involved in antigen processing. Class I MHC molecules are expressed on all nucleated cells, whereas class II MHC molecules are expressed on antigen-presenting cells like macrophages, dendritic cells, B lymphocytes, endothelial cells, and thymic epithelial cells. Expression of MHC gene products is greatly enhanced by cytokines, especially interferon, which stimulates transcription of MHC genes.

Matching the class I and class II MHC genes between the graft and recipient has varying degrees of influence on graft–host interactions and tolerance, differing somewhat with the inherent immunogenicity or tolerogenicity of the organ being transplanted. In kidney transplantation, renal allograft survival directly correlates with the degree of similarity between graft and recipient MHC antigens. Complete HLA matching in liver transplantation is less critical for long-term graft acceptance. Clinically, the HLA-A, HLA-B, and HLA-DR loci are the most relevant for predicting outcome, although the importance of other loci and allelic subtypes is increasingly recognized. Minor histocompatibility antigens are self-peptides derived from nucleotide polymorphisms that differ between HLA identical siblings yet require HLA identity for presentation. These cannot be routinely typed in the laboratory but can greatly influence graft–host interactions in transplantation, especially hematopoietic stem cell transplants.

LABORATORY TESTING FOR COMPATIBILITY IN TRANSPLANTATION

HLA Typing

Histocompatibility between the donor and recipient is primarily defined by genes of the MHC. MHC is a general term for the gene complex encoding the HLA, and hence the two acronyms are used interchangeably in humans. Historically, HLA typing was performed by serologic evaluation, using a panel of anti-HLA antibody containing sera derived from multiparous women. Most clinical HLA laboratories now use DNA-based HLA typing methods. By using the polymerase chain reaction (PCR), polymorphic residues of both class I and class II HLA or MHC molecules can be amplified using primers that bind to the conserved regions of the gene. The precise nucleic acid sequence of the HLA alleles can be accurately determined using sequence-based typing. More commonly, partial amplification of polymorphic residues using sequence-specific primer pairs (PCR-SSP or PCR-SSOP) can identify HLA alleles. Depending on the DNA probe, PCR-based HLA typing is described as either "intermediate-resolution" (beyond the serologic level, but short of the allelic subtype level) or "high-resolution" (allele- or allelic subtype–level typing). The resolution of the HLA typing defines the level of HLA mismatch. Low-resolution serologic typing can identify antigen mismatch (HLA-A2 vs. -A11), whereas high-resolution typing can identify an allele- or allelic subtype-level mismatch (HLA-A*0201 vs. -A*0205).

ABO Blood Typing

ABO blood typing is one of the most important tests in human solid organ transplantation. ABO antigens are primarily expressed by erythrocytes but also can be expressed by platelets and glandular epithelial and endothelial cells. Incompatibility occurs when recipients lacking a certain blood type produce IgM antibodies against that antigen and cause subsequent activation of complement and lysis of transfused incompatible red blood cells. Because ABO antigens are also expressed by endothelial cells, incompatibilities can lead to hyperacute vascular rejection.

In contrast to solid organ transplantation, ABO matching does not directly affect donor selection for allogeneic HSCT. Because inheritance of blood group antigens is independent of HLA antigens, fully HLA-matched donor-recipient pairs are often ABO incompatible. ABO incompatibility requires red blood cell depletion of a stem cell allograft but does not affect myeloid or megakaryocytic engraftment, graft rejection, or graft-versus-host disease (GvHD). Upon engraftment, the recipient transitions to the donor's ABO blood type. During the conversion from recipient to donor blood type, transient hemolysis may occur.

Screening for Preformed Antibodies

Patients awaiting cadaveric organs undergo screening of their blood for preformed antibodies against HLA molecules. These antibodies may be produced by pregnancy, prior blood transfusions, or prior organ transplantation. An aliquot of the patient's serum is mixed in separate wells with cells of at least forty donors assumed to be representative of the donor population. Complement-mediated lysis or flow cytometry with fluorescent-labeled secondary antibodies to human IgG quantifies the number of reactive cells as a proportion of the number of panel cells (percent reactive antibody, or PRA). Because transplantation across a positive cross match can cause hyperacute or acute rejection, patients with high PRAs typically experience longer waiting times on the cadaveric organ donor list. Many centers are therefore currently exploring strategies to remove these antibodies, by plasmapheresis, for example, either preoperatively or perioperatively.

Cross Matching

In solid organ transplants, cross matching is usually done after a potential donor is identified. The recipient's serum is tested for reactivity to the donor's lymphocytes using the previously mentioned complement-mediated lysis or flow cytometric assays. A negative cross match means that there is no recipient antibody that is reactive with donor cells or graft. A positive cross match portends severe rejection if the donor organ is transplanted.

TYPES OF SOLID ORGAN ALLOGRAFT REJECTION

Hyperacute Rejection

In hyperacute rejection, thrombosis of the vasculature occurs immediately after anastomosis of the solid organ graft blood vessels and release of the surgical clamp, which is caused by the presence of preformed antibodies that bind to the endothelial antigens. In the early days of transplantation, ABO incompatibility was the main culprit. Because ABO incompatibility is largely avoided now, hyperacute rejection usually occurs when IgG antibodies react with foreign MHC antigens or lesser-known alloantigens in the endothelium. The latter may be associated with accelerated hyperacute rejection that lasts a few days. Adequate screening for preformed anti-HLA antibodies and

ABO testing should prevent hyperacute rejection.

Acute Rejection

Acute rejection is an inflammatory process affecting the vasculature and parenchyma of the allograft, which occurs a few days to a week after transplantation. Activated T cells can cause direct lysis of the graft or release cytokines that promote inflammation in the allograft. The endothelial cells appear to be the earliest targets for rejection with resultant endotheliitis. A humoral-mediated response causes binding of antibodies to the blood vessel wall with resultant necrosis and occlusion of the arteries.

Chronic Rejection

Fibrosis with intimal thickening and eventual occlusion of medium-sized arteries that supply the graft characterizes chronic rejection. The fibrosis seen in chronic rejection is presumed to be a by-product of previous inflammation from acute rejection or from cytokines that stimulated fibroblast production. Chronic allograft rejection accounts for the majority of allograft failures.

PREVENTION AND MANAGEMENT OF SOLID ORGAN ALLOGRAFT REJECTION

Induction Agents

Induction agents are immunosuppressive drugs given intraoperatively and immediately postoperatively to deplete the T-cell population. OKT3 is a murine monoclonal antibody to the CD3 complex of the T cell, an intrinsic part of the T-cell receptor. The exact mechanism by which T cells are then

cleared from the circulation may occur by FcR-mediated clearance or complement-mediated lysis. OKT3 also blocks the function of killer T cells. Because of its murine origin, recipients often develop anti-murine antibodies precluding subsequent use for rejection episodes. Patients also experience cytokine release syndrome, with release of TNF-α, IL-2, and interferon-gamma into the circulation. Symptoms include fever, rigors, pulmonary edema, aseptic meningitis, and myalgias. Basiliximab (Simulect) and daclizumab (Zenapax) are humanized anti-CD25 monoclonal antibodies directed against the α chain of the high-affinity IL-2 receptor. Such humanized antibodies are engineered to contain a part of the human antibody, rendering them less immunogenic. Alemtuzumab (Campath 1H) is an anti-CD52 monoclonal antibody that is gaining acceptance as an induction agent for steroid-free protocols. This is another humanized antibody, initially designed to treat chronic lymphocytic leukemia. A single dose given intraoperatively should eliminate CD52-positive B and T cells, as well as monocytes and monocyte-derived dendritic cells, from the bone marrow and peripheral circulation. Rituximab (Rituxan) is a monoclonal antibody against the CD20 antigen on B lymphocytes. Originally used to treat non-Hodgkin's lymphoma, it is being used to treat B-cell- or humoral-mediated allograft rejection. Rabbit anti-thymocyte globulin has replaced equine anti-thymocyte globulin as the primary polyclonal antibody to treat acute episodes of solid organ allograft rejection. This drug is made by injecting human lymphocytes into rabbits with subsequent collection and purification of the antiserum. This drug is given for seven to ten days with elimination of T cells from the circulation.

Prolonged lymphopenia occurs after this drug is infused.

Maintenance Immunosuppressive Drugs

The introduction of cyclosporine in 1983 heralded a new era of solid organ transplantation. Five-year graft survival improved dramatically. Cyclosporine is a cyclic peptide from a fungus that binds to cyclophilin, a cellular protein. This complex binds and further inhibits calcineurin and subsequent activation of NFAT (nuclear factor of activated T cells). This prevents IL-2 and other cytokine gene activation. Cyclosporine also promotes TGF-β activation, which may account for the fibrosis noted in allograft parenchyma with prolonged use of this drug. Tacrolimus (Prograf, FK506) is another calcineurin inhibitor similar to cyclosporine. This is a macrolide drug that is more potent than cyclosporine. It binds to an immunophilin, FK506 binding protein, which is involved in the inhibition of calcineurin-mediated IL-2 gene transcription. Like cyclosporine, prolonged use of tacrolimus can cause fibrosis of the allograft parenchyma. Use of tacrolimus has led to fewer solid organ allograft rejection episodes when compared with cyclosporine. Most solid organ transplant centers in the United States have therefore shifted to tacrolimus as the primary maintenance immunosuppressant. Tacrolimus and cyclosporine are fairly similar, however, in preventing GvHD after allogeneic HSCT.

Sirolimus (Rapamune) is another macrolide antibiotic that binds to the FK binding protein and modulates the activity of the mammalian target of rapamycin (mTOR); mTOR inhibits IL-2-mediated signal transduction, resulting in cycle arrest at the G1 to S phase. Sirolimus has replaced cyclosporine and tacrolimus for long-term use in solid organ allografts because of lesser incidence of fibrosis in the allograft parenchyma. Many clinicians and investigators in the field of allogeneic HSCT regard sirolimus as a better drug for long-term induction of host-graft tolerance. Prominent side effects include hyperlipidemia and poor wound healing. In summary, sirolimus blocks the response of B- and T-cell activation by cytokines, while cyclosporine and tacrolimus inhibit production of cytokines.

Azathioprine (Imuran) is a purine analog that inhibits purine nucleotide synthesis and interferes with RNA synthesis. This drug prevents T-cell activation by affecting gene replication and transcription. It is an old drug that continues to play a role in immunosuppression by having fewer side effects and good tolerability by most patients. Mycophenolate mofetil (CellCept) is a reversible inhibitor of the enzyme inosine monophosphate dehydrogenase (IMPDH). IMPDH is a rate-limiting enzyme in the synthesis de novo of purines and production of guanosine nucleotides from inosine. Mycophenolate appears to have selective antiproliferative properties against lymphocytes, which rely on purine synthesis de novo. It is more potent than Imuran and has helped limit the incidence of acute rejection.

Corticosteroids have been mainstay drugs for transplantation since the 1960s. Their mechanisms of action are broad, impairing both the innate and adaptive arms of the immune system. Corticosteroids block cytokine-receptor expression by T cells and inhibit function of antigen-presenting cells. Corticosteroids also cause lymphophenia and prevent migration of monocytes and neutrophils to sites of inflammation. Figure 18.1 illustrates the

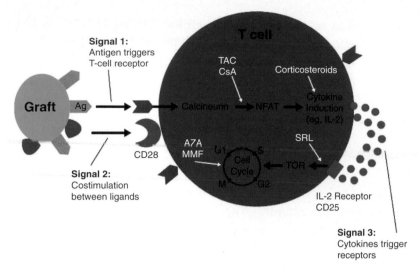

Signal 1:
Antigen triggers
T-cell receptor

T cell

TAC
CsA

Corticosteroids

Graft Ag

Calcineurin → NFAT → Cytokine Induction (eg, IL-2)

A7A
MMF

CD28

G1

Cell Cycle

SRL

TOR

M

G2

Signal 2:
Costimulation
between ligands

IL-2 Receptor
CD25

Signal 3:
Cytokines trigger
receptors

Figure 18.1 T cells of a solid organ transplant recipient (host) recognize antigens on the solid organ graft as foreign and have the potential to mediate graft rejection. Immunosuppressive agents targeting pathways involved in T-cell activation prevent T-cell-mediated graft rejection.

immune cascade and the targets of various immunosuppressive drugs.

Other antirejection drugs are in development, including monoclonal antibodies to adhesion molecules, chemokine receptors, and humanized OKT3. T-cell co-stimulatory blockade and immune modulation using blood transfusions, donor-specific bone marrow infusion, and intravenous immunoglobulin are also in trials.

Standard maintenance immunosuppression consists of at least two or three drugs. The most common combination in solid organ allografting includes tacrolimus, mycophenolate mofetil, and steroids. Hematopoietic stem cell allografts try to avoid steroids as much as possible, and long-term immune suppression as prophylaxis beyond six months is avoided if possible in order not to compromise any graft-versus-tumor (GvT) effect. Steroid-free protocols are gaining popularity in solid organ allografts to avert the long-term side effects of steroid use (i.e., weight gain, diabetes, osteoporosis, hyperlipidemia, and hypertension).

SOLID ORGAN TRANSPLANTATION OUTCOMES

The kidney was the first successfully transplanted human organ. Even when the donor is not an identical twin, patients can do well for some time with grafts from live donors and from unrelated and often totally unmatched cadaveric donors. The half-life of kidney transplants has been increasing and is currently more than ten years. Failures are mainly due to chronic rejection, nephrotoxicity of the calcineurin inhibitor agents, and recurrent disease. Liver and heart transplantation have also provided excellent treatment for many patients. The empiric clinical observation is that livers are more tolerogenic than other solid organ allografts, but the basis for this has not been clearly established. The most common indication for liver transplantation is now hepatitis C, but this almost invariably recurs in the graft and can lead to liver failure irrespective of rejection and other causes of graft loss. The chief complication of heart allografts is chronic rejection, which involves the coronary arteries with accelerated atherosclerosis. There have now been many cases of bilateral lung transplantation with or without the heart; however, the main problem is that the alveoli are particularly susceptible to rejection.

A major conceptual advance in the treatment of diabetes was the successful transplantation of islets of Langerhans by a group in Edmonton led by James Shapiro. The early results were excellent using an immunosuppressive protocol with no steroids and treating patients suffering from hypoglycemia. Most patients required two islet cell donors to reach a euglycemic state. At one year, 80 percent of patients no longer required insulin support. This fell to about 75 percent at two years but deteriorated more quickly thereafter. This study was an important proof of principle that islet cell transplantation could achieve good results. Significant obstacles still remain, however, including the exhaustion of transplanted islet cells, control of chronic rejection, balancing the toxicities of immunosuppressive drugs, and preventing recurrent autoimmune destruction in type I diabetes.

There is continued enthusiasm for the prospect of xenogeneic transplantation of organs and tissues from animals to man, but to date there have been no long-term successes. The best result occurred in the 1960s, when Reemtsma transplanted a kidney from a chimpanzee to a patient who achieved adequate graft function for nearly ten months. There are many difficulties, however, with xenografting. In addition to hyperacute rejection, accelerated rejection, and other immunological factors, there are physiological considerations regarding organ size disparities and whether xenogeneic proteins will function satisfactorily in man.

HEMATOPOIETIC STEM CELL TRANSPLANTATION

HSCT involves the infusion of immature blood-forming cells into the circulation of a patient to reconstitute the recipient's bone marrow. HSCT is a promising form of therapy for patients with certain forms of genetic diseases, specific cancers, and various blood disorders (Table 18.1). The transplanted hematopoietic stem cells (HSCs) may come from the patient (autologous HSCT) or from a different stem cell donor (allogeneic HSCT).

The field of clinical HSCT began in the late 1940s, when experiments in mice showed that shielding of the spleen allowed animals to survive otherwise lethal total-body irradiation. It was not until the seminal publication by E. Donnall Thomas in the 1957 *New England Journal of Medicine*, however, that even transiently successful hematopoietic transplants were first reported in humans; and at least another decade passed before allogeneic marrow grafting really began to have clinical successes. Thomas was later recognized with the 1990 Nobel Prize in Medicine for his pioneering work in HSCT. Outcomes continued to improve through the 1970s as HLA matching became commonplace, allowing expansion of the clinical indications for transplant to patients who did not have end-stage disease and who were in better clinical condition. Further expansion of transplant availability between nonsibling donor-recipient pairs has driven refinements in HLA typing, allowing better matching with high-resolution, DNA-based methods, rather than serologic methods, at the allelic subtype level for class I and II MHC antigens.

Table 18.1 Current Indications for Hematopoietic Stem Cell Transplantation

	Allogeneic	Autologous
Leukemias		
Acute myelogenous	+	±
Acute lymphoblastic	+	±
Chronic myelogenous	+	−
Chronic lymphocytic	+	−
Lymphomas		
Non-Hodgkin's	+	+
Hodgkin's	±	+
Plasma cell disorders		
Multiple myeloma	+	+
Amyloidosis	−	+
Other malignancies		
Germ cell tumors	−	+
Neuroblastoma	±	+
Acquired bone marrow disorder		
Severe aplastic anemia	+	−
Myelodysplastic syndrome	+	±
Myeloproliferative disorders	+	−
Congenital disorders		
Immunodeficiencies	+	−
Wiskott-Aldrich syndrome	+	−
Fanconi's anemia	+	−
Thalassemia	+	−
Sickle cell anemia	±	−
Osteopetrosis	+	−
Storage diseases	±	−

+, established indications; ±, used in small numbers of patients; −, not used.

Hematopoietic Stem Cell Transplant Sources

The stem cell product was originally harvested directly from bone marrow under general anesthesia and used almost exclusively in the allogeneic setting. With the advent of the cytokine era, G-CSF given during recovery from treatment with cyclophosphamide, which spares the actual CD34$^+$ HSCs, has proven effective in mobilizing CD34$^+$ HSCs into the circulation for collection by leukopheresis. These peripheral blood stem cells (PBSC) are now in routine use for autologous transplantation.

G-CSF-mobilized PBSCs, without prior cyclophosphamide treatment, have also largely replaced steady state bone marrow harvesting in allogeneic transplantation. Randomized comparison trial between these two stem cell sources are ongoing. The concentration of CD34$^+$ HSCs in normal resting bone marrow is up to 100 times higher than in peripheral blood. A daily dose of at least 10 μg/kg of subcutaneously administered G-CSF (filgrastim) for four to six days increases the number of CD34$^+$ cells in the blood fiftyfold or higher, or to levels comparable to or greater than those in marrow. One or two peripheral blood leukopheresis collections from G-CSF-primed healthy donors on consecutive days will result in a CD34$^+$ cell collection that is sufficient for the most allogeneic transplants. In the short term, this mobilization regimen is benign, although 80 percent of recipients will develop bone pain and 50 percent develop headaches due to the increased cellularity and turnover of marrow in its closed space (the skull also contains marrow). To date, there have been no long-term safety issues. CD34$^+$ HSCs and their absolute number per kilogram of recipient weight are critical determinants of eventual engraftment, regardless of the stem cell source.

Hematopoietic recovery occurs earlier after transplantation of PBSC than bone marrow, even though long-term engraftment may be similar. This seems due not only to the dose of CD34$^+$ HSCs but also to other lymphocyte subpopulations included in the PBSC graft. An additional advantage of PBSCs, at least in autografts, is the lower risk that PBSCs are contaminated with tumor cells in the bone marrow.

Finally, umbilical cord blood (UCB) is also an enriched source of CD34$^+$ HSCs that is often otherwise discarded if not cryopreserved for future transplantation use. Shelf life is thought to be at least five years, though viable recoveries vary greatly between different cord blood banks. Cell dose has been a major limitation, especially for adults. Pioneering work by Wagner, Barker, and colleagues in this field, however, has established the use of double UCBs to increase cell dose in adults. Interestingly, only one cord establishes long-term engraftment, while the other is lost; and the cord with the larger cell dose does not necessarily persist. Engraftment is much slower than with either PBSC or bone marrow allografts, with particularly notable delays in platelet recovery. Hematopoietic recovery and immunologic recovery are eventually complete and quite robust. Understanding the double-cord biology is an active field of investigation.

Pretransplant Conditioning Regimens

A patient must undergo a conditioning regimen before receiving the HSCT. These regimens fall along a spectrum from fully myeloablative to nonmyeloablative, with reduced intensity regimens in between, and use radiation and/or chemotherapy. These regimens address the two goals of conditioning, which are to provide intensive therapy against the malignancy for which the patient is being treated in the first place and to provide adequate immune suppression to ensure HSC engraftment.

The intensity of the regimen used depends in large part on the aggressiveness of the disease, the remission status, and the degree of HLA matching between donor and recipient (Figure 18.2). Acute leukemias and some high-grade, aggressive lymphomas benefit from fully myeloablative conditioning, which ensures engraftment and protects against recurrent disease. More indolent cancers like low-grade lymphomas rely heavily on the immunologic activity mediated by the allograft against the malignancy (see sections on graft-versus-leukemia/lymphoma, GvL, or GvT) and require only enough pretransplant conditioning to ensure engraftment. Such reduced intensity and nonmyeloablative regimens also extend allogeneic transplant options to individuals who could not withstand the toxicities and side effects of fully ablative conditioning.

Immunological Aspects of Transplantation

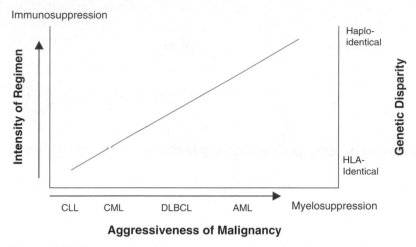

Figure 18.2 The selection of immunosuppressive and myelosuppressive agents used for conditioning patients before allogeneic HSCT depend on the aggressiveness of the disease and the degree of genetic disparity between the donor and host.

Graft-versus-Host Disease

The MHC constitutes one of the most highly polymorphic sets of genes known. From the standpoint of normal biology, this provides a species with a survival advantage by conferring the ability to respond to a myriad of potentially harmful peptide antigens that can be presented by a variety of MHC molecules. This polymorphism is, however, one of the major impediments to allografting because of the risk of GvHD, which is a unique complication of allogeneic HSCT. The organ to be transplanted has immunologic capacity. Hence, one can turn the process of solid organ graft rejection inside out to conceptualize what occurs during a GvH reaction. During GvHD, the engrafted, immunocompetent donor cells recognize the host as foreign and mount an immunologic attack.

The dominant immunologic factors underlying GvHD are the HLA compatibility between donor and recipient and the presence of immunocompetent T cells in the graft. GvHD occurs even between fully HLA-identical siblings, however, because nucleotide polymorphisms differ between such individuals, which are processed and presented by MHC as self-antigens (Figure 18.3). These so-called minor histocompatibility antigens actually require MHC identity between siblings, as this ensures recognition of MHC bearing self-antigen by the correct T-cell receptor in the donor T-cell repertoire. In cases of MHC disparity, which are sometimes used in the absence of a fully matched donor, GvH would additionally target the full alloantigenic disparities themselves. Target organs include those in which antigen-presenting cells reside like the skin, gut, liver, and lung.

There are two forms of GvHD, acute and chronic. Acute GvHD is primarily T-cell and cytokine mediated, whereas chronic GvHD is thought to be B-cell and antibody mediated. Classic acute GvHD typically occurs within the first 100 days after allogeneic HSCT; but persistent, recurrent, or late-onset forms of acute

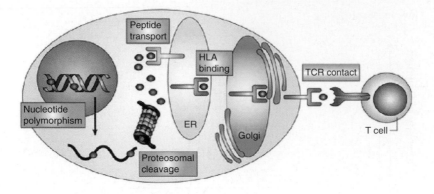

Nature Reviews | Cancer

Figure 18.3 Minor histocompatibility antigens are self-nucleotide polymorphisms that are processed and presented by MHC molecules on the cell surface. Few minor histocompatibility antigens can be typed in the laboratory, and they will differ between otherwise HLA-identical host-donor pairs. T cells recognize these antigens only in the context of MHC identity because the appropriate T-cell receptor must be present in the T-cell repertoire. Reprinted by permission from Macmillan publishers Ltd: Nature Reviews Cancer, Bleakley and Riddell, copyright 2004.

GvHD are more frequently recognized beyond this time point with the increasing use of nonmyeloablative regimens and unrelated donor sources. Chronic GvHD usually occurs beyond 100 days, but an overlap syndrome with features of acute GvHD is also now recognized. Clinical manifestations of acute GvHD can run the gamut from mild skin rash, anorexia, mild diarrhea, or low-grade cholestasis to full-thickness skin sloughing, liters of bloody diarrhea, and severe liver dysfunction with lethal consequences. Chronic GvHD resembles autoimmune diseases, for example, scleroderma, in many of its manifestations. To the extent that DNA-based HLA typing is now more precise and the therapeutic measures available for prevention and treatment of GvHD are more varied, though still imperfect, death due solely to GvHD should be an exceptionally rare event. Treatment of GvHD, however, can involve increasing layers of immune suppression, which can result in serious morbidity or even death.

Unmodified PBSCs seem to carry a greater risk of GvHD, especially chronic, than do bone marrow allografts. The basis for this is largely speculative but remains an area of active investigation. PBSGs are composed of a variety of cellular subsets that may have their own influence on transplant biology. Large numbers of T cells in the PBSC allografts may also increase GvHD risk. This seems unlikely as the sole explanation, however, because when controlled for T-cell numbers, the acute GvHD risk may actually be lower after unmodified PBSC than after unmodified bone marrow allografting. Interestingly, mobilized PBSC grafts induce less acute GvHD than grafts composed of steady state peripheral blood cells, suggesting that there are qualitative differences in T-cell subsets that may carry greater importance than T-cell numbers. UCB does not contain mature or memory T cells. The risk of GvHD mediated by naïve donor T cells sensitized against the host, while not zero, is therefore still considerably less than that which occurs after transplantation of other unmodified transplant products, even for a greater degree of host-donor mismatch.

Prevention of GvHD requires either depletion of T cells from the allograft or pharmacologic prophylaxis to limit sensitization of donor T cells against host antigens. Drugs for GvHD prophylaxis include those used for prevention of solid organ graft rejection such as cyclosporine, tacrolimus, sirolimus, mycophenolic acid, and methotrexate (Figure 18.4). Corticosteroids are used acutely for treatment of GvHD if it occurs; but there are no proven therapies for steroid-refractory GvHD, whether acute or chronic. T-cell depletion is extremely effective in reducing acute GvHD and is more effective in preventing chronic GvHD than is pharmacologic prophylaxis. Techniques to decrease the number of T cells in the HSC allograft have been developed for application in vitro and in vivo. Methods

that achieve less T-cell depletion than others may sometimes require pharmacologic GvHD prophylaxis as well.

Graft-versus-Host Disease and Graft-versus-Leukemia/Lymphoma

It was well after transplants were undertaken in humans that seminal work by Korngold and Sprent in the late 1970s and early 1980s established that donor T cells mediated the onset of acute GvHD between mice that were MHC identical but mismatched for minor histocompatibility antigens. We also now know that T cells are important for the GvL effect. In fact, donor leucocyte infusions (DLI) after allogeneic HSCT can often eradicate minimal residual disease recurrences and convert mixed-to full-donor chimeras. These DLIs are dosed according to their T-cell contents; but the products are usually not purified T cells and therefore contain additional potential effector populations

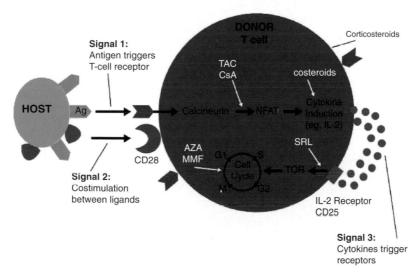

Figure 18.4 Alloreactive T cells of the hematopoietic stem cell (HSC) graft recognize recipient antigens as foreign, and mediate graft-versus-host disease (GvHD) and graft-versus-leukemia/lymphoma. Immunosuppressive agents targeting T-cell activation pathways are administered to modulate the graft response and to prevent or treat GvHD.

like NK cells, which could mediate immunologic reactivity against the residual or recurrent malignancy. Nevertheless, the efficacy of DLI has invoked T cells as at least one of the key, if not the principal, mediators of GvL.

GvHD and GvL are discrete syndromes that may be conceptualized as two circles in a Venn diagram with variable degrees of overlap. Patients who are in complete remission (CR) at the time of transplant, can often receive T-cell-depleted allografts without developing GvHD and suffer no increased risk of relapse (Figure 18.5). In this case, GvL can be easily separated from GvHD. The higher the disease burden going into transplant, however, the higher the acceptable risk for GvHD to maintain the desired GvL effect. Patients who are not in CR at the time of transplant therefore require more overlap between these two processes. Such patients may therefore require a T-cell replete or unmodified allograft, accepting the risk of inducing GvHD to ensure sufficient GvL. The holy grail, however, is to identify antigens that are unique to the malignancy and thus not shared by other target organs (Figure 18.6). This is a formidable challenge because many if not most tumor antigens are self-antigens or differentiation antigens expressed by normal tissue. In the case of hematopoietic malignancies, destruction of normal hematopoiesis when targeting unique leukemia-specific antigens is less problematic when hematopoiesis will be replaced anyway by a functioning allograft.

Important Developments in Supportive Care

In addition to the refinements in HLA typing precision driven by the need to expand donor pools beyond HLA-matched siblings, there have been tremendous advances in the supportive care of patients undergoing transplant. First is the increasingly sensitive and early detection of opportunistic infections like cytomegalovirus, among others. Equally important are the increasingly effective pharmaceuticals for prophylaxis, preemptive therapy, and actual treatment. Similar advances have been achieved in the drugs available to treat fungal infections occurring in the setting of neutropenia before engraftment.

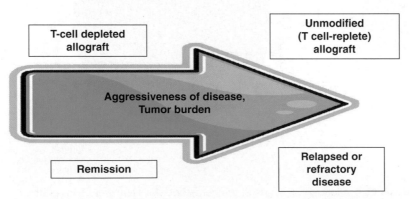

Figure 18.5 Increasing tumor burden and aggressiveness of disease require more overlap of graft-versus-host disease with graft-versus-leukemia/lymphoma/graft-versus-tumor, and hence favor T-cell replete or unmodified over T-cell-depleted allografts.

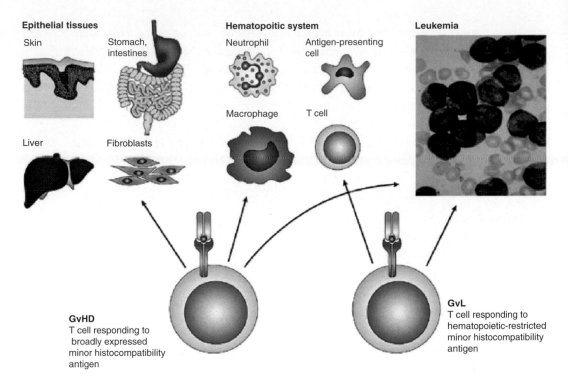

Epithelial tissues

Skin

Stomach, intestines

Liver

Fibroblasts

Hematopoitic system

Neutrophil

Macrophage

Antigen-presenting cell

T cell

Leukemia

GvHD
T cell responding to broadly expressed minor histocompatibility antigen

GvL
T cell responding to hematopoietic-restricted minor histocompatibility antigen

Nature Reviews | Cancer

Figure 18.6 T cells can react against antigens shared by diseased (mediating graft-versus-leukemia/lymphoma, or GvL) and healthy normal tissue (causing graft-versus-host disease, or GvHD). Targeting antigens expressed only by the diseased tissue, and in the case of allogeneic hematopoietic stem cell transplantation, being replaced anyway by the allograft, fosters separation of GvL/GvT from GvHD. Reprinted by permission from Macmillan Publishers Ltd: Nature Reviews Cancer, Bleakley and Riddell, copyright 2004.

FUTURE DIRECTIONS OF RESEARCH

Improved stem cell mobilization reagents for PBSC collections are an active area of interest. Chemokine receptor blockade that alters CD34+ retention in the marrow and allows egress into the circulation has garnered particular attention. Infusing PBSC products free of contaminating tumor cells is important, but purging procedures for autologous PBSC have so far never resulted in better overall survival and hence are considered unnecessary. Tumor contamination is of course not an issue for PBSC collections from healthy allogeneic donors.

Undoubtedly, the next decade will see a shift in clinical HSCT toward nonhemato-

logical diseases. Allogeneic HSCT for solid tumors has received mixed attention and achieved mixed success. The use of HSCT for the therapy of patients with various autoimmune diseases (scleroderma, rheumatoid arthritis, systemic lupus) offers the hope of completely replacing the patient's immune system with an allogeneic HSC graft or "resetting" the immunological clock with a T-cell-depleted autologous HSC graft. Such approaches are still in the realm of clinical trials and not yet standards of care.

A completely new use of stem cells is for tissue remodeling. Animal studies have suggested that stem cells may restore or replace myocardial cells after infusion into the coronary arteries after myocardial damage. Early studies are ongoing in humans to see whether this approach is clinically feasible and effective in patients after myocardial infarction.

As technologies to isolate individual cell populations have improved, adjuvant cellular therapies are also gaining ground. Current protocols are evaluating adoptive cellular immunotherapies using regulatory T cells, viral-specific cytotoxic T cells, mesenchymal stem cells, and natural killer cells.

In addition to HLA, other genetic loci are being evaluated as part of donor selection for allogeneic HSCT. One particular genetic region under consideration is that which encodes natural killer cell receptors. The natural killer cell immunoglobulin-like receptors (KIR) bind HLA epitopes and are encoded by a highly polymorphic gene region similar to the MHC. KIR-HLA combinations have been shown to predict NK cell alloreactivity and survival outcomes for some diseases, including acute myeloid leukemia. KIR genotyping is currently available in most clinical HLA laboratories, although there is insufficient data yet to recommend broad KIR genotyping for selection of unrelated donors. In the rare instances where more than one unrelated donor is available, choice based on KIR genotyping may be reasonable, all else being equal between the donor choices.

BIBLIOGRAPHY

REVIEWS

Appelbaum FR. The current status of hematopoietic cell transplantation. *Annu Rev Med*. 2003;54:491–512.

Barker JN, Wagner JE. Umbilical-cord blood transplantation for the treatment of cancer. *Nat Rev Cancer*. 2003;3(7):526–532.

Bleakley M, Riddell SR. Molecules and mechanisms of the graft-versus-leukemia effect. *Nat Rev Cancer*. 2004;4:371–380.

Copelan EA. Hematopoietic stem-cell transplantation. *N Engl J Med*. 2006;354(17):1813–1826.

Danovitch G. *Handbook of Kidney Transplantation*. Philadelphia, PA: Lippincott Williams & Wilkins; 2005.

Halloran, PF. Immunosuppressive drugs for kidney transplantation. *N Engl J Med*. 2004;351:2715.

Meier-Kriesche HU. Immunosuppression: evolution in practice and trends. *Am J Transplant*. 2006;6(5 Pt 2):1111–1131.

Stuart F, Abecassis MM, Kaufman DB, eds. *Organ Transplantation*. Georgetown, TX: Landes Bioscience; 2003.

LANDMARK PAPERS

Billingham RE, Brent L, Medawar PB. Actively acquired tolerance of foreign cells. *Nature*. 1953;172:603–606.

Gibson T, Medawar PB. The fate of skin homografts in man. *J Anat*. 1943;77:299–310.

Hale DA, Dhanireddy K, Bruno D, Kirk AD. Induction of transplantation tolerance in non-human primate preclinical models. *Philos Trans R Soc B*. 2005;360:1723–1737.

Knechtle SJ. Development of tolerogenic strategies in the clinic. *Philos Trans R Soc B*. 2005;1739–1746.

Korngold B, Sprent J. Lethal graft-versus-host disease after bone marrow transplantation across minor histocompatibility barriers in mice: prevention by removing mature T cells from marrow *J Exp Med*. 1978;148:1687–1698.

Murray JE, Merrill JP, Harrison JH. Renal homotransplantations in identical twins. *Surg Forum*. 1955;6:432–436.

Reemtsma K, McCracken BH, Schlegel JU, et al. Renal heterotransplantation in man. *Ann Surg*. 1964;160:384.

Shapiro AM, Lakey JR, Ryan EA, Korbutt GS. Islet transplantation in seven patients with type I diabetes mellitus using a glucocorticoid-free immuno-suppressive regimen. *N Engl J Med*. 2000;343:230–238.

Thomas ED, Buckner CD, Rudolph RH, et al. Allogeneic marrow grafting for hematologic malignancy using HLA matched donor-recipient sibling pairs. *Blood*. 1971;38:267–287.

Thomas ED, Lochte HL, Lu WC, Ferrebee JW. Intravenous infusion of bone marrow in patients receiving radiation and chemotherapy. *N Engl J Med*. 1957;257(11):491–496.

Index

Insulin-dependent diabetes
mellitus (IDDM), 277–290
animal models of, 278–281
BB rat, 279–280
NOD mouse, 278–279
RIP mice, 280
T-cell receptor transgenic
mice, 280
β cells, 279f, 282–283
antigens for, 282–283
intrathymic negative
selection and, 282
islet-specific response by,
282–283
T cells and, 282
clinical presentation of,
277–278
development rate for, 278f
diagnosis of, 287–289
with immunoassays,
287–288
LADA and, 288
environmental factors for,
284–285
epidemiology of, 278f
etiology of, 283–285, 283f, 287
genetic factors for, 283–284
in immigrant population, in
England, 286f
MS and, 286f
prediabetes and, 288–289
STZ model for, 280–281
treatment for, 289
viruses and, 285, 285f, 287
Integrins, 10
Interferons, 36–37
interleukins, 37
types of, 36–37
Interleukins, 3
cytokine immunomodulation
and, 40–41, 41f
interferons and, 37
psoriasis and, in genomics
for, 167
Intraepithelial lymphocytes, 253
Intrathymic negative selection,
282
Intravenous immunoglobulin
(IVIG), 115

Janeway, Charles, 46

K/BxN model, for RA, 105–106,
181–182
Keratinocytes, 163
Kidneys, 313–314. *See also* Renal
disease
anatomy of, 313
GBM in, 313–315
structure of, 313–314, 314f,
315f

immune injury mechanisms,
316–319
cell-specific, 317, 317t
tissue-specific, 317, 318t
streptococcal cells in, 328f
Killed vaccines, 38
Koch, Robert, 236
Kupffer cells, 18, 45
in liver immunology, 264

LADA, 288
Lambert-Eaton syndrome, 303
Lamina propria lymphocytes, 253
Langerhans cells, 12, 45
in skin, 163
Latent tuberculosis, 235–236
DTH and, 235
Lesions. *See* Antibody-induced
bullous lesions
Leukemias. *See* B-cell type
chronic lymphocytic
leukemia
Leukocyte migration defects,
75–77
symptoms of, 77
Lipopolysaccharide (LPS),
212–213
Live attenuated vaccines, 38
for HIV, 140–141
for TB, 244–245
Liver diseases, 265–274
AIH, 273–274
animal models of, 274
classification of, 273
environmental triggers of,
273
treatment for, 274
HAV, 268
HBV, 265–266
incidence rates for, 265
stages of, 265
vaccines for, 266
HCV, 266–268
biopsy for, 268
incidence rates for, 266–267
pathology of, 267
symptoms of, 267
treatment for, 268
PBC, 269–271
diagnosis of, 269–270
symptoms of, 269
treatment of, 271
PSC, 271–273
clinical presentation of,
271–272
IBD and, 272
symptoms of, 272
treatment of, 273
Liver immunology, 263–264, 264f
Kupffer cells in, 264
LSECs in, 264

Liver sinusoidal endothelial cells
(LSECs), 264
LPS. *See* Lipopolysaccharide
LSECs. *See* Liver sinusoidal
endothelial cells
Lupus cerebritis, 305
Lupus nephritis, 325–326
classification of, 325–326
treatment of, 326
Lymphocytes, 2, 11t
B-cells, 2, 12–13
development/differentiation
of, 2f
flow cytometers and, 25–26
under fluorescein-activated
cell scanner, 25
FACS and, 26, 27f, 28f
GALT and, 253–254
intraepithelial, 253
lamina propria, 253
T$_H$3 cells, 253–254
thymus, 2
Lymphocytic assays, 25–32
with DNA technology, 28–32
for analysis, 28–29
histocompatibility in, 30–31
MHC in, 30–31
microarray, 31–32, 31f
for PCR, 29–30
fluorescein-activated cell
scanner, 25–26
FACS and, 26, 27f, 28f
proliferation, 26–28
Lymphoproliferative syndrome,
54

Macrophages, 17–18
DC, 17–18
immature/mature, 17
macropinocytosis and,
17–18
histocytes, 45
Kupffer cells, 45
Langerhans cells, 45
mature, 18
nonspecific resistance to
infections from, 45
phagocyte deficiencies and,
78–79
TB and, 238–241
effector mechanisms in,
239–241
reactive micromolecules
and, 240
Macropinocytosis, 17–18
Major histocompatibility complex
(MHC), 2, 8–9
adaptive immunity and, 47
antigens and, 9
TNF and, 9
APC and, 8